Pediatric Bioethics

This volume offers a theoretical and practical overview of the ethics of pediatric medicine. It will serve as a fundamental handbook and resource for pediatricians, nurses, residents in training, graduate students, and practitioners of ethics and health care policy. Written by a team of leading experts, *Pediatric Bioethics* addresses those difficult ethical questions concerning the clinical and academic practice of pediatrics, including an approach to recognizing boundaries when one is confronted with such issues as end-of-life care, life-sustaining treatment, extreme prematurity, pharmacotherapy, and research. Thorny topics, such as what constitutes best interests, personhood, or distributive justice, and public health concerns, such as immunization and newborn genetic screening, are also addressed.

Geoffrey Miller is Professor of Pediatrics and Neurology at the Yale University School of Medicine, as well as a member of the Yale Bioethics Center and the Child Neurology Society Bioethics Committee.

D1427358

Pediatric Bioethics

Edited by
GEOFFREY MILLER
Yale University School of Medicine

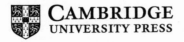

CAMBRIDGE UNIVERSITY PRESS
Cambridge, New York, Melbourne, Madrid, Cape Town, Singapore,
São Paulo, Delhi, Dubai, Tokyo

Cambridge University Press
32 Avenue of the Americas, New York, NY 10013-2473, USA

www.cambridge.org
Information on this title: www.cambridge.org/9780521135948

First published 2010

Printed in the United States of America

A catalog record for this publication is available from the British Library.

Library of Congress Cataloging in Publication data
    Pediatric bioethics / edited by Geoffrey Miller.
       p. ; cm.
    Includes bibliographical references and index.
    ISBN 978-0-521-51798-0 (hardback) – ISBN 978-0-521-13594-8 (pbk.)
    1. Pediatricians – Professional ethics.   I. Miller, Geoffrey, 1947–
    II. Title.
    [DNLM: 1. Pediatrics – ethics. 2. Bioethical Issues. 3. Ethics, Medical.
    WS 21 P3703 2010]
    RJ78.P43 2010
    174'.961892–dc22   2009008942

ISBN 978-0-521-51798-0 Hardback
ISBN 978-0-521-13594-8 Paperback

For Tricia

Contents

Contributors

Stephen Ashwal, M.D.
Distinguished Professor of Pediatrics, Loma Linda University.

G. Kevin Donovan, M.D., M.L.A.
Professor of Pediatrics and Founder and Director of Oklahoma Bioethics Center, Oklahoma University.

Alice D. Dreger, Ph.D.
Associate Professor of Clinical Medical Humanities and Bioethics, Guggenheim Fellow, Feinberg School of Medicine, Northwestern University, Chicago.

Erin Flanagan-Klygis, M.D.
Assistant Professor of Pediatrics and Religion, Health, and Human Values, Rush University, Chicago, and Medical Director of the Rush Pediatric Palliative Care Program.

Joel E. Frader, M.D.
Professor of Pediatrics, Medical Humanities and Bioethics, Northwestern University, Chicago. Former chairman of the Committee on Bioethics of the American Academy of Pediatrics and former president of the American Society of Bioethics and Humanities. Fellow of the Hastings Center.

Christine Harrison, Ph.D.
Director of Bioethics at the Hospital for Sick Children, Toronto, Canada. Former president of the Canadian Bioethics Society and currently chair of the Canadian Paediatric Society Bioethics Committee.

Eva Feder Kittay, Ph.D.
Professor of Philosophy, State University of New York at Stonybrook.

Loretta M. Kopelman, Ph.D.
Professor of Medical Humanities and former chair of the department, Brody School of Medicine, East Carolina University. Founding president of the American Society for Bioethics and Humanities and recipient of the Bartholome Award in Pediatric Ethics from the American Academy of Pediatrics. Former member of the Institute of Medicine and currently a Fellow of the Hastings Center.

Alexandra Kravitt
Intern, University of Pennsylvania Center for Bioethics.

Paul A. Lombardo, Ph.D., J.D.
Professor of Law at Georgia State University's College of Law.

Laurence B. McCullough, Ph.D.
The Dalton Tomlin Chair in Medical Ethics and Health Policy in the Center for Medical Ethics and Health Policy, Baylor College of Medicine, and Professor of Medicine and Medical Ethics. Former president of the Society for Health and Human Values.

Mark R. Mercurio, M.A., M.D.
Associate Professor of Pediatrics and Director of the Pediatric Bioethics Program, Yale University.

Geoffrey Miller, M.A., M.Phil., M.D.
Professor of Pediatrics and Neurology, Yale University. Member of the Yale Bioethics Center and the Child Neurology Society's Bioethics Committee.

Jonathan D. Moreno, Ph.D.
David and Lyn Siljen University Professor and Professor of Medical Ethics and of History and Sociology of Science, University of Pennsylvania. Senior Fellow at the Center for American Progress and a member of the Institute of Medicine.

Edmund D. Pellegrino, M.D.
Chairman, President's Council on Bioethics, Professor Emeritus of Medicine and Medical Ethics, Georgetown University.

Kimberly A. Quaid, Ph.D.
Professor of Medical and Molecular Genetics and Director of the Predictive Testing Program, Indiana University. Member of the Indiana University Center for Bioethics and chair of the Ethical, Legal, and Social Implications Study Section of the National Human Genome Research Institute of the National Institutes of Health.

Angelique M. Reitsma, M.A., M.D.
Associate at the University of Pennsylvania Center for Bioethics.

Lainie Friedman Ross, M.D., Ph.D.
Carolyn and Matthew Bucksbaum Professor of Clinical Medical Ethics and Associate Director, Maclean Center for Clinical Medical Ethics, University of Chicago.

David Sandberg, Ph.D.
Associate Professor of Pediatrics and Child Behavioral Health, University of Michigan.

Sadath A. Sayeed, J.D., M.D.
Instructor in Global Health and Social Medicine, Harvard University, and Neonatologist at the Children's Hospital Boston. Member of the Harvard University Program in Ethics and Health.

Ilina Singh, Ph.D.
Wellcome Trust University Lecturer in Bioethics and Society and Associate Director of BIOS, Centre for the Study of Bioscience, Biomedicine, Biotechnology, and Society, London School of Economics.

Preface

I cannot really define what is meant by the term "bioethics." It seems to mean different things to different people, depending on their situation and perspective. I do appreciate that it encompasses more than norms and codes of conduct for health professionals. Its sources are many and include the heterogeneous tentacles of moral philosophy; the instinctual nature of cultural norms; the development and wrangling compositions of common and statutory law; and lessons from history, the humanities, the social sciences, and the study of human nature. With such broad and variable origins, it is not surprising that the questions that concern bioethics give rise to such vigorous debate, for they entail the age-old arguments about how we might treat each other as individuals, as special or privileged persons, as groups, and within a state, and how these things should be prescribed and proscribed. Underlying all of this is the recognition and government of harmful behavior, potential or otherwise, that has been, is, and evidently will be practiced by human beings, often with the participation of health professionals in clinical and academic medicine. At particular risk from this harm are vulnerable populations such as children. This book presents approaches to this concern that arise in pediatric bioethics. The contributors represent the fields of philosophy, medicine, law, and the social sciences. A broad array of topics is addressed, including theory and principles, genetics and the newborn, therapies, and end-of-life issues. The intention is that from these contributions the reader will be able to derive a good ethical approach to the practice of pediatrics and avoid poorly reasoned responses to ethical questions – responses that are cloaked in misinterpreted word and fashionable phrase. As Hannah Arendt wrote in *Eichmann in Jerusalem: A Report on the Banality of Evil*, "There is a strange interdependence between thoughtlessness and evil."

Geoffrey Miller
Yale University
2009

xiii

A

THE FOUNDATION

Theory and Principles

1

Virtues and Goals in Pediatrics

G. Kevin Donovan and Edmund D. Pellegrino

VIRTUE ETHICS REVISITED

Most physicians, whether they treat children or adults, would not see themselves as having much in common with philosophers. Philosophy is often thought to deal with the abstract, ethereal, or abstruse, whereas medicine is scientific, evidence-based, and goal-directed. Nevertheless, when physicians are questioned, they readily accept that some of the attributes of philosophers are similar to their own. A physician is a seeker of knowledge, one who pursues the application of the right treatment to the right diagnosis for the good of the patient. Doctors tend to be most fulfilled when they have a deep appreciation of both their patients and their profession, the personal interaction as well as the intellectual stimulation of the medical profession. Ultimately, this makes a physician a seeker of truth and wisdom, which is not a bad definition for a philosopher. Although some might shy away from this connection, thinking that to discuss their philosophy of medicine or their philosophy of life would seem somewhat pretentious, most physicians would readily admit to wanting to be a "good" doctor. But what does it mean to be a good doctor? What does it mean to do good in the medical sense? When prodded, we could produce a list of traits that would characterize a good physician. Such lists have been produced before; such traits have been described. The term most often used in these descriptions is "virtue."

Virtue has often been defined as the good character traits of such persons, that is, their disposition to habitually do the things that are right and good. Ultimately, the character of one performing an action is central to the good choice of action. It is the recognition of this truth that has formed the basis of virtue ethics since the time of the ancient Greeks. Aristotle said that "moral virtues are states of character, a disposition to excellence that makes one a good man and causes him to perform his function well."[1] As one of us has pointed out, virtue is the most ancient, durable,

3

and ubiquitous concept in the history of ethical theory. This is so because one cannot completely separate the character of a moral agent from his or her acts, the nature of those acts, the circumstances under which they are performed, or their consequences. Virtue theories focus on the agent – on his or her intentions, dispositions, and motives – and on the kind of person the moral agent becomes, wishes to become, or ought to become as a result of his or her habitual disposition to act in certain ways.[2]

Although the concept of virtue was both durable and ubiquitous in theories of ethics from the Greeks to more modern times, it always had its deficiencies. Conceptual difficulties inherent in the concept of virtue itself led to challenges to a theory of virtue ethics and its gradual falling into disfavor, as described by Alasdair MacIntyre.[3] Virtue ethics was supplanted by other approaches following the Renaissance and the Age of Reason. Part of this was a result of the disarray of normative ethics in general, and part was due to problems with virtue-based ethics in particular. Virtue ethics does not emphasize principles, rules, duties, or concrete prescriptions. It does not, therefore, tell us how to resolve specific moral dilemmas. It says only that a virtuous person will be predisposed to act in accord with the virtue appropriate to the situation. For many, following this circular reasoning feels like trying to nail Jell-O to the wall. If a good thing is that which a virtuous person would do, then a virtuous person is one who would do the good. We must define either what is good or what a virtuous person is in order to avoid this circularity, and it is just these definitions that have challenged philosophers throughout the ages. Moreover, virtue theory cannot stand alone, any more than can other normative theories, without some concept of what kind of person the moral agent is, or is striving to become. For instance, a deontology-based ethic would focus on the act itself, whether it is right and good. But the individual is judged only by whether his or her moral conduct is in accord with a universal norm – for example, utility, justice, or beneficence. It sheds little light on the intention of the moral agent and ignores important aspects of the interaction, such as virtue or caring. A more consequentialist approach relies on an outcome that maximizes good for the most people, balancing goals and resources and considering the needs of everyone affected. In this way, we expect to produce the greatest good for the greatest number. Such a focus on good outcomes is very appealing to those trained in medicine and public health. Difficulties arise in the attempt to find agreement on which values should be maximized, and we begin to see that the values of the moral agent are not inconsequential. If the goal is to maximize happiness, then both the definition of happiness and the interplay between the (virtuous) person and the production of happiness, for oneself and for others, becomes problematic if this approach is used alone.

In the development of virtue ethics, it was necessary to examine the connection between virtue and happiness. Are people virtuous in order to be happy, or are they happy because they act virtuously – is virtue truly its own reward? Is virtue to be pursued for its own sake or for "excellence" or "nobility"? In Western culture, a synthesis of classic and medieval philosophy derived a sustained answer to this. Thomas Aquinas developed a virtue-based ethics that began with the same elements as Aristotle's. He saw truth as the end point of the natural intellectual virtues, and the good of humans as the end, or "telos," of the natural moral virtues.

To this, he added the virtues of faith, hope, and charity, as defined by Christian theology. There existed an objective moral order in which human nature could be understood by human reason and that thereby defined the telos of human activity. For the Greek philosophers, the telos was natural happiness, but it was understood by Aquinas to be supernatural happiness, achieved by union with God. Virtues, then, were traits that habitually disposed humans to act in accord with the objectives or ends of human nature. The virtues were seen as having normative force, not because they were admirable in themselves, but because they would predispose one to achieving those desired ends, the good of human beings. Beginning at the time of Enlightenment, these sources of morality were challenged and the ancient Greek philosophies were devalued. Virtues were replaced by competing concepts – for example, rights (Locke), duty (Kant), moral sentiment (Hume), and consequences or utility (Bentham and Mill). Even when these other concepts were considered, the question of the character of the agent could not be entirely ignored, and so the importance of the virtuous person was never entirely discounted. Nevertheless, in the present day it is unlikely that the concept of virtue ethics could be widely accepted in society, given the lack of agreement on a definition of human good or the proper telos of human activity.

VIRTUE ETHICS AND MEDICINE

The concept of virtue as a normative theory for medical ethics paralleled the history of the concept of virtue in general ethics, yet it persisted from the time of the Hippocratic oath well into the 20th century. In the past generation, cultural and societal changes have led to an emphasis on consumerism, diminished trust in authority figures such as physicians, and an emphasis on autonomy-based relationships on the part of patients. These were closely linked to a weakening of the moral consensus that had provided the basis of professional ethics, and the growth of alternative approaches to ethics, such as principle-based ethics, and more particular approaches based on feminist ethics, narrative, and caring. Consequently, the dominance of virtue in medical ethics has diminished.

The absence of a generally accepted norm of virtue ethics in general ethics need not prevent a return to virtue in professional ethics.[2] There are good reasons to suppose this is possible. First, there is growing dissatisfaction with the incompleteness of principle-based ethics, one that is guided solely by reference to the principles of autonomy, beneficence, and justice. This approach fails to account for the complexity of moral problems in medicine or to consider the need for compassion and humility in human interactions.[4] Such theories require a more solid and expansive base in a philosophical system in order to achieve normative force. Moreover, there is a common understanding that the individual character of the physician, or bioethicist, cannot be left out of the moral equation. The kind of person doing the analysis or performing the action will have an effect on the action that is chosen no matter which theoretical approach is being employed. Finally, in the domain of professional ethics, unlike general ethics, there still exists a real possibility of agreement on generally acceptable ends – the goals of medicine.

GOALS

In an attempt to define the values at the core of medicine and to reach some consensus on the goals of medicine, a report was produced by an international project of the Hastings Center.[5] Leaders representing 14 countries, primarily but not exclusively Western democracies, published their perspectives on the proper priorities. They acknowledged the differences between general societal goals and a specific professional ethic, stating, "Medicine must have its own vital life and its own clear direction. It should listen to what societies want. ... yet in the end, it must chart its own course in partnership with society." They listed four goals for medicine:

- The prevention of disease and injury and the promotion and maintenance of health
- The relief of pain and suffering caused by maladies
- The care and cure of those with a malady and the care of those who cannot be cured
- The avoidance of premature death and the pursuit of a peaceful death

They considered these goals to be universally valid because of our common human nature, the inescapable fact of illness, pain, and suffering, and the growing universalization of scientific knowledge and medical skills. In doing so, they also rejected too broad a concept of health, such as defined by the World Health Organization (1947). Rather than attempt to ensure "complete physical, mental, and social well being," their definition focused on medicine as a response to a malady of the individual. Thus, they returned the focus to the doctor–patient interaction, while at the same time acknowledging that medicine as a profession is distinct and "must have its own internal compass and abiding values ... resting upon its traditional and largely universal goals."

In fact, the work of this international group can be summarized and condensed into a single concept: the goals of medicine must serve the good as found in and defined by the doctor–patient relationship. In the doctor–patient relationship, most would agree that the proper end point should be the good of the patient. The good of the patient has been characterized by an action that is both right and good: *right* according to medical standards of effectiveness, achievability, and likelihood of providing a beneficial outcome, and *good* according to the desirability of this benefit, as judged by patients' values.[6]

VIRTUE ETHICS IN PEDIATRICS

If such a general goal of medical activity can be agreed upon, then those attributes that lend themselves to it may be seen in light of this goal. Virtues specific to medical activity can be described in this context and serve as instrumental goods that lead to the ultimate goal of the medical interaction, the good of the patient. Therefore, a professional virtue is defined in terms of the end point of the clinical encounter. "Healing is the activity specific to nursing and medicine. Those dispositions that impact the capacity to heal well are the virtues of medicine, nursing, dentistry, and the like. They are the virtues internal – in MacIntyre's sense – to the practice.[3] Possession of these internal virtues defines the good nurse or physician."[2] We have attempted a listing of such virtues and considered their application to the practice of pediatrics. Not everyone will agree with what is included, what is omitted, and why. Such lists are notoriously difficult to compile and cannot be thought of as all-inclusive. Therefore, one should feel free to add one's own choices to our list of virtues and propose even better examples of their application.

THE CARDINAL VIRTUES

The virtues wisdom, fortitude, temperance, and justice are considered cardinal (from Latin for "hinge") by Plato and Aristotle, in that all the others hinge on these four. They are not the only or even the highest virtues, but are essential for the existence and functioning of other virtues.[7]

Prudence, or Wisdom: Solomon asked for an understanding heart, and prudential wisdom is essential for the discerning physician. To come to the proper conclusions while weighing alternatives in the midst of clinical uncertainty requires good judgment; similarly, wisdom guides us in weighing apparent conflicts among values and virtues and selecting the best course for the good of the patient. This can be even more problematic in the care of children, where parental preferences may or may not reflect the good of the child and the patient's values may not have had the opportunity to mature. It is considered proper to look to parents for decisions about what is good for a child. Although we act as if a suitable proxy can exercise the autonomy of the nonautonomous child, this is not altogether an unreasonable fiction. The definition of "autonomy" is not only "self-will," but also "respect for others." In this sense we defer to parents or other appropriate proxies to make decisions for those without this capacity, not applying the patient's (nonexisting) values, but acting in their best interests (see Chapter 3). In such cases, balancing multiple interests will require a great deal of prudential wisdom.

Courage: Here we define courage not as physical bravery, but as fortitude or strength of character. In the clinical setting, our judgment about diagnosis or treatment may not be in perfect accord with those around us. Abraham Lincoln said, "Be sure you're right, then go ahead." The first half of his maxim requires prudential wisdom, the latter, courage. It is no less a necessity in the face of moral dilemmas, especially when one's convictions place one against the tide in order to protect the vulnerable infant or child. A need for moral courage may arise in many disputes involving vulnerable children in such areas as truth telling (Chapter 6), brain death (Chapter 18), and feeding and caring for the severely brain damaged. On such occasions, we may at times find ourselves at odds with colleagues and families. Other virtues, such as humility, should temper our action, but at times we must stand fast, particularly because children are unable to speak adequately for themselves.

Moderation, or Temperance: This is a daily requirement for those who deal with potentially rowdy children, noncompliant parents, or the general frustrations of the health care system. It may seem at times that all physicians, and particularly those who deal with children, must behave as "super-adults." Such self-restraint is often necessary to maintain a workable doctor–patient relationship. It is needed and justified even more when the patient is a vulnerable child, and it is the parents who are demanding, noncompliant, or unreliable. We must restrain ourselves, having chosen to care for children even when their caretakers choose to act like children.

Moreover, Aristotle's "moderation in all things" should also guide us in seeking a necessary balance between the demands of our professional and personal lives.

Justice: To deal with each patient equally is to render according to his or her needs, treating like cases alike but different cases differently. In the relationship with a specific patient, the needs of distributive justice in society become secondary to the needs of that individual and the requirement for a healing action directed at his or her condition.

Nevertheless, the requirements of justice will also propel us to make improvements in the health care delivery system, for the good of all, as well as our particular patients. This is governed in part by the next virtue.

Fidelity: In professing to be able and willing to help in a medical relationship, the physician makes a commitment to ensuring that his or her interests coincide with or defer to the needs of the patient. This commitment creates the trust without which a healing relationship cannot function. This commitment manifests itself in ways large and small: in being responsive to the child's needs and those of the parents, even when this is inconvenient; in truth telling; and in the maintenance of professional skills and competence.

Benevolence: Making the good of the patient one's intention is the sine qua non of the doctor–patient encounter. It is the virtue that underlies the principles of beneficence and nonmaleficence. It starts with the Hippocratic promise to do no harm, but extends into every treatment, every action, every test ordered or unnecessary intervention avoided. Because the younger and more vulnerable child relies on us to define and pursue what is right and good, this bedrock of benevolence will guide our actions on behalf of all, from the smallest (Chapters 8 and 10) to the more mature, from tested treatments (Chapter 15) to those being developed (Chapters 5, 9, and 13).

Altruism, or Effacement of Self-Interest: This is a virtue that draws many to the practice of medicine in the first place, motivates them to get up in the cold and dark of night, and to provide care to the needy. It is often leeched out of the individual in the process of medical training.

Compassion: Closely coupled to the previous two virtues, and flowing from them, compassion enables us to keep in mind the humanity of the sufferer, to avoid both callousness and a coldly intellectual approach to the treatment of his or her disease. We especially must maintain compassion for children, who are often not responsible for their medical predicaments, and try to avoid facile judgments about those who may be.

Humility and Intellectual Honesty: Last but not least, humility is the lynchpin of constant learning. Physicians are given pride of place in a medical hierarchy and often come to believe it is their duty and privilege to make the right decision for patients. It may become difficult to admit that they sometimes just do not know what is medically correct. In such cases, the doctor may err by keeping too narrow a focus, blaming treatment failures on the family's noncompliance, or stubbornly repeating the same diagnostic or therapeutic mistake. We may fail to listen to the patient or may fail to seek wiser counsel. Such pride comes at a cost, but the patient pays for it.

To all of these, Aristotle would have added gentleness, friendliness, and wittiness.[1] The first two are treasured virtues in a pediatrician, but we are pleased with the last one as well. We firmly believe that gentle humor is a good antidote for a child's anxiety and even serves to alleviate the monotony of medical routine. It should never be hurtful or sarcastic, and self-deprecating humor is the best of all.

The restoration and maintenance of virtue as a guiding force in professional ethics is not only possible, but vital. It depends on those who want to become virtuous, who are willing to ask themselves at each critical juncture, "Is this action compatible with the kind of physician I want to be?"

To many, this will be the determinative question; unfortunately, for some it will remain irrelevant. The practice of medicine will depend heavily on the former, those reflective and introspective souls who are determined to seek the best in themselves and for the profession. It was with such people in mind that this ancient Greek saying was printed in the journal *Pediatrics* more than a decade ago:

A doctor has opportunities for studying human nature which are given to no one else, wherefore a philosopher ought to begin his life as a doctor, and a doctor should end his life by becoming a philosopher.

References

1. *The Ethics of Aristotle: The Nichomachean Ethics.* Thomson JAK, trans. New York: Penguin; 1976:22–24.
2. Pellegrino ED. Toward a virtue-based normative ethics for the health professions. *Kennedy Inst Ethics J.* 1995;5:253–277.
3. MacIntyre A. *After Virtue: A Study in Moral Theory.* Notre Dame, Ind: University of Notre Dame Press; 1984:187.
4. Fiester A. Why the clinical ethics we teach fails patients. *Academic Med.* 2007;82:684–689.
5. The goals of medicine: setting new priorities [special supplement]. *Hastings Cent Rep.* 1996;26:S1–S27.
6. Pellegrino ED, Thomasma DC. *For the Patient's Good: The Restoration of Beneficence in Health Care.* New York: Oxford University Press; 1988.
7. Kreeft P. *Back to Virtue: Traditional Moral Wisdom for Modern Moral Confusion.* San Francisco: Ignatius Press; 1992:59–69.

2

Contributions of Ethical Theory to Pediatric Ethics

Pediatricians and Parents as Co-fiduciaries
of Pediatric Patients

Laurence B. McCullough

INTRODUCTION

It might at first appear that pediatric ethics is sui generis, but it is a mistake to think so. Consider the well-known clinical ethical concept of pediatric assent. This ethical concept was pioneered in the 1980s by Sanford Leikin[1,2] and endorsed in 1995 by the American Academy of Pediatrics.[3] Pediatric assent recognizes that minor children cannot be accorded the legal right of informed consent but that older minor children, especially adolescents with chronic diseases, are capable of adult-like decision making about the clinical management of their diagnoses. The ethical content of the concept of pediatric assent is that, to the extent that their capacity for decision making and its exercise is adult-like, children should, with very few exceptions, be treated as having authority over themselves. Assent might appear to be unique to pediatrics, but it is not.[3] It also bears on the authority that should be given to decision making and its exercise by older patients with the diminished decision-making capacity that results from progressive dementing disorders.[4] In other words, the ethical concept of geriatric assent should guide decision making with geriatric patients who lack intact decision-making capacity.

Rather than being understood to be sui generis, pediatric assent should be understood to be professional medical ethics applied to the specialty of pediatrics and its subspecialties. The core ethical concept of professional medical ethics is the ethical concept of the physician as fiduciary of the patient.[5,6] In this chapter, I will show that pediatricians have the fiduciary ethical obligation to protect and promote the health-related interests of children. I will also show that parents are in an ethically parallel relationship with their child when their child is a patient. Parents also have the fiduciary obligation to protect and promote the health-related interests of their child who is a patient. Parents also have a fiduciary obligation to protect and promote the other, non-health-related interests of their child who is a patient. In order to make good on these claims about pediatric ethics as professional medical ethics, I will provide a historical account of the origins of the ethical concept of the physician as fiduciary of the patient. I will then explain how the ethical concept of being a fiduciary also applies to the parents of a child who is a patient and identify the major clinical implications of this concept in professional medical ethics.

THE ORIGINS OF THE ETHICAL CONCEPT OF THE PHYSICIAN AS FIDUCIARY OF THE PATIENT

Two giants of the modern period in the history of English-language medical ethics invented the ethical concept of the physician as fiduciary of the patient and therefore invented medicine as a profession: the Scottish physician-ethicist John Gregory (1724–1773) and the English physician-ethicist Thomas Percival (1740–1804). Many physicians take the view that medicine as a profession can trace its roots in Western history back to Hippocrates and the Hippocratic oath. However, the distinguished historian of medical ethics Robert Baker has shown conclusively that the idea that the history of medical ethics is but a footnote to the Hippocratic corpus does not withstand close scrutiny.[7,8] Indeed, the Hippocratic oath and its accompanying ethical texts are marked by a deep and unresolved tension between entrepreneurial self-interest and a nascent concept of medicine as a life of service to the sick. In the subsequent history of medicine, this tension was resolved in actual clinical practice very largely in favor of entrepreneurial self-interest. The ethics of entrepreneurial medicine were contractual, in which the well-to-do sick contracted for services from physicians, surgeons, apothecaries, female midwives, and other sorts of practitioners. The latter did not have any concept of an obligation to protect the sick. That work was left to the sick themselves. Entrepreneurial medicine was governed by the very familiar ethics of the marketplace, *caveat emptor.*

Gregory[9] (1772) and Percival[10] (1803) should be credited with having been the first in the history of Western medical ethics to see that entrepreneurial medicine was morally perilous both for the sick and for medical practitioners. They therefore set out to transform entrepreneurial medicine into the profession of medicine and did so by inventing the ethical concept of the physician as fiduciary of the patient.[11] It is crucial to appreciate the context in which Gregory and Percival invented the concept of the physician as fiduciary of the patient as the intellectual basis for the transformation of medicine into a profession.

Medical practice and medical experimentation in eighteenth-century Britain and its North American colonies was thoroughly entrepreneurial. Dorothy and Roy Porter, prominent historians of eighteenth-century British medical ethics, provide a landmark account of this medical world of practitioners and the sick.[12] There was then no stable medical curriculum and no licensure (except for the efforts, usually not successful, of the royal colleges to use their power of licensure to create monopolistic control of the medical marketplace); there were no third-party payers and no regulation of drugs and devices. Many practitioners plied the medical trades, including university-trained physicians, apprentice-trained surgeons and apothecaries, female midwives, who competed fiercely with the male "midwives" (physicians who practiced obstetrics, using the new technology of forceps), and many so-called irregulars (less politely, quacks).

The sick routinely undertook self-diagnosis and self-treatment (self-physicking, it was then called). Many did so out of economic necessity, because only the well-to-do could afford physicians' and surgeons' fees. (Physicians and surgeons complained, often and bitterly, about the failure of their moneyed customers to pay them.) The sick also self-physicked because they did not trust practitioners intellectually – to know what they were saying and doing – or morally – to put the interests of the sick first and their own financial and other self-interests second.

Such mistrust was remarkably well founded. There were almost as many concepts of health and disease, and remedies for the latter, as there were practitioners. The intellectual foundations of medicine, which we take for granted in the era of evidence-based medicine, were in terrible condition. This medical marketplace was oversupplied and so competition was fierce, especially given that the outcome of failure to compete successfully was poverty, unless one married very well and one's wife brought to her marriage a considerably dowry. Physicians therefore acted rationally on the basis of self-interest. They did what they could to stand out, including adopting "little peculiarities" of dress, speech, and manners.[9] It was essential to master the accoutrements of being a gentleman (women were not yet admitted to the study and practice of medicine), because those who retained one's services came from a higher social class and held and wielded the power of the purse over physicians.

In a contractual practice of medicine, the well-to-do sick paid the piper and called the tune. As a consequence, the well-to-do sick had power over physicians; physicians had little or no power over the sick. The great shibboleth of bioethics, the systematically paternalistic physician who controlled the sick with overweening power, simply did not exist in the private practice of medicine.

The situation of the sick poor who were admitted to the newly created infirmaries differed. Gunther Risse provides a compelling account of these new hospitals for sick members of the working class.[13] These hospitals were created by the employers of what would come to be known as the workplaces of the industrial revolution. The infirmaries provided free medical care for the men, women, and children whom these industrialists employed. The "trustees," as they were known, provided an annual "subscription," or budget, for the hospital. The trustees deliberately underfunded the hospital, to put pressure on its lay managers – physicians were not in charge – to control costs. Modern insurance companies did not invent this practice, although they have brought it to an exquisite state of development.

The infirmaries served the sick poor who were considered worthy. Physicians were appointed by the trustees to serve as "faculty" of the infirmary. The faculty were not paid. However, physicians gladly accepted – indeed, sought out – such an appointment, because it brought with it the stamp of approval of the leading lights of the new, wealthy and politically ever more powerful social class. This approval could be, and was, used to build one's private practice, just as a "clinical" appointment to an academic department of pediatrics is used by private-practice pediatricians today.

The worthy poor were sharply distinguished from the unworthy poor. The latter placed themselves in this social and ethical category of opprobrium because they were willfully lazy and shiftless and thus had brought poverty on themselves. They were not admitted to the infirmaries, for their own moral good. This sharp distinction between those who were worthy and unworthy among the sick poor came across the Atlantic Ocean to the British American colonies, and it is with us still, although we do not use the phrase "unworthy poor" any more in polite society. In the United States we have Medicare and the Veterans Health Affairs system for the worthy and Medicaid for the unworthy. Political support for the former two programs is strong, while for the latter program it is chronically weak, reflecting with precision 18th-century moral categories that create obstacles to medical care for indigent children who, by any stretch of the imagination, cannot be judged to have brought their medical indigence on themselves.

The trustees had several motives for creating the infirmaries. These included their interest in advancing their social and political standing vis-à-vis the landed aristocracy. As a consequence, the trustees wanted their infirmaries to meet with social approval, and they knew that low mortality was essential not only for the infirmaries, but also their benefactors, to achieve such approbation. Entrepreneurial physicians since the time of Hippocrates understood how to achieve this goal: one had to become very good at the prognosis of incurable, life-taking conditions so that one could in a timely, self-interested fashion declare a case incurable and withdraw. By thus routinely abandoning the dying, physicians would almost certainly avoid being blamed for the ensuing death. This standard was articulated as late as the early 18th century by Friedrich Hoffmann (1660–1742) in his *Medicus Politicus*, the politic doctor.[14,15] The trustees took this lesson to heart and instructed lay managers – physicians were not to be entrusted with this important rationing task – to deny admission to the sick with "fever," a catchall diagnostic category of conditions whose outcome was very likely to be death, even with treatment. This self-interested segmenting of the medical market worked. In a hospital with no scientific or clinical concept, and therefore no effective practice, of infection control, mortality was very low.

The benefactors of the infirmaries did not trust physicians and surgeons to control the most expensive resources in the hospital: the drugs, fortified wines, and beers in the formulary. These they put under the control of apothecaries, thus making physicians accountable to non-physicians.

In these new hospitals, physicians gained a kind of power over the sick that they did not have in their private practices treating the well-to-do sick. The worthy sick poor, who thought of themselves as "inmates" at the infirmaries, worried about the abuses of the power of physicians and surgeons, for example, for the purposes of conducting experiments with their newly invented secret remedies or nostrums, an abuse that Gregory attacked.[9]

Gregory based his medical ethics on David Hume's (1711–1776) principle of sympathy.[11,16,17] Sympathy, a constitutive component of human nature, involves the capacity of each morally well-formed human being to enter into and experience the sufferings of others and therefore to be motivated routinely to relieve and prevent such suffering. On the basis of Humean sympathy, Gregory thought that the plight of the sick, resulting from the crisis of intellectual and moral distrust, whether the sick were well-to-do or worthy poor, was not acceptable. Moreover, Gregory was very concerned that the entrepreneurial, self-interested practice of medicine introduced biases that disabled clinical judgment and decision making, calling into question the very competence of physicians.

Gregory therefore starts his medical ethics by addressing the problem of competence on the basis of the philosophy of science and medicine of Francis Bacon (1561–1626). Bacon had already called for medicine to be based on "experience," that is, the rigorously collected and described results of natural and designed experiments. In effect, Bacon called for medicine to become evidence-based, a call that medicine is now fully answering five centuries after it was issued.[11]

Before Gregory, physicians routinely used the word "profession" to describe themselves. However, they used this word in a self-interested way: to distinguish themselves from practitioners who had not attended a university and received a "regular" education (a dubious claim on its face, given the absence of a stable medical curriculum) and to claim that their uneducated competitors – surgeons, apothecaries, and "irregular" practitioners – were therefore inferior practitioners.

Gregory set out to give the word "profession" content, both intellectual and moral. In doing so, he put in place the first two of the three components that constitute the ethical concept of the physician as fiduciary of the patient and therefore of medicine as a profession: *Physicians should become and remain scientifically and clinically competent.* In contemporary terms, this means that physicians should practice according to the intellectual and clinical discipline of evidence-based medicine. When physicians do so, they justifiably invite the sick to trust them intellectually, to know what they are saying and doing. Gregory was well aware that the sick did not trust their physicians intellectually and were justified in their intellectual distrust. Becoming scientifically and clinical competent means that physicians gain intellectual authority for their clinical judgments about patients' health – its preservation through primary prevention and its restoration through secondary and tertiary prevention in response to disease and injury. The scientific and clinical competence of physicians is confined to health, understood in biopsychosocial terms.[17] Physicians set themselves up for entirely preventable ethical conflict when they fail to stay within the bounds of their professional expertise and authority. This has important implications for pediatric ethics, as explained later in this chapter.

Gregory also introduced the second component of the ethical concept of the physician as fiduciary of the patient and therefore of medicine as a profession: *Physicians should commit themselves to the protection and promotion of the health-related interests of the sick as their primary concern and motivation and keep self-interest systematically secondary.* The ethical concept of the physician as fiduciary of the patient therefore requires considerable self-sacrifice. The ethically justified limits of the professional virtue of self-sacrifice thus becomes a central topic for professional medical ethics.

The first two components of the ethical concept of the physician as fiduciary of the patient are expressed in the core professional virtue of integrity. Professional integrity obligates physicians to practice medicine, conduct research, and teach according to standards of intellectual excellence (the first component of the concept of the physician as fiduciary of the patient) and standards of moral excellence (the second component of the concept of the physician as fiduciary of the patient).

Gregory gestured in the direction of the third component of the ethical concept of the physician as fiduciary of the patient and therefore of medicine as a profession when he excoriated the "corporation spirit" of the organized medicine of his own day, that is, the royal colleges operating under the auspices of a royal charter. The royal colleges were essentially merchant guilds that existed and conducted themselves primarily for the sake of the financial and political interests of their members in gaining and holding market share. The self-interested nature of the royal colleges was reflected in their "moral statutes" (*statuta moralia*) or rules of conduct. These included prohibitions against attacking brother physicians in public so as not to injure the profession, that is, impair guild members' ability to present an attractive public face to their potential customers among the well-to-do.[11]

Percival gets the credit for picking up on Gregory's gesture and explicitly expressing it in conceptual terms. Percival did so in his discussion of the ethics of determining when a physician or surgeon should retire from practice. He provided insightful analysis of intellectual skills such as an acute memory and the ability to reason by analogy from present to past cases and, for surgeons, skills such as "quickness of eye-sight, delicacy of touch, and steadiness of hand, which are essential to the skilful performance of operations."[10] This passage is especially moving in light of the fact that Percival by then had become blind and had retired from medical practice, thus following and exemplifying his ethical analysis and argument. He concluded:

Let both the physician and surgeon never forget, that their professions are public trusts, properly rendered lucrative whilst they fulfil them; but which they are bound, by honour and probity, to relinquish, as soon as they find themselves unequal to their adequate and faithful execution.[10]

This introduced the third component of the ethical concept of the physician as fiduciary of the patient and therefore of medicine as a profession: *Physicians should maintain, strengthen, and pass on medicine as a public trust for the benefit of present and future patients.*

Gregory and Percival were the first in the history of Western medical ethics to use the word "patient" rather than the phrase "the sick" – for the Latin *aegrotus*, which is used in previous texts. In doing so, they drew an important implication from the ethical concept of medicine as a profession. Until medicine became a profession, a process that started with Gregory and Percival and still has a long way to go if critics such as Rothman are correct,[18] there are no physicians, just medical and other practitioners. By consistently implementing the three commitments of the concept of the physician as fiduciary, medical practitioners become professional physicians. In other words, the profession of medicine is not a given that comes down to us robustly intact from the oath of Hippocrates. Rather, the profession of medicine exists as a function of the collective clinical judgments, decisions, and behaviors of physicians. External entities such as payers do not create the profession of medicine, and they cannot destroy or injure it. Physicians are fully in charge of both and should hold themselves accountable for both.

When there are professional physicians, the sick become patients. They can and should trust professional physicians both intellectually and morally. The older, contractual relationship between the sick and hired practitioners has been re-formed into a physician–patient relationship as a fiduciary relationship of protection and promotion of the patient's and research subject's health-related interests.

THE ETHICAL CONCEPT OF PARENTS AS FIDUCIARIES
OF THEIR CHILD WHO IS A PATIENT

The moral relationship between parents and their child who is a patient directly parallels that of the pediatrician–patient relationship: *Parents are the fiduciaries of their child who is a patient.* It is crucial to appreciate that, as laypersons, parents cannot completely fulfill the first criterion of being a fiduciary, having the competence to protect and promote the health-related interests of their child who is a patient. To be sure, parents have some competence in this arena, but their expertise pales in comparison with that of the pediatrician. It follows that, for parents to be able to properly fulfill their fiduciary obligation to protect and promote the health-related interests of their child who is a patient, they need to defer to the evidence-based clinical judgment of pediatricians. In other words, *the pediatrician and parents are co-fiduciaries of the child who is a patient.* Pediatricians therefore have the obligation, in the informed-consent process with parents, to present all of the medically reasonable alternatives to them, that is, all technically possible and physically available clinical management plans that have a reliable evidence base of expected net clinical benefit. As fiduciaries of their child who is a patient, parents are ethically free to select any one of such medically reasonable alternatives. They are not ethically free to reject all medically reasonable alternatives, because doing so is not consistent with protecting and promoting the child's health-related interests.

In making decisions about which medically reasonable alternative to accept for the clinical management of their child's condition, disease, or injury, parents should, as fiduciaries of their child who is a patient, identify and consider the non-health-related interests of their child. No special competence is required for them to do so. Pediatricians should keep in mind that, as professional physicians, they have no special competence to make judgments about the non-health-related interests of the patient who is the child of parents charged with the ethical obligation to protect the health-related and *other* interests of their child who is the pediatrician's patient. Parents' discretionary judgment about how to fulfill their fiduciary obligations to their child who is a patient should therefore be respected by the pediatrician. The assumption that pediatricians have the competence and therefore authority and power to judge and reject parental exercise of fiduciary obligations to protect and promote the non-health-related interests of their child who is a patient sets the pediatrician up for entirely preventable ethical conflict. Professional integrity imposes the discipline on pediatricians of recognizing that their professional expertise and therefore authority and power extend only to the health-related interests of a child who is a patient.

CLINICAL IMPLICATIONS OF THE ETHICAL CONCEPT OF PEDIATRICIANS AND PARENTS AS CO-FIDUCIARIES OF PEDIATRIC PATIENTS

There are two ethically justified constraints on the respect that the pediatrician owes to parental discretion, and both originate in professional integrity. Both constraints originate in the fact that failing to prevent death and to prevent serious, far-reaching, and irreversible loss of health imperils all of the child's non-health-related interests. The first constraint therefore originates in the pediatrician's fiduciary obligation to protect the life of the child who is a patient when there exist medical interventions that are reliably expected to preserve the child's life at a reasonable cost of disease-related and iatrogenic morbidity, impaired functional status, pain, distress, and suffering. The second constraint originates in the pediatrician's fiduciary obligation to protect the health of the child who is a patient when there exist medical interventions that are reliably expected to prevent serious, far-reaching, and irreversible loss of the patient's health at a reasonable cost of disease-related and iatrogenic morbidity, impaired functional status, pain, distress, and suffering. Parents do not have the right to obligate pediatricians to act in ways that are inconsistent with professional integrity, and the purpose of these two constraints is to protect the limited, ethically justified assertion of professional integrity.

Pediatricians should assert these constraints in a respectful but firm fashion. The best way to do so is to ask parents to reconsider a decision that, as a matter of professional integrity, the pediatrician should not accept. The pediatrician should also be willing to make strong recommendations, to influence parental decision making. If these measures fail, pediatricians should be clear that they will not accept the parents' decision and explain the evidence base for not doing so. Further measures to protect professional integrity and enforce the parents' fiduciary obligation to protect the health-related interests of their child who is a patient as the necessary condition for protecting the non-health-related interests of their child include referral for ethics consultation or to the institutional ethics committee, initiation of civil action to obtain appropriate court orders, or notification of child protective services in one's legal jurisdiction.

The reader will have noticed the use so far of the phrase "the patient who is a child." While perhaps somewhat awkward and certainly uncommon in clinical discourse, the phrase is important because it reminds us that the ethical concept of the co-fiduciary responsibility of pediatricians and parents is limited to the clinical setting. This concept does not bear on the larger question of whether parents should make their child a patient, that is, when parents are obligated to seek medical care for their child. This question should be addressed through institutions for making and enforcing public policy, that is, legislatures and courts. The public policy issue concerns whether the above two constraints on parental discretion over a child who is a patient should also apply – and be enforced through the power of the state – when they apply to the discretion of parents over a child who is not yet a patient, that is, who has not been brought to a pediatrician or other health care professional for medical care. The two constraints are surely relevant, and so pediatricians have a crucial contribution to make to public policy deliberations. However, there are other ethical issues, especially concerning the justification for the use of intrusive and potentially psychosocially destructive state power, that go far beyond professional medical ethics.

CONCLUSION

Ethical theory contributes to pediatric ethics by calling for the proper intellectual classification of pediatric ethics: it is a species or specialty of professional medical ethics. As professional medical ethics, pediatric ethics rests on the conceptual foundations of three ethical concepts: the pediatrician as fiduciary of the child who is a patient, parents as fiduciaries of the child who is a patient, and pediatricians and parents as co-fiduciaries of the child who is a patient. The ethical concept of the pediatrician as fiduciary of the pediatric patient is limited by the competence of medicine to address health-related interests. The ethical concept of parents as fiduciaries of pediatric patients has a wider scope, because it concerns both health-related and non-health-related interests of the child who is a patient. In the context of co-fiduciary responsibility for pediatric patients, there are two ethically justified constraints on parental authority and power over pediatric patients that originate in professional integrity.

References

1. Leikin S. Minors' assent or dissent to medical treatment. *J Pediatr.* 1983; 102:169–176.
2. Leikin S. Minors' assent, consent, or dissent to medical research. *IRB.* 1989; 15:1–7.
3. American Academy of Pediatrics, Committee on Bioethics. Informed consent, parental permission, and assent in pediatric practice. *Pediatrics.* 1995; 95:314–317.
4. Molinari V, McCullough LB, Workman R, Coverdale JH. Geriatric assent. *J Clin Ethics.* 2004;15:261–268.
5. McCullough LB, Chervenak FA. *Ethics in Obstetrics and Gynecology.* New York: Oxford University Press; 1994.
6. McCullough LB. The ethical concept of medicine as a profession: its origins in modern medical ethics and implications for physicians. In: Kenny N, Shelton W, eds. *Lost Virtue: Professional Character Development in Medical Education.* New York: Elsevier; 2006:17–27.
7. Baker RB. Deciphering Percival's code. In: Baker R, Porter D, Porter R, eds. *The Codification of Medical Morality: Historical and Philosophical Studies of the Formalization of Western Medical Morality in the Eighteenth and Nineteenth Centuries. Volume One: Medical Ethics and Etiquette in the Eighteenth Century.* Dordrecht: Kluwer Academic; 1993:179–211.

8. Baker RB. Medical propriety and impropriety in the English-speaking world prior to the formalization of medical ethics: introduction. In: Baker R, Porter D, Porter R, eds. *The Codification of Medical Morality: Historical and Philosophical Studies of the Formalization of Western Medical Morality in the Eighteenth and Nineteenth Centuries. Volume One: Medical Ethics and Etiquette in the Eighteenth Century.* Dordrecht: Kluwer Academic; 1993:15–17.

9. Gregory G. *Lectures on the Duties and Qualifications of a Physician.* London: W Strahan and T Cadell; 1772. Reprinted in McCullough LB, ed. *John Gregory's Writings on Medical Ethics and Philosophy of Medicine.* Dordrecht: Kluwer Academic; 1998:161–245.

10. Percival T. *Medical Ethics: Or a Code of Institutes and Precepts, Adapted to the Professional Conduct of Physicians and Surgeons.* London: J Johnson & R Bickerstaff; 1803.

11. McCullough LB. *John Gregory and the Invention of Professional Medical Ethics and the Profession of Medicine.* Dordrecht: Kluwer Academic; 1998.

12. Porter D, Porter R. *Patient's Progress: Doctors and Doctoring in Eighteenth-Century England.* Stanford, Calif: Stanford University Press; 1989.

13. Risse GB. *Hospital Life in Enlightenment Scotland: Care and Teaching at the Royal Infirmary of Edinburgh.* Cambridge: Cambridge University Press; 1986.

14. Hoffmann F. *Medicus Politicus, sive Regulae Prudentiae secundum quas Medicus Juvenis Studia sua et Vitae Rationem Dirigere Debet.* Geneva: Fratres de Tournes; 1749.

15. Jonsen AR. *A Short History of Medical Ethics.* New York: Oxford University Press; 2000.

16. Hume D. *A Treatise of Human Nature (1739).* Norton DF, Norton MJ, eds. Oxford: Oxford University Press; 2000.

17. Engel GL. The need for a new medical model: a challenge for biomedicine. *Science.* 1977;196:129–136.

18. Rothman DJ. (2000). Medical professionalism: focusing on the real issues. *New Engl J Med.* 2000;342:1283–1286.

3

Using the Best-Interests Standard in Treatment Decisions for Young Children

Loretta M. Kopelman

Controversies sometimes exist about how to make good treatment decisions for infants and young children. For example, consider the following:

Case 1: Baby T was born at 32 weeks gestation and, as predicted in prenatal screening, had (non-mosaic) trisomy 13 and a semi-lobar holoprosencephaly as well as microencephaly. The only indication that she is conscious is that she reacts to painful stimuli by crying and withdrawing, and with an increased heart rate. Her teenage parents, however, are angry and distrustful. They do not believe the doctors, nurses, and members of the ethics committee who agree that when Baby T is conscious she is in considerable pain and that her life-prolonging treatments have no prospect of improving her condition but merely of prolonging her dying. Although carefully and compassionately counseled before and after Baby T's birth about her condition, her parents insist that they want "everything done" because they believe their daughter will be "perfectly normal."

Holoprosencephaly is a disorder that arises from the failure of the embryonic forebrain to divide correctly. Consequently, the lobes of the cerebral hemisphere do not form properly. A spectrum of severity exists depending on the extent to which the lobes form, ranging from most severe to nearly normal. Those with the most severe form die at birth, and all are mentally retarded. Baby T has a severe case, but not as severe as that of children in whom a single-lobe brain structure exists.

Studies show that most adults would not want to prolong children's lives with maximal life-saving interventions if, like Baby T, they faced an existence of severe and intractable pain.[1-8] Comfort care and relief of pain and suffering are of primary importance in palliative care for adults, even if this results in a shorter life.

Baby T's young parents, like other guardians, have the legal authority to make medical decisions for their child whether or not this is what most adults would choose for themselves. In some jurisdictions, these same underage parents who are authorized to make complex medical decisions for their children cannot make them for themselves because they have not reached the age of majority.* What is noteworthy about this case is that all parties believe that they act in Baby T's best interests. Parental demands for health care for their child do not mean they will get it. Doctors in the United States, however, are reluctant to discontinue life-support care for infants without parental consent even if it seems harmful, in part because of policies concerning who is authorized to make decisions for children and how they must be made. Parents have considerable discretion to judge what is in their child's best interests, but they also have duties to provide them with acceptable care. This duty is part of the standard that has come to be known as the best-interests standard. It is a relatively new policy.

The policy that dominated for centuries, including well into the 20th century, was that children were the property of their parents or guardians, who were authorized to make all decisions for them. For example, Thomas Hobbes, a major figure in philosophy in the 17th century, wrote:

Children therefore, whether they be brought up and preserved by the father, or by the mother, or whomsoever, are in the most absolute subjection to him or her, that so bringeth them up, preserves them. And they may alienate them, that is, assign his or her domination, by selling or giving them in adoption or servitude to others; or may pawn them for hostages, kill them for rebellion, or sacrifice them for peace, by the law of nature, when he or she, in his or her conscience, think that to be necessary.[9]

From the vantage point of the 17th century, the most surprising feature about this statement was that Hobbes gave authority to women as well as men. This view of children as property disappeared as the 20th century advanced and another standard emerged, namely, the best-interests standard.

The best-interests standard was introduced to undercut policies that children (and other incompetent persons) were property of their guardians and to give children's interests *some* weight.[10-13] Judges, physicians, lawmakers, teachers, and others increasingly used it as a guide for making decisions for persons lacking decision-making capacity.[10-13] Consequently, with the introduction of the best-interests standard, parents were restricted to making decisions that did not abuse, neglect, or endanger their children, and clinicians could turn to the courts if parents' decisions seemed unreasonable. Today, if a father wishes to treat his bacterial pneumonia with herbal tea, he is at liberty to do so, but he has no right to make this decision for his child. Guardians still have considerable discretion unless they abused, neglected, or endangered their wards, in which case the courts have the authority to take custody temporarily or permanently.

In what follows, the best-interests standard is analyzed on the basis of how this complex guide for decision making for young children (and other

---

* For example, this is the case in North Carolina. As with any other parent, however, custody of their child can be removed temporarily or permanently in some conditions, as discussed later in the chapter.

incapacitated or incompetent persons) is used and why it is important. After discussing problems with other analyses, I will argue that this three-part analysis avoids the pitfalls of incoherence, vagueness, and subjectivity of other formulations. Properly understood in terms of its use by doctors, judges, and others, it offers clear guidance about how to protect persons lacking decision-making capacity. In the final section, I will argue that the best-interests standard should be adopted for persons of all ages for reasons of consistency, compassion, and justice and that there should not be one rule for infants and another for the rest of us.

REJECTING INTERPRETATIONS OF THE BEST-INTERESTS STANDARD REQUIRING WHAT IS IDEAL

The best-interests standard has been discussed frequently in the medical, legal, and bioethics literature, but it is given different meanings by different authors. In the bioethics literature, it has been widely interpreted as requiring decision makers to do what is *ideal*. For example, this interpretation is found in two highly influential works. First, in discussing how surrogate decision makers *must* reach decisions for nonautonomous patients, Tom L. Beauchamp and James F. Childress write:

Under the Best Interests Standard a surrogate decision maker must determine the highest net benefit among the available options, assigning different weights to the interest the patient has in each option and discounting or subtracting inherent risks or costs. The term *Best* is used because the surrogate's obligation is to maximize benefit through a comparative assessment that locates the highest net benefit. The Best Interests Standard protects an incompetent person's wellbeing by requiring surrogates to assess the risks and benefits of various treatments and alternatives to treatment.[14]

Second, Allen E. Buchanan and Dan W. Brock offer a similar analysis of the best-interests standard:

The Best Interests Principle states that a surrogate is to choose what will best serve the patient's interests, in other words, that which will maximally promote the patient's good. ... Thus, according to the Best Interests Principle, the surrogate must try to determine the net benefits to the patient of each option, after assigning weights reflecting the relative importance of various interests affected when subtracting the "cost" from the "benefits" for each option.[15]

Both formulations of the best-interests standard are problematic because they sometimes require what is *impossible*. It might be best or ideal if each of six patients receives a kidney transplantation, but if only one kidney is available, they all cannot have it. There is an old saying in ethics that "ought implies can," meaning that one cannot have a duty to do the impossible. Since these formulations of the best-interests standard sometimes require the impossible, they cannot capture the meaning of this practical standard.

Moreover, even when it is possible to provide what is ideal, the best-interests standard as analyzed by Buchanan and Brock and by Beauchamp and Childress could result in a guidance principle that is *too* individualistic. (A full discussion of these criticisms and responses to them can be found elsewhere.)[16] Moving a family from Utah to New York in order for a patient to receive marginally more effective treatments could cause the rest of the family to suffer from the disruption of the relocation and possible bankruptcy. A family is not and should not be required to ignore all interests to provide what is ideal for one member.

This formulation has also been criticized as vague and subjective. Critics question how we can really know what is ideal and charge that we probably just fall back on our own intuitions and biases about what is best to do. For example, Baby T's parents believed that they were doing what was best by keeping her alive so she could get well and have a normal life. In the next section, I offer a different analysis of the best-interests standard, arguing that it is a practical guide that does not require what is ideal, but what is reasonable, and that it offers guidance that is not excessively individualistic, vague, or subjective.

ANALYZING THE BEST-INTERESTS STANDARD IN TERMS OF WHAT IS REASONABLE

In what follows, I offer an analysis of the best-interests standard for making decisions based on its use.[12,17–19] People can, of course, define terms as they wish, but if a standard is meant to be useful it must serve a certain purpose. The purpose of the best-interests standard is to offer good and practical guidance about how to make decisions for those unable to make them for themselves. Beginning with the assumption that the analysis of the best-interests standard should reflect how it is used, I offer a three-part analysis that does not require setting aside all others' interests or providing what is ideal; rather it requires what is reasonable given the options. I argue that this analysis avoids the pitfalls of incoherence, vagueness, and subjectivity that characterize other formulations. In the final section, I will argue that the best-interests standard should be adopted for persons of all ages for reasons of consistency, compassion, and justice and that there should not be one rule for infants and another for the rest of us.*

---

* Portions of the next sections are adapted from Kopelman LM, The best interests standard for incompetent or incapacitated persons of all ages. *Journal of Law, Medicine and Ethics.* 2007;35:187–196, and Kopelman LM, A new analysis of the best interests standard and its crucial role in pediatric practice. William G. Bartholome Award in Ethical Excellence, American Academy of Pediatrics. Available at: http://aap.org/sections/bioethics/KopelmanSpeech2007.pdf.

The best-interests standard should be analyzed in terms of three necessary and jointly sufficient conditions, or so I will argue. These conditions are stated and discussed in the following paragraphs.

First, decision makers should use the best available information to assess the incompetent or incapacitated person's immediate and long-term interests and set as their prima facie duty that option (or from among those options) that maximizes the person's overall or long-term benefits and minimizes burdens.

This condition is a prima facie duty (or all-things-considered obligation) because it can be overridden by higher duties. The first condition may seem to have similarities to the analyses of Beauchamp and Walters and Buchanan and Brock, yet there are important differences. It is a prima facie duty, is only one of three necessary conditions, and does not require what is ideal but what is reasonable given the options. It might be best for someone who is dying to have a scarce resource, but there may be a higher duty to give it to someone who can recover. This first condition is relatively easy to use when informed people of goodwill agree about what information is salient, which goals and values are relevant, and how to achieve these goals and to rank the potential benefits and risks (including their nature, probability, and magnitude). If a child has bacterial pneumonia, there is overwhelming evidence that he or she should be treated with antibiotics immediately. Parents who claim herbal tea is just as good as or better than antibiotics cannot support their claims. What is good, bad, better, or best for patients is not just what anyone thinks but should be judged on objective scientific, medical, and other rational grounds. In the case of Baby T, the parents are mistaken that their child will become normal. Thus, this first condition has objective features about what is best or worst based on what we ought to believe given the evidence.

In addition to having objective features, this first condition has subjective features whereby people's values or goals may shape decisions about what is best or worst so long as they do not abuse, neglect, or endanger their ward. Because people may have very diverse values and goals, they may rank potential benefits and risks differently, with the result that they reach different conclusions about what is best for someone. People's subjective views about the value of extending the life of someone who is permanently unconscious, for example, may play an important role in deciding whether certain lifesaving interventions are appropriate. Thus, the first condition has objective as well as subjective features, but this is not the whole story; two other necessary conditions exist.

Second, decision makers should make choices for the incompetent or incapacitated person that must at least meet a minimum threshold of acceptable care; what is at least good enough is usually judged in relation to what reasonable and informed persons of goodwill would regard as acceptable were they in the person's circumstances.

This condition acknowledges that people sometimes make different choices in deciding what is best for those lacking decision-making capacity, but it requires them to select options at least meeting a minimum threshold of ethically, legally, or socially acceptable care. What is ethically acceptable may, of course, differ from what is legally or socially acceptable. For example, as noted, in the late 19th century, advocates for children increasingly argued that children should not be viewed as property and that it should be illegal to abuse, neglect, or endanger them.

Like the first condition, the second has both objective features (what choices are minimally acceptable to reasonable and informed persons of goodwill) and subjective features (personal views about what is acceptable). The objective features of the second condition are the thresholds of acceptable care or what is morally, legally, or socially a "good enough" decision. Parents who believe herbal therapies are adequate to treat their child's bacterial pneumonia are endangering their child on objective grounds. Choices should be assessed in terms of considered judgments concerning medicine, science, and duties to children.

The best-interests standard is an umbrella principle in the sense that it can be used differently in different situations. For example, what is acceptable from a legal perspective may differ from moral or medical recommendations. For example, it is not illegal for parents to have their children tested for untreatable, later-onset diseases like Huntington disease or Alzheimer disease, yet they will have a difficult time finding geneticists willing to test children for such diseases. Their professional organizations recommend against it, and most see this testing as infringing on the child's right not to know; they point out that many at-risk adults prefer not to know if they are likely to get diseases like Huntington or Alzheimer disease.[18] Parents are given considerable legal authority and up to a point may let children stay up late, watch hours of television, eat junk food, and not do their homework. In short, a decision that is good enough from a legal perspective may be far from medically or morally ideal.

The best-interests standard should not, however, be merely regarded as the "good enough" standard, since this important guidance standard should set a worthy goal for action; that is, if possible, choices should be better than merely acceptable. For example, this guidance principle directs doctors to provide the best available option for their patients, not merely what is barely good enough.

From a legal perspective, family members are permitted to decide what is best for incompetent or incapacitated relatives unless they neglect, abuse, or endanger them. Because guardians have considerable discretion, they can make decisions that take the interests of others into account. Parents must get medical care for a child having a severe asthma attack, but they have no duty to bankrupt themselves to provide the best surgeon in the world for one child at the expense of the interests of all other family members. If one is guided by how the best-interests standard is used, it is a mistake to conclude that it is excessively individualistic and excludes all other people's interests other than the needs of the patient. Moreover, as noted, this standard would be incoherent and self-defeating if it required the best for everyone.

This second condition also has subjective as well as objective features. It has subjective features in the sense that decision makers' values and views can shape decisions about what is a reasonable or acceptable option. Both families of infants favoring comfort care and families of infants favoring highly experimental care for their dying relatives may make different decisions so long as they are morally, socially, or legally acceptable choices. Decision makers can use their own values to decide what is best for their child, but their decisions cannot fall below a certain threshold of acceptable care. Everyone does not have to agree that decision makers' choices are best, just that they are objectively reasonable or good enough.

The meaning of the best-interests standard is shaped by the contexts in which it is used. These include established rights of and duties to people who lack decision-making capacity. For example, in medicine the best-interests standard is linked to duties related to providing incompetent and incapacitated persons with good patient care. These duties are related to people's rights to get care consistent with established standards of care and practice guidelines (not necessarily what is ideal). In law the best-interests standard is often used to find good (not necessarily ideal) placements for children in custody decisions in divorce cases or in situations where children are abused, neglected, or endangered. Establishing policies about how to treat others helps specify how to understand the best-interests standard when it is used in different contexts and answer charges that it is vague or means whatever anyone thinks it means.

CAPTA'S BABY DOE RULES: A CHALLENGE TO THE BEST-INTERESTS STANDARD

Some critics of the best-interests standard contend that it offers too little protection, especially for infants less than 1 year of age. They argue that it is so vague it merely invites decision makers to choose whatever they happen to think is best.* Some also argue that decision makers will not put the interests of the infant first or may place insufficient value on the lives of people with disabilities.[12] The death of a baby in 1982 fueled these criticisms and caused a policy change for infants under 1 year of age; the infant who died came to be known as "Baby Doe."

Case 2: Baby Doe had been born with trisomy 21 and could not be fed by mouth because he had esophageal atresia. His parents would not authorize the lifesaving

---

* In addition to Reagan and former attorney general Koop, Hilary Rodham Clinton also criticizes this standard as vague.

operation. Baby Doe's pediatrician sought a court order to remove parental custody at least temporarily and authorize the surgery. The Indiana courts, however, supported the family's decision, and while an appeal was being made to the United States Supreme Court, Baby Doe died.

Upon learning about the death of Baby Doe, the Reagan administration decided that more protections for imperiled infants were needed. It promulgated an interpretation of civil rights law that came to be called "Baby Doe rules." This interpretation was later struck down by the Supreme Court.[20] The current Baby Doe rules,[21] which are essentially similar, are amendments to the Child Abuse Protection and Treatment Act (CAPTA) that establish federal requirements for states to receive grants.[22] These regulations concern the treatment of extremely ill, premature, or terminally ill infants under 1 year of age. They require all infants to receive maximal lifesaving treatment (including all appropriate medications, feeding, and hydration) unless in the reasonable medical judgment of clinicians one of the following exceptions is met:

(i) the child is "chronically and irreversibly comatose";

(ii) "treatment would merely prolong dying, not be effective in ameliorating or correcting all of the infant's life-threatening conditions, or otherwise be futile in terms of the survival of the infant"; or

(iii) "the provision of such treatment would be virtually futile in terms of the survival of the infant and the treatment itself under such circumstances would be inhumane."[21] (For a full statement, see Box 3.1.)

Box 3.1. The current Baby Doe rules were enacted in 1984 and went into effect in 1985. They are funding requirements for states to receive child abuse funds, regulated by the states and technically optional. The key portion states:

[The withholding of medically indicated treatment is] the failure to respond to the infant's life-threatening conditions by providing treatment (including appropriate nutrition, hydration, and medication) which, in the treating physician's (or physicians') reasonable medical judgment, will be most likely to be effective in ameliorating or correcting all such conditions, except that the term does not include the failure to provide treatment (other than appropriate nutrition, hydration, or medication) to an infant when, in the treating physician's (or physicians') reasonable medical judgment any of the following circumstances apply: (i) The infant is chronically and irreversibly comatose; (ii) The provision of such treatment would merely prolong dying, not be effective in ameliorating or correcting all of the infant's life-threatening conditions, or otherwise be futile in terms of the survival of the infant; or (iii) The provision of such treatment would be virtually futile in terms of the survival of the infant and the treatment itself under such circumstances would be inhumane [DHHS, 1985:1340.15(B)2].

Although either set of Baby Doe rules, if followed, would have required the lifesaving surgery for Baby Doe, so would have the best-interests standard if it had been properly used.* With a relatively easy operation, the infant could have had a meaningful life. Moreover, the Baby Doe rules were immediately seen as troubling by neonatologists and pediatricians belonging to the American Academy of Pediatrics (AAP). In a survey done shortly after they were enacted, many reported that these rules ignored parental consent, caused overtreatment, and failed to take into account the infant's suffering unless the infant was dying. In reviewing one case, nearly a third of the physicians responded that CaPTA's Baby Doe rules would lead them to act contrary to the infant's best interests.[12,17,23,24]

In 2002 Wisconsin gave CAPTA's Baby Doe amendments their first and only review by an appellate state court. In *Montalvo v. Borkovec* the court ruled that a baby's parents had no role in consenting to or refusing maximal treatment because the child was not dying or comatose.[25] This ruling reflects the letter and spirit of the drafters of both sets of Baby Doe rules, namely President Reagan[26] and Attorney General Koop;[27] it also mirrors the view of other advocates who claimed the Baby Doe–type rules were needed to stop individualized interpretations about what was best for infants.[28,29] This ruling contravenes claims that the second set of Baby Doe rules (the CAPTA amendments) offered more flexibility than the first.[12]

ONE STANDARD FOR PERSONS OF ALL AGES

Adults reject CAPTA's Baby Doe–style rules for themselves. For example, the President's Council on Bioethics, when writing its report for the care of elderly persons with dementia, ardently defended the best-interests standard and rejected inflexible rules that give families few options.† The President's Council favored families and clinicians having flexibility and making individualized and compassionate decisions for the incapacitated elderly. One of the council's final recommendations is: "The goal of ethical

---

* CAPTA's Baby Doe rules were passed by Congress with the critical support of the American Academy of Pediatrics (AAP) and other organizations. While some leaders of the AAP supported both sets of Baby Doe rules, others believed the second set of rules were less stringent than the first and compatible with the best-interests standard because they included the words "reasonable medical judgment." While the words "reasonable medical judgment" appear in CAPTA's Baby Doe rules (see Box 3.1), this did not allow parents and physicians to decide on their own what is "reasonable." Doctors could employ reasonable medical judgment in applying only the three exceptions. The rules limit the use of reasonable medical judgment to assessing whether infants are dying or chronically and irreversibly comatose, or what medications or other procedures are needed to sustain life. For further discussion see Kopelman LM, Are the 21-year-old Baby Doe rules misunderstood or mistaken? *Pediatrics.* 2005;115:797–802.

† The President's Council uses the best-care standard for the legal standard and the best-interests standard for its expression in a medical context.

care giving in a clinical setting is not to extend the length or postpone the end of a patient's life as long as is medically possible, but always to benefit the life the patient still has" (p. 212).[3] The council makes it clear that decision makers should weigh benefits and burdens in another of its final recommendations: "The clearest ethical grounds for foregoing life sustaining treatment are an obligation to avoid inflicting treatments that are *unduly burdensome to the patient being treated* and an obligation to avoid treatments that are not at all (or not any longer) efficacious in obtaining a desired end" (p. 213, emphasis in original).[3] The recommendations for making medical decisions for incompetent adults match long-standing recommendations for flexibility, individualized decision making, and careful attention to quality of life in making medical decisions for children and infants by the AAP, the Nuffield Council, and other organizations.[3,30–32]

In what follows I will argue that *CAPTA's Baby Doe rules should be rejected and the best-interests standard should be used for persons of all ages.* Accordingly, recommendations and principles like those offered by the President's Council for the elderly based on the best-interests standard should not exclude infants and should also guide decisions in the care of incapacitated people of all ages.

Moral Requirements

A necessary condition of *moral* judgments is the consistency requirement that one treat others as one wants to be treated. So unless adults support a Baby Doe–type policy for themselves should they become incapacitated, they should not adopt such rules for others – in this case for infants under 1 year of age. CAPTA's Baby Doe rules restrict the kind of prudent judgment and particularized clinical judgment that are recommended by the President's Council, the AAP, and other organizations with a rigid approach to decision making; moreover, most adults want flexibility and individualized decision making for their surrogates if they should become incapacitated and reject Baby Doe–type policies for themselves.[1–8] The Supreme Court was also critical of the first set of Baby Doe rules, finding them to be inflexible, to ignore the role of surrogate consent, and to require overtreatment of some patients.[*] In contrast, the President's Council recommends that families and clinicians should be able to make a prudent decision based on the needs of the particular patient in the particular setting. Thus, the CAPTA's Baby Doe policy is unfair to infants and seems to violate a necessary condition of morally justifiable judgments by singling out one

---

[*] The Supreme Court in *Bowen v. American Hospital Association* so judged the first set of rules and the neonatologists the second set (see Kopelman LM, Kopelman AE, Irons TG, Neonatologists judge the 'Baby Doe' regulations. N Engl J Med. 1988;318:677–683). But I have argued that both sets are substantially similar.

group for rules others do not want. This judgment is reinforced when we consider issues of justice.

Justice

As a matter of justice, we should treat similar cases similarly and different cases differently where the similarities and differences are relevant. Yet CAPTA's Baby Doe rules offer a different guidance principle for infants, singling them out for an inflexible policy that adults reject for themselves. Thus, in fairness, the policies for all, young and old alike, should be the same unless someone can make a good case that age is a relevant consideration.

Some have argued that age is relevant because older patients losing capacity are on a well-understood trajectory and a mistake would not be a mistake for a lifetime, while errors in the care of an infant might make the difference between a brief and a long life. Yet in some situations the trajectory and outcomes are equally clear, such as in the case of Baby T, who had severe holoprosencephaly and other anomalies (Case 1).

Some conclude that to be fair to infants who are so young, we should pursue long shots, even a 1 in 1,000 chance to save them. Yet if adults reject this policy for themselves, good reasons should be given for adopting it for infants. Established guidelines for adults do not require that every lifesaving option be pursued unless the person is irreversibly comatose or dying; rather, they show that adults generally want flexibility and options, with their family and clinicians deciding for them if they cannot choose for themselves. They do not generally want to pursue every small chance to maintain a poor quality of life.*

Others have argued that special rules are needed to protect infants because parents have not fully bonded with them; they often cite as proof two cases, that of Baby Doe (Case 2) and that of an infant known as "the Hopkins baby" (a case that many believe occurred at Johns Hopkins Hospital but that, as we shall discuss, was a composite of three cases).[33,34]

Case 3: The "Hopkins baby" was born with trisomy 21 and a duodenal atresia that made feeding by mouth impossible. When the parents refused corrective surgery, the clinicians accepted their decision and the baby died. It took 10 days for the baby to die of dehydration and starvation.

Despite their similarities, there are some important differences between these two cases. Baby Doe was a real baby and the events discussed actually happened in 1982. In contrast, the world came to know about the Hopkins baby by means of a film that was really an account based on stories about three infants who died in the 1960s.[34] In 1971 the chair of the Pediatric

---

* These considerations were raised by members of the President's Council on Bioethics when I testified on December 8, 2005, in Washington, DC.

Department at Johns Hopkins University, Robert Cooke, made this film without clarifying that the case presented was a composite; he showed it widely, and it had a profound impact on the debate over how to treat imperiled newborns.[34] In the film the pediatricians, unlike those in Baby Doe's case, do not challenge the parents' decision. Although the Hopkins baby was not real, the biases, legal precedents, misunderstanding, ignorance, and underdeveloped policy that permitted nontreatment decisions for such babies were real and resulted in bad decisions. Unwarranted views about people with trisomy 21 needed to change and did change in the intervening decades as more was learned about this genetic condition. Unequivocally such infants would be treated today. If the parents objected to providing an infant with lifesaving interventions, a court order would routinely be obtained in many countries to take custody of the child away from the parents so the courts could give permission for such interventions.

There is danger in basing policy on a few cases, especially those from decades ago. Unjustifiable decisions can be found for people of all ages. Moreover, medicine has changed radically in the intervening decades since the Hopkins baby and Baby Doe died. New medicines, procedures, interventions, outcome studies, and intensive care units have resulted in radically different views about what is best for adults as well as infants. Finally, the assertion that special rules are needed for infants because clinicians and parents disvalue disabled infants should be backed by substantial proof and not just by anecdotes. Yet no data have been offered for such sweeping conclusions.

If no compelling justification exists for treating infants differently, and I can find none, then as a matter of justice rules like CAPTA's Baby Doe rules should be rejected as a guidance principle for decision making for persons lacking decision-making capacity.

Compassion

The current tough cases in neonatal intensive care units bear no resemblance to Baby Doe or the Hopkins baby. Rather they often represent conflicts between honoring the requirements of CAPTA's Baby Doe rules and those of the best-interests standard. As noted, shortly after the Baby Doe rules went into effect, nearly a third of the neonatologists in reviewing one case responded that the Baby Doe rules would lead them to act contrary to the infant's best interests.[23]

Consider the following case, which is somewhat similar to Case 1 and illustrates a conflict between what is required under the CAPTA's Baby Doe rules and the best-interests standard:

Case 4: Since birth, 10-month-old R.D., who has a diagnosis of holoprosencephaly, has reacted only to painful stimuli. R.D. is admitted to the hospital for failure to thrive and found to have renal failure of unknown cause. Doctors determine that his kidney disease can be managed with renal dialysis but not cured. His doctors and nurses wonder if renal dialysis is required, optional, or contraindicated given his underlying condition.

Because R.D. is not dying, can survive with treatments, and is not in an irreversible coma, the Baby Doe rules require maximal lifesaving treatments. Yet, as noted, the evidence shows that this is not the decision that most adults would want for themselves when facing a choice between prolonging a life with severe and intractable pain and a more comfortable but shorter life.[3] Comfort care and relief of pain and suffering are of primary importance in palliative care.[6–8] CAPTA's Baby Doe rules, however, unlike the best-interests standard, would not allow families and physicians the discretion to make comfort care primary unless treatment were virtually futile in terms of survival.[12,13] Unlike Baby T in Case 1, the baby in Case 4 is not dying. Yet the CAPTA's Baby Doe rules allow no consideration of suffering in making decisions unless the person is dying.

In Case 1 angry and unrealistic teenage parents refused to hear that their child would be anything but perfectly normal. In the end, the health care professionals did not challenge the competency of the parents in the courts, but tried to win their confidence. Patience, good communication, and help from the parents' minister and aunt, who was a nurse, helped win enough of their trust that they were willing to strike a compromise. Eventually the parents admitted that they believed their child would be well and normal on the date she was supposed to have been born, the due date they had been given months before, now 10 days away. Everyone agreed to provide all maximal treatment until that date, and then lifesaving treatments would be discontinued in favor of comfort care. The baby died on that date.

Many organizations, councils, and committees recommend prudence and flexibility; they allow the withdrawing or withholding of maximal care for reasons other than the CAPTA's Baby Doe rules (impending death, irreversible coma, or the judgment that treatments are virtually futile in terms of survival and are therefore inhumane).[1–8] The President's Council, unlike the CAPTA's Baby Doe rules, permits consideration of pain and not just when the treatment would be virtually futile in terms of survival.[3] The President's Council considered a case strikingly similar to Case 4. Neither patient was dying or comatose and both needed dialysis to live, although the infant also had intractable pain. The elderly patient had severe dementia and became agitated and confused upon leaving her home; yet the council judged that families should be able to decide not to provide dialysis in such cases.

The President's Council's defense of the best-interests standard encourages individual evaluations of the burdens and benefits of treatment to the person and rejects a one-rule-fits-all approach to medical decision making. Using the council's principles and finding that life for this infant is only a burden, parents and clinicians should have the option to decide if it is in the baby's best interests to make comfort care primary and not perform dialysis.

CONCLUSION

The analysis of the best-interests standard given herein is based on its purpose and use. It does not require decision makers to select the ideal option or one that maximizes all benefits and minimizes burdens for the incompetent person. Such a requirement would be individualistic and incoherent. Moreover, it is not vague when seen as part of traditions such as those in law or medicine that interpret and specify acceptable and reasonable choices for incompetent persons who cannot choose for themselves.

The best-interests standard should be used to protect people of any age who lack decision-making capacity. It offers objective guidance, including, for example, how to resolve disputes by seeking better information and clarity, but also leaves room for decision makers' subjective views as long as their choices are reasonable. It instructs surrogates to maximize benefits and minimize hazards in making decisions for the person and set that as their prima facie duty (the first condition); while this ranking may reflect decision makers' personal preferences, it must also be objectively justified as an acceptable ranking of potential benefits and risks. It should also meet considered thresholds of acceptable care (the second necessary condition) and established duties to and rights of people (the third necessary condition). Using this standard, decision makers should select what they view as the best available option, and their choice need not be ideal or exclude the interests of others. Yet their decision should be challenged if it is unreasonable or fails to meet minimally acceptable care thresholds.

Unlike CAPTA's Baby Doe rules, the best-interests standard permits, within morally, legally, and socially sanctioned limits and established duties, the sort of compassionate and individualized medical decision making adults want for themselves. This stance is also widely supported by policymakers, including those of the AAP and the President's Council.[1–8,30–32] Important guidelines for making medical decisions for sick and imperiled adults lacking decision-making capacity recommend that guardians and clinicians use the best-interests standard to find compassionate, reasonable, and acceptable choices suiting the situation.[1–8] It is unfair and morally unjustifiable to impose on others rules we do not want for ourselves. A necessary but not sufficient test of how we should treat others is how we want to be treated. To the extent possible, the same discretion about what is permitted, required, and forbidden for older persons with diminished capacity should apply to infants. If it is justifiable to foster individualized decision making by families and clinicians that focuses on the benefits and burdens to the particular patient in making decisions for older persons, we should also allow this for infants. If there are times when adults want comfort care and palliation to be the primary consideration, we should also allow this for infants. For reasons of consistency, compassion, and justice, the best-interests standard should be adopted for persons of all ages, and there should not be one rule for infants (CAPTA's Baby Does rules) and another for the rest of us.

References

1. Steinhauser K, Christakis N, Clipp E, McNeilly M, McIntyre L, Tulsky J. Factors considered important at the end of life by patients, family, physicians, and other care providers. *JAMA*. 2000;284:2476–2482.
2. Singer P, Martin D, Kelner M. Quality end-of-life care: patients' perspectives. *JAMA*. 1999;281:163–168.
3. President's Council on Bioethics. *Taking Care: Ethical Care Giving in Our Aging Society*. Washington, DC: President's Council; 2005.
4. National Hospice Organization. *Standards of a Hospice Program of Care*. Arlington, Va; National Hospice Organization; 1990.
5. Byock IR, Caplan A, Snyder L. Beyond symptom managements: physician roles and responsibilities in palliative care. In: Snyder L, Quill TE, eds. *Physician's Guide to End-of-Life Care*. Philadelphia: American College of Physicians, American Society of Internal Medicine; 2001.
6. Faull C, Carter Y, Daniels L. *Handbook of Palliative Care*. 2nd ed. Malden, Mass: Blackwell; 2005.
7. Lynn J, Schuster J, Kabcenell A. *Improving Care for the End of Life: A Sourcebook for Health Care Managers and Clinicians*. New York: Oxford University Press; 2000.
8. Doyle D, Hanks G, Cherny N, Calman K. *Introduction: Oxford Textbook of Palliative Medicine*. 3rd ed. Oxford: Oxford University Press; 2004:1–4.
9. Hobbes T. *Elements of Law* (1640); 23(8). Many editions of this work exist. An electronic version can be found at: http://etext.lib.virginia.edu/toc/modeng/public/Hob2Ele.html.
10. Goldstein J, Freud A, Solnit AJ. *Beyond the Best Interests of the Child*. New York: Free Press; 1973.
11. Krause HD. *Family Law in a Nutshell*. 2nd ed. St. Paul, Minn: West; 1986.
12. Kopelman LM. Are the 21-year-old Baby Doe rules misunderstood or mistaken? *Pediatrics*. 2005;115:797–802.
13. Kopelman LM. Rejecting the Baby Doe rules and defending a "negative" analysis of the best interests standard. *J Med Philos*. 25th Anniversary Issue. 2005;30:331–352.
14. Beauchamp T, Childress J. *Principles of Biomedical Ethics*. 6th ed. Oxford: Oxford University Press; 2008:138.
15. Buchanan AE, Brock DW. *Deciding for Others: The Ethics of Surrogate Decision Making*. Cambridge: Cambridge University Press; 1990:94.
16. Kopelman LM. The best-interests standard as threshold, ideal, and standard of reasonableness. *J Med Philos*. 1997;22:271–289.
17. Kopelman LM. The best interests standard for incompetent or incapacitated persons of all ages. *J Law Med Ethics*. 2007;35:187–196.

18. Kopelman LM. Using the best interests standard to decide whether to test children for untreatable, late-onset diseases. *J Med Philos.* 2007;32: 311–330.
19. Kopelman LM, Kopelman AE. Using a new analysis of the best interests standard to address cultural disputes: whose data, which values? *Theoret Med Bioethics.* 2007;25:373–391.
20. *Bowen v. American Hospital Association,* 106 S. Ct. 2101 (1986).
21. U.S. DHHS 1985: 1340.15[b]2 – Final Rules. Federal Register.
22. U.S. Child Abuse and Treatment Act.
23. Kopelman LM, Kopelman AE, Irons TG. Neonatologists judge the "Baby Doe" regulations. *N Engl J Med.* 1988;318:677–683.
24. Kopelman LM, Kopelman AE, Irons TG. Neonatologists, pediatricians and the Supreme Court criticize the "Baby Doe" regulations. In: Caplan AL, Bland RH, Merrick JC, eds. *Compelled Compassion.* Totowa, NJ: Humana Press; 1992:237–266.
25. *Montalvo v. Borkovec.* WI App 147; 256 Wis. 2d 472; 647 N. W. 2d 413 (2002).
26. Reagan R. *Abortion and the Conscience of the Nation.* Nashville, Tenn: Thomas Nelson; 1984.
27. Koop CE. The challenge of definition. *Hastings Cent Rep.* 1989;19(Suppl. 1): 2–3.
28. Murray TH. The final anticlimactic rule on Baby Doe. *Hastings Cent Rep.* 1985; 85:5–9.
29. Robertson JA. Extreme prematurity and parental rights after "Baby Doe." *Hasting Cent Rep.* 2004;34:32–39.
30. Oh W, Blackmon L, American Academy of Pediatrics, Committee on Fetus and Newborn. The initiation or withdrawal of treatment for high-risk newborns. *Pediatrics.* 1995;96:362–364.
31. Kohram A, Clayton E, American Academy of Pediatrics, Committee on Bioethics. Guidelines on foregoing life-sustaining medical treatment. *Pediatrics.* 1994;93:532–536.
32. American Academy of Pediatrics, Committee on Bioethics. Ethics in the care of critically ill infants and children. *Pediatrics.* 1996;98:149–153.
33. Gustafson JM. Mongolism, parental desires, and the right to life. In: *Perspectives in Biology and Medicine.* Vol. 17. Chicago: University of Chicago Press; 1973:529–530. Reprinted in: Beauchamp TL, Childress JF, eds. *Principles of Biomedical Ethics.* New York: Oxford University Press; 1979:267–268.
34. Jonsen AR. *The Birth of Bioethics.* New York: Oxford University Press; 1998.

4

The Moral and Legal Status of Children and Parents

Sadath A. Sayeed

Certain festivals will be established by law at which we shall bring the brides and grooms together. ... As the children are born, officials appointed for the purpose ... will take them.[1]

INTRODUCTION

Children and their parents are, of course, intimately related. Many of our most closely held values and personal preferences flow, and indeed much of our moral identity arises, from our experiences in familial life. Socrates recognized this in *The Republic* and proposed that the bond be immediately severed as one means to secure a more just society for all citizens of the state. It might be tempting to dismiss this radical suggestion as an anti-quated idea of Greek philosophy, but we would be short-changing ourselves by doing so. Through provocation, Socrates and Plato challenge us to think deeply about the nature of human good, the purpose of human life, and as a consequence, about procreation, child rearing, and the role of parents and the state in acting as responsible custodians for future generations. They further remind us that any descriptive account of the moral and legal status of children and parents must be built on certain core assumptions that, however widely shared, may or may not ultimately prove justifiable. A modest goal for this chapter is to introduce these concerns to the reader without presuming conclusive answers.

THE MORAL STATUS OF CHILDREN AND PARENTS

It seems sensible to start our discussion with some common intuitions about families that find expression in our developed social norms. First, we largely accept that children enter the world partly pre-wired, but not entirely pre-formed, and are thrust onto a continuum of sensory experi-ence that matures over time to help generate interests, preferences, and values. Second, we largely accept that most persons who are also parents are uniquely positioned and motivated to positively fill these experiences through their caregiving. Finally, we largely believe that it is no trivial moral matter that most parents love their children more deeply than anyone else and that they most often *willingly* enter the domain of parenting prepared to sacrifice their own interests for the sake of their children in ways they would not (nor be expected to) do for others. These foundational beliefs are succinctly captured in a recent United States Supreme Court opinion:

The law's concept of the family rests on a presumption that parents possess what a child lacks in maturity, experience, and capacity for judgment required for making life's difficult decisions. More important, historically it has recognized that the natural bonds of affection lead parents to act in the best interests of their children. As with so many other legal presumptions, experience and reality may rebut what the law accepts as a starting point.[2]

In a pluralist society like the United States, it is further accepted that there is no singular path to human flourishing. There is harm we might all agree is best avoided, but beyond that, there is no singular prescription for success. What generally follows is that we more or less accept that there is no exclusive path by which to rear our offspring. Here, as in most liberal democracies, parents can raise their children as Mormons or as atheists, to develop a love of jazz piano or NASCAR racing, to excel at mathematics or carpentry:

Reasonable people disagree both about the nature of the good life and about the how to prepare children to lead it. Consequently, although there is consensus that certain practices are harmful to children, it is much more common to find a practice is controversial but reasonable: many parents think it harmful, many others think it beneficial, and there are reasoned arguments on each side.[3]

The conservative scholar Leon Kass points to a further complexity regarding what is best for our children:

Even were we to agree that it were desirable that our children be well-behaved, excellent in their studies, or able to handle disappointment, there are tough questions about which means are best suited to these ends.[4]

Genuine indeterminacy about our children's best ends and the means to achieve them helps buttress a societal predisposition to allow parents some elbow room to raise kids as they see fit.

However, even as we are prepared to acknowledge a reasonable basis for ambiguity and imprecision in determining what is best for children, we are reluctant to abdicate all notions of responsibility, that is, to throw up our hands and yield unfettered authority to parents. This is hardly a postmodern epiphany; consider the prescient claim of the 17th-century political philosopher John Locke:

The Power, then, that Parents have over their Children, arises from that Duty which is incumbent on them, to take care of their Offspring, during the imperfect state of Childhood. To inform the Mind, and govern the Actions of their yet ignorant Nonage, till reason shall take its place, and ease them of that Trouble, is what Children want, and the Parents are bound to.[5]

More recently, the philosopher Gerald Dworkin has argued:

There is ... an important moral limitation on the exercise of ... parental power, which is provided by the notion of the child eventually coming to see the correctness of his parent's interventions. Parental paternalism may be thought of as a wager by the parent on the child's subsequent recognition of the wisdom of the restrictions.[6]

In these commentaries written more than 300 years apart, we see a core moral constraint that is meant to peck at the foot of anyone bearing responsibility for child rearing. The fact is that most children will outgrow their dependent states; most children eventually become capable of autonomous self-governance, free to accept or reject their parents' worldviews. As such, childhood can be conceptualized as a gradual process of physical and mental separation, of individuation and self-identification.

Law professor Dena Davis amplifies the moral "ought" that follows from the ubiquitous biological fact that children outgrow their dependent states:

Morally the child is first and foremost an end in herself. Good parenthood requires a balance between having a child for our own sakes and being open to the moral reality that the child will exist for her own sake, with her own talents and weaknesses, propensities and interests, and with her own life to make.[7]

Davis is sharply critical of parental decisions that purposefully appear to permanently close off opportunities for children. A paradigmatic example involves "choosing" a pre-fetus known to carry a gene that generates certain future phenotypic disability such as deafness. Whatever posited benefit the child may perceive to gain from growing up in a nurturing and loving family that celebrates the rich culture found in deaf communities, Davis argues, cannot totally justify the harm done by deliberately narrowing the child's future life prospects. Nontrivial interests of the child are being sacrificed for her parents' happiness. Put more provocatively, the child has become little more than *instrumental*, being used as a means to her parents' ends.

The force of this moral worry about using children as a means to our ends need not reach all the way back to pre-birth reproductive choices by would-be progenitors. There can be legitimate concern about some deliberate decisions by parents that appear to narrow children's life prospects after they are born. Consider the long-standing controversies involving families and religious cults in the United States. Although our laws have tended to tolerate children being brought up in such isolated communities, partly on the assumption that exposure to religious ideas and devotional life are not inherently harmful activities, our qualms about such practices of indoctrination are not entirely absent. Fanatical parents may not use the forbidden "sticks and stones," but if their efforts to inculcate so severely limit a child's exposure and understanding that, once arriving at maturity, she needs years to re-engage with modernity, we might not rest comfortably believing no real harm has been done. No doubt, what counts as serious and substantial psychological injury is notoriously much harder to measure than physical harm, but this difficulty in quantification does not deny its existence.

Taken to an extreme, the claim that children ought to be regarded as moral ends in and of themselves, that they "are deserving of respect and are not to be objectified,"[8] can serve as a conceptual basis to critique a host of controversial parenting choices. Some child advocates have even called for state licensing of parents: "Society must be much more proactive in assuring that only people who can properly raise children are allowed to become and remain parents."[8] For such theorists, the opportunity to rear children is not a right or a trump over almost all other considerations, but rather a contingent and temporary grant of authority, a custodial privilege capable of quick revocation. The moral issue is cast in terms of "justice across generations":

[This] calls for a metaphor of dynamic stewardship, in which power over children is conferred by the community, with children's interests and their emerging capacities the foremost consideration. Stewardship must be earned through actual care-giving, and lost if not exercised with responsibility.[9]

Such radical conceptualizations of the proper relationship between children and parents are obviously not without criticism. An extreme (and anachronistic) reaction has us retreating back to an Old Testament–like understanding of proper parent–child relationships, where blind obedience to parental will is the commanded norm and, for example, where capital punishment is authorized for children who curse or rebel against their parents.[10] A more sophisticated response capitalizes on the widely held intuition that preservation of the psychic bond between parents and their children is of utmost moral importance:

The influences of some parental authority and responsibility are inevitable in view of the natural dependence of children. Rather than inhibiting optimal child development, however, this element of the parent–child relationship may be the child's most valuable source of developmental sustenance. ... Children have many special needs that must be met in their quest for maturity and independence. The most critical of these needs is a satisfactory and permanent psychological relationship with their parents.[11]

Here the claim is not that we should discourage children from realizing their future independence and maturity; rather it is that the only means to ensure such a successful transition and passage into adult life is by making parental authority "sovereign."[11]

[Children] struggle to attain a separate identity with physical, emotional, and moral self-reliance. These complex and vital developments require the privacy of family life under the guardianship by parents who are autonomous. ... When family integrity is broken or weakened by state intrusion ... [t]he effect on the child's developmental progress is invariably detrimental.[12]

Thus, the reasoned push-back from the overtly "child-centered" model for evaluating the rights and responsibilities of parents focuses our attention on the perceived consequences for the child's welfare when parental authority is questioned or undercut by others. This argument boils down to an empirical claim about the inevitably worse outcomes for children who lose a vital parental connection through the interference of nonfamilial "child liberators."

Unfortunately, just as we face difficulty in measuring the degree of harm in the case of controversial child-rearing practices, we face difficulty in substantiating the evidentiary claim that the detrimental effects on children are too overwhelming when parental bonds are severed by the state. In fact, just as we know that some young adults find their voice and begin to flourish capably once freed from an oppressive child-rearing regime, we also know from experience that not all children are destined to suffer irreparable psychic damage when they are separated from wantonly neglectful parents. Still, few seriously dismiss the importance of stable and enduring relationships between parents and their children, and any realist will sensibly cast a skeptical eye at the available alternatives the state or communities to date have been able to consistently provide.

To summarize, then, if we remain steadfast in prioritizing the liberty-loving, autonomous individual in our normative outlook, we set ourselves up for inescapable moral tension in thinking about the ideal relationship between parents and their children. Children become adults, and this implies that any control parents have over their children is necessarily temporary. It means that children will eventually have the opportunity to reject their parents' worldviews. It further suggests that there may be times when we should be prepared to limit parental dominion over a child when the latter's ongoing welfare is in doubt. The controversy centers around what should constitute sufficient harm to children such that we are prepared to intercede on behalf of these vulnerable individuals. There is a real cost to interceding that cannot be lightly dismissed, and we have yet to generate broadly appealing, socially constructed alternatives. The reader is perhaps best served by recognizing the absence of convincing empirical evidence to support the more strident arguments from any advocacy camp about the ultimate consequences for children of our action or inaction. The strongest claims from both child "liberationists" and family "sovereignists" appear too sweeping.

THE LEGAL STATUS OF CHILDREN AND PARENTS

The tension reflected in competing moral understandings of the proper relationship between parents and their children bubbles to the surface in modern American law:

> Legislatures nor courts have developed a coherent philosophy or approach when addressing questions relating to children's rights. ... The absence ... is not surprising. The status of children in society raises extremely perplexing issues. The demand for children's rights calls into question basic beliefs of our society. ... Most legal and social policy is based on the beliefs that children lack the capacity to make decisions on their own and that parental control of children is needed to support a stable family system, which is crucial to the well-being of society. ... On the other hand, our society is unwilling to treat children merely as the property of adults.[13]

Transparent recognition of the problems we face in socially constructing the optimal relationship between children and their parents nowadays disguises a historical tendency in American law to grant tremendous deference to parents in almost all family matters. Despite the conceptual basis offered by John Locke prior to the founding of the United States, the realization of substantive legal rights for children is a relatively modern occurrence. Indeed, before the 20th century, children *were*, arguably, more akin to property than persons in the eyes of the law.

While it is true that parents were not free to destroy children as they might personal property, the law did little to discourage valuing them primarily as economic commodities. In 1836, the first state child labor law was passed in the United States and required only that all children in Massachusetts under the age of 15 working in factories attend a minimum of three months of school.[14]

> In 1900, one out of every six children between the ages of ten and fifteen worked for wages. One-third of the workforce in southern textile mills was children aged ten to thirteen.[15]

Political resistance to legislative attempts to regulate child labor was fierce at the turn of the century, and a public alarm was sounded to combat creeping communist ideology and the destruction of sacred family autonomy.[15] Federal efforts to gain control of and regulate child labor were not successful until 1938 after passage of the Fair Labor Standards Act.[16] Contemporaneously, evolving normative ideas about the moral status of children helped spur the creation of the American juvenile court system. The first state juvenile court system was established in 1899 in Illinois, and the model spread relatively quickly, with 46 states establishing a separate adjudicatory system for minors by 1925.[16] Before its establishment, child "delinquents" were treated no differently than their adult counterparts, being forced into adult prisons for punishable behaviors.

It is worth emphasizing here that the federal Constitution and the Bill of Rights make no explicit mention of children or parental rights and responsibilities. While perhaps tempting, it is a historical mistake to assume that the treasured liberties held by adult citizens of the United States automatically transferred to children upon ratification of these documents by the Constitutional Congress. Indeed, it was not until a trio of United States Supreme Court opinions were delivered in the first half of the 20th century that the legal rights and responsibilities of children and parents began to be addressed at a constitutional level. These three cases are essential to understanding how modern American jurisprudential thought has come to define the relationship between children, parents, and the state.

Two cases, *Meyer v. Nebraska*[17] and *Pierce v. Society of Sisters*,[18] vindicated parental rights "to direct the upbringing and education of children under their control,"[18] the latter case specifically denying states the authority to compel mandatory attendance at public schools. The *Pierce* opinion memorably states:

The child is not the mere creature of the state; those who nurture him and direct his destiny have the right, coupled with the high duty, to recognize and prepare him for additional obligations.[18]

In *Meyer*, the Court even went so far as to specifically reject the Platonic ideal of subordinating family sovereignty to the needs of the state: "[T]heir [Greek] ideas touching the relation between individual and state were wholly different from those upon which our institutions rest."[17]

The third case, *Prince v. Massachusetts*,[19] involved a custodial adult guardian and her 9-year-old niece, both of whom were Jehovah's Witnesses. Together, they preached on the street and handed out literature to passers-by, despite having been warned on a prior occasion that such activity was in violation of state child labor laws. Before the Supreme Court, the primary question involved to what extent two constitutional liberty interests – first, religious freedom specifically protected by the First Amendment and, second, a basic right of parents to raise their children free from interference – could be circumscribed by a state's *parens patriae* power. The *parens patriae* power was a traditional and established legal mechanism inherited from British law that granted government the authority to protect those persons who were deemed especially vulnerable or incapable of caring for themselves.

Prince is a landmark opinion, and distinct from its two predecessors, in decisively affirming the authority of the state, on suitable occasions, to intervene in family life. Interestingly, the Court did not reject the *Meyer–Pierce* line of reasoning, but instead modified its earlier position:

[T]hese decisions [*Meyer* and *Pierce*] have respected the private realm of family life which the state cannot enter. But the family itself is not beyond regulation in the public interest. ... and neither rights of religion nor rights of parenthood are beyond limitation. … The state's authority over children's activities is broader than over like actions of adults.[19]

Thus, if *Meyer* and *Pierce* are best understood to be constitutional vindications of parental rights, *Prince* cautions against excessive exuberance. In the eyes of the Supreme Court, children clearly have cognizable interests that are separable from those of their parents.

Child advocates have long celebrated the *Prince* opinion because it definitively establishes a basis for legally questioning controversial parental activity that might harm children. The opinion is also perhaps the legal pronouncement best known to many pediatricians because of the following rhetorical flourish:

Parents may be free to become martyrs themselves. But it does not follow they are free, in identical circumstances, to make martyrs of their children before they have reached the age of full and legal discretion when they can make that choice for themselves.[19]

The Court's concern for children in *Prince* is not countenanced merely in negative terms. Not only are parents obliged to avoid martyring their children, to avoid negligent or reckless endangerment, but they along with society have positive duties:

A democratic society rests, for its continuance, upon healthy, well-rounded growth of young people into full maturity as citizens, with all that implies. It may secure this against impeding restraints and dangers, within a broad range of selection.[19]

Thus, the justification for allowing the state to intervene in family matters not only stems from the moral separability of the child's interests from the parents', but also is based on the fact that the very existence of society depends on a continual replenishment of capable adult citizens. Perhaps, we can see in this language the footing for an argument about "dynamic stewardship" and "justice across generations."[9]

Importantly, since the *Prince* decision, American courts have never seriously doubted whether children enjoy independent legal rights. The decision helped lay the groundwork for the landmark desegregation decision, *Brown v. Board of Education*,[20] which specifically granted to children equal protection under the laws guaranteed by the Fourteenth Amendment. Around a decade later, the due process rights under the same amendment were similarly secured in another opinion, *In re Gault*,[21] a case involving a 15-year-old juvenile who had been committed to a state institution until the age of 21 without the benefit of adequate adjudicatory procedures. Today, it may seem odd that establishing children's legal rights in the United States required a long struggle by dedicated advocates over a hundred years. The fact that our laws have evolved over time to better reflect enlightened normative ideas about children speaks to the power of social and political movements. To the extent that our developed laws can and do reflect broad moral consensus, they represent society's ultimate, and arguably most powerful, expression of how we ought to regard the lives of children.

Nevertheless, the pragmatic utility of law today to assist in resolving many acute pediatric bioethical dilemmas at the bedside remains decidedly equivocal. Part of the reason resides in the fact that symbolism contained in opinions like *Pierce* is, at best, an ideal approximation. We should not fool ourselves into believing that we *know* what circumstances actually suffice to suggest the impermissible martyrdom of our children. The resolution of specific controversial cases involving children and their mental and physical health requires attention to the particular details, to the messy context in which the drama is being played out. By necessity, judges must pass authoritative judgment on whether actual or proposed conduct, behavior, or decisions are sufficiently harmful or risky to warrant punishment or prevention. Not surprisingly, judges, just like the rest of us, are apt to disagree on occasion. Consider the outcome in two more recent state cases involving parents who refused on religious grounds to treat their children with conventional cancer therapy.[22,23] In one instance, a 3-year-old child was thought to stand a 40% chance of cure, and in the other, a 12-year-old was thought to have a 25–50% chance of long-term survival. The court in the former case sided with the parents' decision and emphasized the risks and adverse effects of the treatment itself and the statistical likelihood that it would fail.[22] The court in the latter case said nothing about the risks of treatment and ordered the treatment over the objections of the parents.[23]

How do we explain such seeming legal inconsistencies? Students of law, perhaps more so than students of medicine, are comfortable living with conceptual ambiguity:

[R]ules and principles of ... law have never been treated as final truths, but as working hypotheses, continually retested in those great laboratories of the law, the courts of justice. Every new case is an experiment; and if the accepted rule which seems applicable yields a result which is felt to be unjust, the rule is reconsidered. It may not be modified at once, for the attempt to do absolute justice in every single case would make the development and maintenance of general rules impossible; but if a rule continues to work injustice, it will eventually be reformulated. The principles themselves are continually retested; for if the rules derived from a principle do not work well, the principle itself must ultimately be re-examined.[24]

Thus, for students of law, each new bioethical case represents an opportunity to revisit earlier established characterizations of harm, benefit, justice, and other necessarily abstract terms. The job in the courtroom is to convincingly make the facts of a particular case fit the logic of the controlling principles. Here, it cannot be overemphasized that both facts and laws are subject to *human* construction and interpretation. Judges, regulators, and juries, like physicians, parents, and ethicists, are all influenced by a constellation of historical and concurrent social and cultural forces, and all invariably must emphasize some details or ideas over others in rendering an opinion about any particular case. In the words of the early-20th-century Supreme Court jurist Oliver Wendell Holmes, "The life of the law has not been logic; it has been experience."[25]

In the context of pediatric health care, we now appreciate that a prudential goal for judges and state authorities is to respect (i.e., avoid interfering with) reasonable decisions made by parents on behalf of their children and/or minors who demonstrate the capacity to maturely speak for themselves. It is important to note that, when we grant some significant legal space for reasonable differences of opinion, we necessarily create the opportunity for a clash between closely held values. Thus, we are now in the habit of debating what kinds of choices parents make for their children or child-rearing conduct should be questioned by the state. And in the case of older children, we are now in the habit of debating when the preferences of these adults-in-the-making ought to be honored regardless of parental opinion. It should not be surprising that judicial decisions that touch on core pediatric bioethical dilemmas occasionally appear to be inconsistent. It should not be surprising that states map inconsistently in providing adolescents either in statutory or in common law with the opportunity for general emancipation, limited emancipation, and/or mature-minor exceptions in the medical decision-making context. While a lack of uniformity may be lamentable from the standpoint of predictability, it reinforces the observation that a pluralist society like the United States is not likely to resolve through law a deep, underlying substantive moral debate about whether, when, and how the state ought to regulate the relationship between children and their parents.

Another, less obvious limitation of law in productively resolving pediatric bioethical dilemmas can be seen by evaluation of the infamous *Baby K* case.[26] In this case, the hospital sought declaratory legal relief to avoid the provision of stabilizing life-sustaining treatment to an anencephalic child were she to present in the future to the emergency room in respiratory distress. The involved medical community argued that such treatment was futile and/or inhumane given the child's neurological status. The mother of the child desired such interventions if and when necessary to maintain life. The district court of eastern Virginia relied on, among other things, a "plain language" interpretation of the applicable federal statute, the Emergency Medical Treatment and Labor Act (EMTALA), and held that treating physicians would be required to provide the needed treatments to stabilize the child or risk statutory violation. Not surprisingly, this decision has been derided by many as a paradigmatic instance of the law's insensitivity to clinical ethics.

Arguably, however, a more complete accounting of the judicial decision would acknowledge that a judge must attend not only to the bioethical issue at hand, but also to the implications of his or her judgment for our system of legal adjudication as a whole. This does not necessarily mean that the decision was decided satisfactorily from the standpoint of what was "best" for Baby K, the providers, or the hospital; rather it redirects our attention to other important social values that are introduced once a bioethical controversy enters the courtroom. Respect for the principles of statutory construction, respect for controlling precedent, and deference to higher authorities of law are each independent and critical considerations that a judge must attend to in formulating a legal opinion. Adhering to the accepted, formal rules of judicial interpretation is something society has a profound interest in seeing our judges do – as such an assurance promotes our confidence in our legal system. In deciding *Baby K*, a judge could reasonably justify a problematic bioethical outcome by respecting what he or she understood to be the clear command of the U.S. Congress in enacting EMTALA, by not reading more into the statute than was transparently there.

This is not to say that such a sentiment actually motivated the judge in the case, but instead to suggest why some, if not most, lawyers could look at the decision and accept it *as a matter of judicial construction of statutory law*. Physicians, on the other hand, will have a much harder time swallowing such a legalistic explanation because they tend to focus on the core bioethical problem that brought the case to the courtroom in the first place: an essentially brainless child was being subjected to lifesaving treatments that she could never evince an interest in receiving. What is crucial for our discussion is to appreciate that the deciding judge could have been sympathetic to the physicians' moral worry, and perhaps even harbored doubt about the benefit of such interventions, but nevertheless found that a source of *legal* remedy is not to be found in EMTALA. Taken further, a thoughtful decision might direct the dissatisfied to the proper source of remedy: the legislature. If physicians want to change what their professional obligations consist of in cases such as this, they need to push their representative lawmakers to make for that precise allowance. Either the relevant law itself must be changed through amendment, or another source of controlling law must be successfully invoked to warrant a different judicial opinion.

The point of this exercise is to highlight a demonstrable disconnect between those in clinical medicine who sincerely seek an acceptable moral solution at the bedside and our judicial system, which is charged with providing an acceptable legal solution for all of society. Commenting on the law's inherently conservative nature and its need to serve as a reliable guidepost for future behavior in order to promote social stability, the preeminent Supreme Court jurist Benjamin Cardozo stated nearly a century ago:

> [The] work of modification is gradual. It goes on inch by inch. Its effects must be measured by decades and even centuries. Thus measured, they are seen to have behind them the power and the pressure of moving glacier.[24]

Cardozo's commentary highlights an important tension we must recognize in any discussion relating law to clinical ethics: the former is fundamentally a tool of governance and therefore subject to procedural constraints and pragmatic limitations of implementation and execution. The latter is fundamentally about how our conduct and actions can best be justified at the bedside of a patient. The two do not always share the same end purpose. As Cardozo suggests, and *Baby K* shows, the timeline for meaningful change in law is often incongruent with pressing ethical needs in clinical medicine.

Admittedly, it may be hard in the abstract to take seriously the idea that our legal institutions might someday collapse if judges don't follow the rules. But perhaps more modestly, it should not be beyond us to understand there are separable and important procedural considerations that must be taken into account when law and legal institutions are harnessed to resolve medical ethical dilemmas. We may even need to remind ourselves on occasion that we all benefit from the maintenance of a reliable, robust, and predictable system of authoritative dispute resolution that is capable of evolving, albeit slowly. Regardless, a willingness to accept occasional bedside injustice for the sake of a greater societal or institutional "good" is one reason most clinical bioethicists appear to agree on one thing: the machinery of the law should be employed only as a last resort when it comes to resolving acute bedside dilemmas.

The law's real and sometimes imagined limitations help explain our reticence to engage its help to resolve many pediatric bioethical dilemmas. In tracking the history of American family law, Professor Carl Schneider notes that despite the remarkable and undeniable power to regulate parent and child relationships bottled up within the *parens patriae* doctrine, society seems perpetually reluctant to wield it.[27] He suggests three reasons for this: first, we believe family life is private life and, therefore, subject to a sense of personal privilege and a right of noninterference; second, we believe interceding in family life to protect vulnerable parties actually risks further injuring the party the law seeks to protect (e.g., through deprivation of psychological bonds of affection); and finally, we believe the remedies that can be offered to rectify familial problems themselves are not particularly effective deterrents in situations where other social pressures have much greater influence over parental conduct. Schneider concludes:

The [state] tradition of non-interference persists not only because we fear the state's power, but also because we doubt the state's efficacy. The state's retreat from direct regulation of some areas of family life has reinforced the popular belief that "you can't enforce morality." And that retreat has encouraged people to believe that family law's ultimate goals of permitting, inspiring, and sustaining decent relations between ... parents and children can be secured – if society can secure them – only through comprehensive and costly social services and social reform.[27]

Thus, despite the high-minded rhetoric of the *Prince* opinion, today we sensibly remain tempered in our expectations of the law as it relates to children and families. Even as that watershed opinion set the stage for the

United States to put forever behind the days of unregulated child labor or of ignoring other blatantly harmful parental practices, government institutions today are still not much interested in defining "high duties" beyond the *de minimis*. State authorities do not routinely check up on parents to make sure such high duties are meaningfully fulfilled. As Chief Justice Burger intimated in the *Parham* opinion[2] quoted earlier in this chapter, the legal default is to presume that parents do right by their children, and it is only for lived experience to tell us otherwise. We really need no further proof of the descriptive veracity of his opinion than the current system of child welfare and protection in the United States. It is largely a reactionary (excluding educational mandates) model; that is, typically, only when someone bears witness and publicly objects to the perceived maltreatment of children will the apparatus of the state wake up to consider intervention. We remain a long, long way from licensing parents to be parents.

Professor Schneider's comments point to a further complexity in considering the moral and legal status of children and parents. Health care providers, teachers, and other similarly professionally placed adults have been legally deputized to act as watchmen over society's children, but as any thoughtful child advocate knows, this is no straightforward task – for it takes us right back to the gray area of debating what is best for children and what is the best means to achieve agreed-upon ends. The task is further complicated by the fact that, as deputies, we bear intimate witness to the social determinants of child health that more often have little to do with parents behaving irresponsibly and more to do with the background conditions of poverty and poor education that conspire to limit a parent's ability to fully meet the needs of the child. The complete story is rarely as simple as a "neglectful" mother failing to bring her son his asthma medication during a particularly bad broncho-spastic episode that needs more than home inhaler treatment. Too often, it is that she cannot afford to move out of a place that exacerbates her child's chronic condition, she cannot afford child care for her other children, nor does she have the extra money to take an unreliable bus to get to the clinic to get her son seen in a timely manner. If she calls 911, she is treated unceremoniously and may even be asked to foot part of the outlandishly expensive bill. We risk oversimplification in categorizing much lamentable parental conduct in black-and-white terms; a more complete picture of what we ought to think of as harm must pay attention to what the surrounding community has or has not done to assist the most disadvantaged parents among us to do right by their children.

A deeper appreciation of the social determinants of the status of children and parents also helps to explain the limitation of the world's most enlightened and dramatic effort to better secure the legal status of children in recent times. In 1989, the United Nations published the Convention on the Rights of the Child.[28] This remarkable document enumerates dozens of specific rights for children and responsibilities for member states as a formal means to promote and guarantee the welfare of all children under the age of majority. Interestingly, all member nations have ratified this convention except the United States and Somalia, making it the most widely ratified human rights treaty in history. The reasons for its failure to be accepted in the United States are complex, but a fascinating hint of the resistance harkens back to the turn of the 20th century and the fight against child labor laws: "[The convention is] the tool of a powerful feminist–socialist alliance that has worked deliberately to promote a radical restructuring of society."[29] Less ideologically driven arguments that have discouraged the adoption of the convention in the United States are based on a concern about its potentially untoward impact on our well-developed domestic family laws.

Regardless of its political fate in this country, a more critical issue regarding the convention pertains to its general enforceability. When one speaks of legal rights and responsibilities such as those contained in the convention, we are necessarily led to a pragmatic consideration of implementation. It is one thing to claim a right to some good, and quite another to back that claim with the sanction of a recognized state authority in order to ensure free exercise of the right. The First Amendment's guarantee of freedom of speech by itself would be of little import if there wasn't an effective means to vindicate such liberty interests when threatened. It is important to recognize that the UN convention provides no authority to force nations into compliance with its terms. As example, Article 24 of the convention states:

State parties recognize the right of the child to the enjoyment of the highest attainable standard of health and to facilities for the treatment of illness and rehabilitation of health.[28]

Yet we know that millions of destitute children in developing nations die each year from easily treated diseases, treatment for which is available to financially better off children whose families can afford to pay within those same countries. Similarly, by one estimate, in the year 2000, more than 250 million children were forced into labor and exploited for profit,[22] yet the convention specifically protects children from "economic exploitation and from performing any work that is likely to be hazardous or interfere with the child's education, or to be harmful to the child's ... development."[28]

Countries signing the convention are required to report on their progress to a UN committee in meeting its substantive requirements, but no formal mechanism for addressing individual complaints exists. That the convention commands broad acceptance is a major achievement – its nearly universal ratification surely emblemizes a welcome normative trend regarding the legal status of the world's children. But the gap between the declaration of children's rights and their effective enforcement remains appallingly wide in most countries. It is here where a more robust discussion of the social determinants of child health matters most. We can continue to talk about the moral and legal status of children in academic halls and in international assemblies, but unless and until we more determinedly focus on the socioeconomic conditions that systematically marginalize many children and their families, much of our discussion might continue to be mistaken for empty rhetoric by those suffering on the ground.

CONCLUSION

In conceptually outlining the moral controversy surrounding the status of children and parents and briefly tracing the historical evolution of the legal status of children, this chapter is meant to provide a foundation for considering the numerous, more specific pediatric bioethical controversies discussed elsewhere in this book. Law, particularly in a pluralist society, is ill suited to the task of comprehensively quashing entrenched moral disagreements about the nature of family life. One enduring dilemma we face is: if we really believe that children are separable from their parents, and ideally should be entitled to a free and open future, we must cast a suspicious eye on custodial activity that purposefully and demonstratively narrows future mental and physical prospects. Yet if that is an essentially moral proposition, it is distinctly different from the following legal question: when should our suspicion translate into state action? An answer to this question requires a definitive characterization of the conduct or decision in question as harmful or not. Almost all pediatric bioethical controversies taken to the courtroom nowadays turn on an intractable disagreement about how best to understand the posited harm to the child. For many children in the world, the whole idea of debating the nature of their harm in a courtroom remains fanciful. Arguably, our social, lived experiences with and among children offer our most vital source of normative inspiration.

References

1. *Plato's Republic.* Grube G, trans. Indianapolis: Hackett; 1974.
2. *Parham v. J.R.,* 442 U.S. 584, 1979.
3. Gilles SH. Christians, leave your kids alone! *Constitutional Commentary.* 1999; 16:149–212.
4. President's Council on Bioethics. *Beyond Therapy: Biotechnology and the Pursuit of Happiness.* Pre-publication version. Washington, DC; October 1983.
5. Locke J. *The Second Treatise of Government.* Peardon T, ed. London: Macmillan; 1986.
6. Dworkin G. Paternalism. *Monist.* 1972;56:64–74.
7. Davis D. Genetic dilemmas and the child's right to an open future. *Hastings Cent Rep.* 1997;27:7–15.
8. Eisenberg HA. "Modest proposal": state licensing of parents. *Conn Law Rev.* 1994;26:1415–1452.

9. Woodhouse B. Hatching the egg: a child-centered perspective on parents' rights. *Cardozo Law Rev.* 1993;14:1747–1865.
10. Exodus 21:15; Deuteronomy 21:18–21.
11. Hafen B. Children's liberation and the new egalitarianism: some reservations about abandoning youth to their "rights". *BYU Law Rev.* 1976;605–658.
12. Goldstein J, Freud A, Solnit A. *Before the Best Interests of the Child.* New York: Free Press; 1979.
13. Wald M. Children's rights: a framework for analysis. *UC Davis Law Rev.* 1979;12:255–282.
14. Child Labor Public Education Project. Available at: http://www.continuetolearn. uiowa.edu/laborctr/child_labor/about/us_history.html. Accessed October 24, 2008.
15. Woodhouse B. Who owns the child? *Meyer* and *Pierce* and the child as property. *William and Mary Law Rev.* 1992;33:995–1122.
16. Abrams D, Ramsey S. *Children and the Law: Doctrines, Policy, and Practice.* 2nd ed. West Group; 2003.
17. *Meyer v. Nebraska,* 262 U.S. 390, 1923.
18. *Pierce v. Society of the Sisters of the Holy Names Jesus and Mary,* 268 U.S. 510, 1925.
19. *Prince v. Massachusetts,* 321 U.S. 158, 1944.
20. *Brown v. Board of Education of Topeka, Shawnee County, Kan.,* 347 U.S. 483, 1954.
21. *In re Gault,* 387 U.S. 1, 1967.
22. *Newmark v. Williams,* 588 A.2nd 1108 (Del 1991).
23. *In re Hamilton,* 657 S.W. 2nd 425 (Tenn 1983).
24. Cardozo B. *The Nature of the Judicial Process.* New Haven, Conn: Yale University Press; 1921.
25. Holmes O. *The Common Law* (1881).
26. *In re Baby K.,* 832 F. Supp. 1022 (E.D.Va.1993).
27. Schneider C. Moral discourse and the transformation of American family law. *Mich Law Rev.* 1985;83:1803–1880.
28. United Nations Convention on the Rights of the Child. ILM 1989;28: 1448–1453.
29. Fagan P. How UN conventions on women's and children's rights undermine family, religion, and sovereignty. *Heritage Found Rep.* 2001;1407:1–3.

5

The Ethics of Pediatric Research

Jonathan D. Moreno and Alexandra Kravitt

In general terms, the ethics of adult participation in research is fairly straightforward: adults must consent to being the subjects of research and, in doing so, assert their autonomy in determining the discretionary use of their bodies. But unlike adults, children cannot give such consent. Many have not yet matured sufficiently to understand the risks and benefits of participating in a study, and they are not yet fully able to weigh the pros and cons of participation for themselves or to contribute to new knowledge that may help future generations of children. Yet there is a consensus that children's participation in research may be ethically justifiable under certain conditions.

There is ample reason for caution. The history of research with children reveals that the interests of child participants were not always protected and that in some cases researchers exploited children. In the past 40 years, however, the United States has developed guidelines and regulations to protect children from serious and unnecessary risks and to safeguard their best interests. While these standards are intended to be as straightforward as are regulations for adults, there is still room for misinterpretation and controversy.

HISTORICAL PERSPECTIVES

Most documentation of pediatric research was scant until the 18th century. In fact, most pediatric writing until the late 1600s focused on simple observations, folklore, and trial and error. The physiology of children and adolescents was not explored at this point, and infant and maternal mortality rates were consistently high. During the 17th century, there was a rebirth of medicine, and physicians took an interest in children and their ailments.[1] This great interest in disease led to the introduction of a smallpox vaccine in the 18th century. The first immunization trials were performed on slaves and children. In 1796, Edward Jenner vaccinated his 1-year-old son with cowpox to see if it offered immunity to smallpox. Later, Jenner experimented with his inoculation on other children in his village. Unlike many other researchers of his time, however, Jenner discussed the risks with his subjects and attempted to minimize them. He did not seem troubled by the fact that he used children in his breakthrough experiments, because he strived to create a vaccine that would be of great benefit to children and society. In 1802, Jenner's vaccine was tested on 48 children residing in an almshouse.[2]

Pediatric medicine became thoroughly recognized in the 19th century, leading to the creation of pediatric hospitals.[3] The establishment of an environment with a group of individuals within a certain age range gave researchers a stable population with which to experiment. These institutions, along with orphanages, had frequent and rapid outbreaks of viruses, making children desirable candidates for research. Like most research of the time, there was little or no concern about securing parental permission or the child's assent, and most people considered the societal benefits of research on children to outweigh the risks that were imposed.[1] After the exploitation of children as laborers during the industrial revolution, the early 1900s saw greater interest in child welfare and children's health problems. Unlike Jenner, investigators of the early 20th century rarely discussed the risks or discomfort associated with research. Subjects were often children of economically disadvantaged parents, were abandoned, or resided in orphanages. The initiation of World War II created a rushed incentive to perform research on children in order to assist with the well-being of soldiers overseas. Both Allied and Axis forces expanded research exponentially throughout this period. Scientists at Nazi concentration camps performed horrifying and dehumanizing experiments on adults and children. These experiments often resulted in extreme suffering, disability, and, most often, death. Josef Mengele, a German SS officer and a physician at Auschwitz-Birkenau, was particularly interested in twins and dwarfs.[4] He dissected live infants, castrated boys without the use of an anesthetic, and even sewed two Gypsy children together in an attempt to create Siamese twins. Most of his subjects died during his procedures or shortly thereafter due to infection, and none of them had the capacity or opportunity to refuse participation.

Following World War II, studies were conducted at Willowbrook State School in New York, home to mentally impaired children. In the studies, researchers deliberately infected children with viral hepatitis in order to study the natural course of the disease and, it was hoped, develop a prophylaxis. Willowbrook was overcrowded and unsanitary, which optimized the transmission of hepatitis and its incidence. Critics of the Willowbrook experiment argue that the infection of healthy children amounted to the exploitation of an institutionalized and vulnerable population.[5]

The Tuskegee Syphilis Study was initiated in 1932 by the U.S. Public Health Service to investigate the progression of syphilis in 400 black men in Alabama. The Tuskegee study did not involve children, but its exposure focused the public eye on the exploitation of vulnerable populations in the research setting.[6] Other experiments in which children were exploited include Dr. Henry Heiman's attempt, at the end of the 19th century, to produce gonorrhea in a 4-year-old "idiot" with chronic epilepsy as well as a 16-year-old "idiot."[7] (Patients with mental illnesses were readily exploited.) After their invention, physicians used x-rays to study the development of the fetus in utero. Earlier, in 1896, Dr. Arthur Wentworth performed spinal taps on 29 children to determine if the procedure was harmful.[7] In essence, history has shown that children have been mistreated, exploited, and violated as research subjects.

REGULATIONS ON PEDIATRIC RESEARCH

In 1947, 23 Nazi medical doctors and bureaucrats were tried in Nuremberg, Germany, for crimes committed in the form of medical experiments in concentration camps. Concerned about the apparent absence of an internationally recognized standard of human experimentation ethics, the Nuremberg judges formulated what posterity has come to know as the Nuremberg Code. The first principle of the code states that "the voluntary consent of the human subject is absolutely essential. This means that the person involved should have legal capacity to give consent."[8] The judges addressed research with adults only, vetoing research on children and arguing that children lack the legal capacity to make informed decisions. In 1964, Nuremberg's concern with "healthy volunteers" was overridden by the World Medical Association Declaration of Helsinki. While Nuremberg was regarded as a response to horrifying and unjust research performed in concentration camps, Helsinki addressed the hazards of under-researched treatments.[9] It also differentiated between therapeutic research (procedures administered on the basis of evidence that intervention may benefit research participants individually) and nontherapeutic research (procedures that are administered without therapeutic warrant, solely to answer the scientific question at hand).[10] Furthermore, Helsinki allowed both types of research to be performed on a minor with consent from the minor's representative.[7] In 1974, Congress created the National Commission for the Protection of Subjects of Biomedical and Behavioral Research, which is known more succinctly as the National Commission. The National Commission made recommendations concerning research regulation.[1]

Two central figures in the pediatric research ethics debate included Paul Ramsey and Richard McCormick. In 1975, Ramsey, a Protestant theologian, suggested strict compliance with the Nuremberg Code, asserting that there should be a complete ban on research with children, unless that research offered the prospect of direct benefit to the child.[11] While Ramsey held to strict prohibition on nontherapeutic research with children, Richard McCormick, a Catholic theologian, argued that research with children is not only morally permissible but morally obligatory to improve the health and well-being of children; parental consent is enough to safeguard the interests of the individual child.[12] Another view was held by Diana Baumrind, a research psychologist, who in 1978 introduced the concept that a child's participation in research should be encouraged as a morally socializing event. Parents should have their children participate in research to introduce them to altruistic values. Current federal regulations concerning research with children are a compromise between the proposals of Ramsey and McCormick.[4]

The National Commission introduced the Belmont Report, one of the most influential documents concerning research ethics, in 1979.[1] This report declared three key principles. The first stipulated that, in research, there must be respect for persons. According to the report, respect has two components: "first, that individuals should be treated as autonomous agents, and second, that persons with diminished autonomy are entitled to protection." Furthermore, "[r]espect for the immature and the incapacitated may require protecting them as they mature or while they are incapacitated,"[13] referring to children and others who lack the ability to provide consent. Informed consent, parental permission, and the minor's assent are the practical applications of the Belmont principle of respect for persons. The second Belmont Report principle concerns beneficence, which is understood to be the ethical requirement to, first, "do no harm" and, second, to "maximize possible benefits and minimize possible harms."[13] Finally, the report requires justice, which is understood to be "fairness in distribution" of the burdens and the benefits of the research enterprise.[13] The Belmont Report provides the framework on which ethical decisions concerning pediatric research are based.

Following the Belmont Report, Congress adopted in 1981 the "Policy for Protection of Human Research Subjects" of the Department of Health and Human Services (DHHS). This document was revised in 1991 and is now known as the "Common Rule" and codified as 45 CFR 46. The Common Rule instructs institutional review boards (IRBs) to ensure that the risks to subjects are minimized and that these risks carry reasonably equal weight in relation to the anticipated benefits. In 1983, Subpart D, "Additional Protections for Children Involved as Subjects in Research," was added. An IRB must determine which of the following categories of research apply to the proposed study:

45 CFR 46.404: Research involving greater than minimal risk to the children.
45 CFR 46.405: Research involving greater than minimal risk but presenting the prospect of direct benefit to the individual child subject involved in the research.

45 CFR 46.406: Research involving greater than minimal risk and no prospect of direct benefit to the child subjects in the research, but likely to yield knowledge about the subject's disorder or condition.

45 CFR 46.407: Research that the IRB believes does not meet the conditions of the above (404–406), but finds that the research presents reasonable opportunity to further the understanding, prevention, or alleviation of a serious problem affecting the health/welfare of children.[14]

In following these rules, IRBs assess whether or not a physician is morally permitted to offer enrollment in a clinical trial to his or her patient. The conventional answer is that a physician is morally permitted to offer enrollment when the administration of therapeutic procedures in a clinical trial is consistent with competent medical care. Nontherapeutic procedures do not offer therapeutic benefit to participants, so IRBs must weigh the risks, which are limited to a "minor increase over minimal risk." The IRB reviewing the study should be able to conclude that the risks to the study subjects are minimized and consistent with a sound procedure. Furthermore, it must determine whether the risks are reasonable in relation to the knowledge potentially gained.

An IRB may routinely rely on the moral intuition of board members in order to promulgate these rules, and reliance on individual intuition may result in inconsistent decisions among IRBs.[10] For example, an IRB must determine whether a research study would pose greater than minimal risk to the child. "Minimal risk," as defined by the code of federal regulations 45 CFR 46.102, entails "that the probability and magnitude of harm or discomfort anticipated in the research are not greater in and of themselves than those ordinarily encountered in daily life or during the performance of routine physical or psychological examinations or tests." Yet this definition does not specify the risks of daily life, nor does it describe what "direct benefit" or "minor increase over minimal risk" encompasses. Therefore, much depends on how each IRB defines "minimal risk."[15]

To apply the "risks of daily life" standard, it may appear that IRBs must first determine the amount of risk in the daily lives of the children who might be in the study, in order to have a basis for comparing the risks of a certain research proposal. Yet this "individualized risk" interpretation would allow researchers to expose some individuals to greater risks because they may already face greater risks in their daily lives. Many researchers and IRBs consider the process of determining who has greater daily risks – and therefore who is more suitable for a study – to be exploitative and manipulative. A more common standard for assessing minimal risk is the objective interpretation. This standard refers to the risks of average healthy people's daily lives. The Council for International Organizations of Medical Sciences takes a different route: it concludes that those unable to consent may be involved in nontherapeutic research that will not directly benefit them only when the risks are equal to or less than those "associated with routine medical and psychological examinations of such persons."[16] This definition, however, is also controversial. Another guideline, the "charitable participation" standard, establishes that individuals should participate in research that does not offer them direct benefit only when the risks of the study do not exceed the risks of charitable activities that are acceptable for those individuals in their daily lives. For example, for average healthy American children, the activity that poses the greatest risk of death in their daily lives appears to be riding in a car. If a child were to ride in a car as part of his or her participation in a charitable activity, the mortality risks allowed under the charitable participation standard would be the same as those allowed under the risks of daily life.[17] There is little guidance for how an IRB should interpret minimal risk when assessing a proposed study; the concept is vague and holds different contextual meanings.

COMPETENCE, PERMISSION, AND ASSENT

In the United States, individuals under the age of 18 are considered minors. A competent adult is presumed to have an adequate level of decisional capacity and is therefore granted the right to decisional autonomy. While adults are presumed to be competent, minors are presumed to be incompetent, without any decisional capacity. Until minors reach the majority age, they are legally dependent on their parents or guardian. Exceptions are made for emancipated minors – for example, members of the armed forces or those who are not financially dependent on their parents – a point to which we shall return later.

In the medical setting, a competent adult must give informed consent to be treated or to participate in a study. Informed consent is derived from the duty to respect personal autonomy. With minors, however, the state assumes that the child is not competent to make autonomous decisions concerning medical treatment, so parental permission takes the place of informed consent. The process of enrolling a child in research is not limited to parental permission; the child's assent should also play a significant role in the decisional process if, in the IRB's view, the child is capable of providing assent. Obtaining assent consists of informing the minor of his or her condition and of the test or treatment proposed, and then asking the minor whether he or she is willing to undergo that test or treatment.

While the requirement for assent is necessary to show respect for the child, assent is basically a statement of preference.[18] The main difference between assent and consent is that while the willingness of the minor to participate in the study is given great weight, the treatment may proceed against the wishes of the minor if the parent or guardian gives his or her permission.[19] Parental permission is not always required of both parents. An IRB may determine that one parent's permission is sufficient under 46.404, minimal risk, or 46.405, providing direct benefit to the child. The permission of both parents is required when research is approved under 46.406, if there is a minor increase over minimal risk and no prospect of direct benefit to the child. Exceptions to having both parents give permission include situations in which one parent is deceased, unknown, incompetent, or unavailable. One may argue that permission by two parents provides greater protection for the child than the permission of only one parent, but there may be a caveat here: both parents must be *willing* to sign for the child's participation in research. Given that 3,742 American children are born to unmarried women everyday, it may be too difficult for the other parent to consent even if he is known and competent. Many single parents fear that the second parent will refuse to give permission because of interpersonal antagonism; their refusal may not have to do with the best interests of the child.[15]

We assume that parents provide permission for the treatment seemingly in the best interests of the child, for the right of parental permission is founded on the values of parenting and of preserving the intimate bond within the family. Parents have authority over their children when it comes to medical care. Children do not always know what is in their best interests, and it is assumed that parents do know their child's best interests. Yet it does not follow from this premise that parental duty is always to decide based on the best interests of their child; it is contestable that a child's best interests are most efficiently served by parental permission. There may be conflicting interests with the best interests of the child. For example, parents may have other children and the interests of one child may conflict with the interests of another. The parents may also have other duties that conflict with the best interests of the child. While parents are not the rightful *owners* of their children (in this day and age, one cannot be owned by another person), the child's best interests will follow from the values of parenting. Children are the products of their parents, but since they are their own functional beings, parents do not have ownership rights over their child as an artist may have over his painting. Parents are protectors of their children but do not have ownership rights that would allow them to treat their children as if they were material products.[20]

A child's assent cannot be overridden if the treatment or the study is for nontherapeutic purposes, even if there is no breaching of minimal risk. Consider the case of a physician who asked a father and his son if he could take a small blood sample from the child for his research. The physician explained that the research was not for the child's therapeutic benefit, that taking blood would hurt only a little and would not create long-lasting harm. The father gave his permission, but the son refused to do so. The father demanded that the researcher take the sample:

This is my child. I was less concerned about the research involved than with the kind of boy I was raising. I'll be damned if I was going to allow my child, because of some idiotic concept of children's rights, to assume he was entitled to be a selfish, narcissistic little bastard.[5]

A commentator on this case argues that the father was not teaching his son altruism, but was merely being a dominant force. He contends that a child's dissent should be respected so he has some ability to be autonomous.[15]

Our society promotes intimate family relationships, for we share ourselves with those to whom we are closest. In order to preserve family intimacy, many believe that parents should make decisions for their children. Yet in order to have intimacy in a family, parents ought to also be open to the opinions of their child and the pediatrician. This openness promotes an even stronger familial bond. Parents may put inappropriate demands on their child and the pediatrician. Parental love is central, but sometimes the love is so strong that it promotes a motivation that does not actually lead to meeting the child's best interests. Strong love may lead parents to demand a treatment or test for a child that may be unpleasant or extreme. Therefore, many argue that the decision to include a child in research should be reached only when the doctor sees that the interests of the child and the parents have been separated.[20]

INFORMING PARENTS AND CHILDREN ABOUT RESEARCH

Problems relating to competence on both the parent and child side of consent are compounded by those arising in relation to the provision of information. One of the most significant challenges of the research setting is the ability of the doctors or investigators to impart information about the study to the parents and their child in the clinical setting. Parental comprehension of most aspects of research is judged to be poor. Perhaps it is difficult for them to understand the language used in the design of the study, and this difficulty may be magnified in a setting where the child or parents are upset, confused, or ill. Society in general suffers from a lack of understanding of research methodology. This lack of understanding may prevent parents or children from consenting to research, or it may allow them to enter into a study that they may not have wanted to enter. Despite signing the consent form, participants may later complain that they did not understand the full implications of the consent.[21]

A study done by Eric Kodish and his colleagues investigated how researchers explained randomization to parents whose children were candidates for enrollment in pediatric leukemia treatment trials. The authors reported that 50% of the parents interviewed did not understand the concept of randomization (50% did not understand that their child's treatment would be selected by random assignment), while 18% of the parents did not know that they could refuse to have their children participate in the study, and 20% did not know that they could withdraw their child from the study at any time. Parents of a lower socioeconomic status were less likely to understand the concept of randomization than were parents of a higher socioeconomic status.[22]

Despite Kodish's results and other evidence indicating poor understanding on the part of parents and children, successful consent procedures can be implemented if good-quality and accessible information is available to them. Some studies have shown that providing an information sheet or leaflet has improved their understanding. More research is needed on competent children's comprehension of information relating to research and how to best inform children. Although children may be given leaflets and brochures about a study, there is little evidence that reading material is the best way to inform them. Videos and education through the media and at school could also be valuable in informing children about research and its methodology.[23]

THE RESPONSIBILITY OF INVESTIGATORS AND IRBS

In some cases, researchers can be perceived as placing their own inquisitiveness and the interests of their institutions above the interests of the research subjects and the communities to which they belong. While there is room for researchers and their institutions to increase their respect for research protection policies, specific scandals and failures do not indicate that the system of oversight is naive or corrupt. The case of *Grimes v. Kennedy Krieger (KKI)* is an instructive example of an alleged lack of oversight and underestimation of the interests of minor subjects. In a two-year study (1993–1995), researchers at KKI, a Baltimore-based child's health facility and research institution associated with Johns Hopkins University, set out to measure the effectiveness of differing levels of lead abatement procedures in housing. The U.S. Environmental Protection Agency and local Maryland organizations funded the study in order to determine how much rental property owners would need to invest in order to reduce lead exposure to children. A total of 108 Baltimore rental properties were classified into five groups of varying lead abatement with two control groups. Over the two-year period, the researchers measured and compared lead dust levels collected in the housing with lead levels in blood samples drawn from the children living in those homes. Informed consent was obtained, and parents were kept up-to-date about their child's blood levels and the results of lead dust collection in their houses.[24]

Two families involved in the study brought cases against KKI. The Maryland Court of Appeals allowed the parents of the minor children to bring a negligence lawsuit against KKI for lead-related injuries acquired during the study. The parents claimed that KKI designed a study that placed their children at an unnecessary risk and that KKI had discovered dangerous lead conditions in their houses but delayed reporting the test results. Furthermore, they claimed that KKI had failed to completely and accurately inform them about the hazards and risks of the study. The Maryland judges expressed concern that the study's consent forms did not clearly explain the risk that the children would likely ingest lead dust particles that could be extremely hazardous to their well-being. In addition, the court was concerned that such studies have the potential to exploit economically disadvantaged populations because they have limited access to lead-free housing. One of the main conclusions reached by the appeals court was that, in the state of Maryland, a parent cannot consent to a child's participation in nontherapeutic research that involves *any* risk of damage to the child's health.[25] The case of *Grimes v. Kennedy Krieger* brought two important lessons into the spotlight: first, all risks of the research must be disclosed in the consent form, and second, parents must be made aware of any new risks that are discovered during the course of the study. If researchers are not able to convince the research population that their study is acceptable, they must reevaluate and revise their proposed research until the community's concerns are minimized. Also, researchers must place the interests of their research subjects above their own study's interests as well as the interests of their institution.[24]

SELECT POPULATIONS

Adolescents

The adolescent population consists of persons who are approximately 10–21 years of age. Adolescents face social pressures, the development of cognitive skills, and hormonal changes that promote high-risk behaviors that may have negative long-term health consequences, such as violence, risky sexual activity, and substance abuse. Consequently, adolescents are a particularly interesting population for researchers to investigate. Most adolescents are considered minors without the competence of adults; competence in this sense is not necessarily an indication of decisional capacity, but a legal term that gives individuals "adult" status. Several standards are used to determine decisional capacity: evidencing a choice, understanding the facts involved in a choice, manipulating information, and appreciating the nature of the information and applying it to one's personal situation. An individual's decisional capacity depends on his or her ability to evaluate the risks and benefits of a certain situation and make an autonomous decision. Children and adolescents develop decisional capacity in different stages; minors have differing abilities when it comes to risk–benefit evaluation.[19]

Jean Piaget evaluated the stages of mental development in children and adolescents. The final and most important stage of development is the "formal operations stage," where children and adolescents between the ages of 11 and 13 develop the ability to think abstractly and hypothetically, which would be required in order to choose between options and consent to treatment. Some individuals do not reach this stage until much later, even into adulthood. As a result, it may be concluded that there is no one age at which all individuals develop decisional capacity to consent to treatment or a study. The current 18 years of age policy does not take into account the individuals between the ages of 13 and 18 who may have reached the formal operations stage and therefore have the cognitive ability to consent. Findings from other studies show that many adolescents under the age of 18 do indeed possess elements of decisional capacity that are necessary for providing consent.[26]

As a result of these data, the decisional role of older minors has changed in certain contexts. In its 1978 report, the National Commission emphasized the need to recognize and respect the wishes of children as they cognitively mature.[21] State laws require parental permission for most forms of treatment for minors, but there are exceptions to these laws that allow adolescents to receive treatment or participate in a study without their parents' permission or even their knowledge. There are three major exceptions: emancipated minors, mature minors, and medically emancipated minors.

Emancipated minors are treated by the law as though they have already reached the age of decisional capacity and are no longer under the care of their parents or guardians. In the past, minors have become emancipated when they married or enrolled in the military. Today, courts have also ruled that minors may be considered emancipated if they live apart from their parents, if they are are financially independent, and if their parents no longer care for them. Once emancipated, minors may consent to their own medical treatment or enrollment in studies, though this ability is not explicitly stated in all state laws.[2]

The concept of "mature minor" has evolved as a means for minors with an adequate level of decisional capacity and understanding of their medical situation to consent to treatment or participation in a study. This statute applies to minors who are not emancipated from their families but demonstrate the ability to understand the risks and benefits of a treatment and the ability to provide consent. The mature-minor doctrine, unlike the emancipated-minor doctrine, applies only to specific medical decisions. In most states, the standards for identifying a minor as mature include marriage, pregnancy, or status as a minor parent. In other states, emancipation is one means of being declared a mature minor.[15]

Medically emancipated minors are minors who may be treated by their physicians for medical conditions without the involvement of their parents. This permits an adolescent to seek care if he or she has a sexually transmitted disease, has a mental illness, suffers from substance abuse, or requires treatment pertaining to pregnancy and contraceptives. Physicians have begun to make attempts to involve minors who are terminally ill or at the end of life in the decision-making process in order to increase their comfort in these final stages.[19]

These exceptions allow researchers to obtain waivers of parental permission; 45 CFR 46.408 (c) permits an IRB to waive parental involvement in research.[27] The National Commission emphasized the "special needs of adolescents," particularly the need for improved treatment of problems involving sexual health and drug use. The commission argued that requiring parental permission for research participation in these types of studies would make it difficult for certain types of research to take place due to the sensitive nature of the material and the reluctance of adolescents to request parental permission to participate in these studies. Studies that involve drug use, mental health, sexual activity, and pregnancy have the potential to improve adolescent health, but it is difficult to enroll participants because they do not feel comfortable obtaining permission from their parents.[27] Unfortunately, IRBs rarely invoke the option of waivers for research involving adolescents. This is perhaps due to the fact that IRBs interpret the appropriate uses for a waiver in different ways, and some IRBs would waive parental permission while other boards would require permission for the same studies. There is little federal guidance on how an IRB should allow for a waiver. In 1995, the Society for Adolescent Medicine released guidelines that encouraged IRBs to utilize waivers, but these guidelines did not greatly influence IRB decision making. In 2003, the society re-released these guidelines, emphasizing the urgent need for research with adolescents, yet it appears that many IRBs still do not make waivers more available.[27] The lack of waivers for research with adolescents represents an obstacle to research that could be very beneficial to adolescent health and well-being.[19]

Wards

The final section of Subpart D addresses research with wards. A "ward" refers to a child who has no parental or legal guardian to provide permission for enrollment in a study. A ward may be in an institution or in foster care. 45 CFR 46.409 permits wards to be enrolled in research that has the prospect of direct benefit or offers no greater than minimal risk. Under 45 CFR 46.409 (a), however, research that involves a minor increase over minimal risk or research approved by the DHHS may be conducted on a ward only if the research is related to the child's status as a ward or is conducted in "schools, camps, hospitals, institutions, or similar settings in which the majority of children involved as subjects are not wards."[14] Research with wards also requires the appointment of an advocate for the child's interests.

Neonates

While the philosophical guidelines for research with neonates are similar to those for any other child, there are some subtle differences. In 2001, Subpart B – Additional Protections for Pregnant Women, Human Fetuses and Neonates Involved in Research – was revised and codified as 45 CFR 46.201–207, which concerns nonviable neonates or neonates whose viability is uncertain. The main purpose of Subpart B is to regulate research involving pregnant women, fetuses, and nonviable fetuses after birth. A nonviable neonate is defined in 45 CFR 46.202 (e) as "a neonate after delivery that, although living, is not viable," and in 45 CFR 46.202 (h) "viable" is defined as "being able, after delivery, to survive (given the benefit of available medical therapy) to the point of independently maintaining a heartbeat and breathing."[14] Researchers face a great difficulty, as much neonatal research involves extremely premature neonates with questionable future viability. For neonates in this uncertain state, Subpart B attempts to ensure that research is delayed until there is a prospect of enhancing the probability of long-term viability or that the knowledge obtained by making the neonates research subjects cannot be gained by any other means.[1]

PAYMENTS FOR PARTICIPATION IN RESEARCH

Enticing potential research participants with money is not a new practice. In a study conducted in the 1800s, William Beaumont, an army physician, provided one of his subjects with lodging, food, and $150 for a year of participation. Walter Reed paid volunteers $100 in gold to participate in his study of the transmission of yellow fever in the 19th century. Those who contracted yellow fever received another $100, which was paid to their heirs in the event of their death. Today, enticing individuals to participate in a study is common. Only 11% of IRBs have reported *not* having approved pediatric trials that offered payment.[28]

There are two categories of monetary enticement: payments that dissolve barriers to research participation (reimbursement) and payments that provide inducements to participate in research (inducements). Reimbursement is an offer of payment that is intended to cover the costs directly related to participation in the study. These may include the costs of parking, travel, meals, lodging, and child care that a family might incur. These are expenses that would not exist if the family had chosen not to participate in the study. Reimbursement sometimes includes payments intended to cover lost wages, but only if the recipient has lost income because of time lost at work. Reimbursement for lost income is not always available or appropriate.[29]

Inducements, on the other hand, are payments that encourage potential research subjects to enroll in a study. Under this category, there are three types of inducement payments: compensation payments, appreciation payments, and incentive payments. Compensation payments are intended to remunerate parents and children for their time and for the inconvenience of participation, yet this payment is not intended to replace lost wages. Appreciation payments are bonuses given to a child as a thank you after he or she has participated in research. Finally, incentive payments are offered to encourage or entice an individual to enroll in a study. Monetary enticements that are offered on the completion of a study have been shown to be more effective than money offered at regular intervals throughout the study. All three types of inducement payments go above and beyond reimbursement and provide a positive incentive to enroll in a study.[29]

A major concern about reimbursement and inducements is that of coercion and undue influence. Of course, coercion should be avoided at all costs, yet the legal manifestation of research ethics is silent on the issue of subject payment, allowing for much discretion for interpretation by researchers and IRBs. The Belmont Report indirectly addresses the issue, noting that "the element of informed consent requires conditions free of coercion and undue influence."[14] President Clinton's National Bioethics Advisory Commission observed that monetary incentives might create undue influence on persons who are economically disadvantaged. Its 2001 report recommends that IRBs scrutinize payments offered to enrollees, and even reduce payments if necessary. 45 CFR 46 makes no direct reference to research payments other than the fact that the possibility of coercion and undue influence must be minimized. 45 CFR 46.111 cautions investigators and IRBs to provide safeguards when subjects are vulnerable to coercion because of being economically or educationally disadvantaged.[14]

In pediatric research, it is important to recognize that what may be an undue influence on an adult for his or her own participation in research is different from the undue influence of a parent making a decision on behalf of a child. Payments for participation in a study require much caution when children are not in a position to provide valid consent. Children must trust others to safeguard their interests, but payment options have the potential to distort decision making, enticing parents to consider monetary issues and not the well-being and best interests of the child as they consider enrollment. Inducement payments can distort a parent's perception of the risks and benefits of entering a child in a study. IRBs must be careful that parents are not tempted to use their child as a means to the end of financial benefit. One solution to this problem has been suggested by the American Academy of Pediatrics: the nondisclosure of payments other than reimbursement might resolve the problem of undue influence. If any valuable consideration is to be provided to the child, perhaps in the form of a toy store gift certificate, it is best not discussed before the completion of the study.[30] Of course, under that arrangement the incentive value of payments will be eliminated, and the reason for their being offered

Section One - Subpart A; and Section Three - Parental Permission and Child Assent

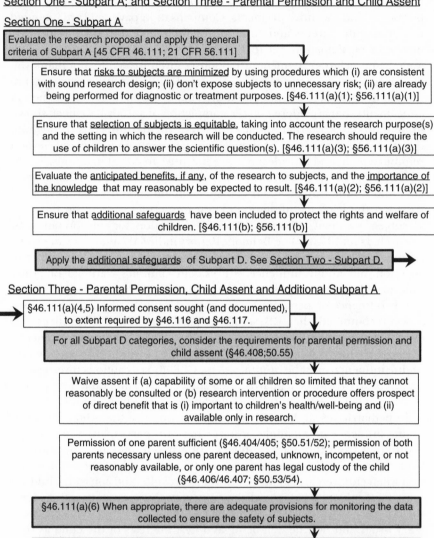

FIGURE 5.1. Algorithm for pediatric protocol analysis (Subparts A and D – 45 CFR 46 and 21 CFR 50). The content of this document does not represent the official views or policies of the Office for Human Research Protections, the Federal Drug Administration, or the Department of Health and Human Services. The content represents solely the advice and views of its author, Robert M. Nelson.

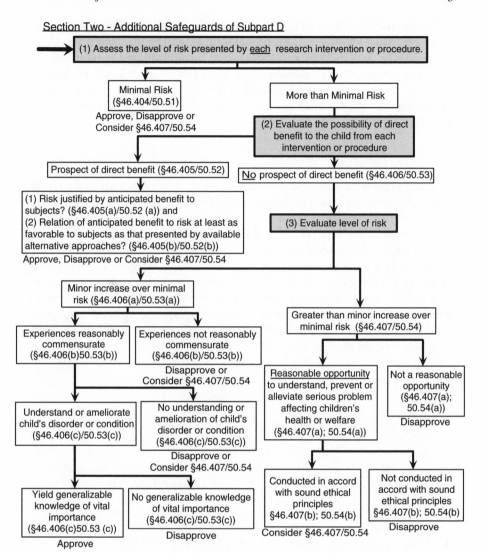

Section Two - Additional Safeguards of Subpart D

(1) Assess the level of risk presented by <u>each</u> research intervention or procedure.

Minimal Risk
(§46.404/50.51)
Approve, Disapprove or
Consider §46.407/50.54

More than Minimal Risk

(2) Evaluate the possibility of direct
benefit to the child from each
intervention or procedure

Prospect of direct benefit (§46.405/50.52)

<u>No</u> prospect of direct benefit (§46.406/50.53)

(1) Risk justified by anticipated benefit to
subjects? (§46.405(a)/50.52 (a)) and
(2) Relation of anticipated benefit to risk at least as
favorable to subjects as that presented by available
alternative approaches? (§46.405(b)/50.52(b))
Approve, Disapprove or Consider §46.407/50.54

(3) Evaluate level of risk

Minor increase over minimal
risk (§46.406(a)/50.53(a))

Greater than minor increase over
minimal risk (§46.407/50.54)

Experiences reasonably
commensurate
(§46.406(b)50.53(b))

Experiences not reasonably
commensurate
(§46.406(b)/50.53(b))
Disapprove or
Consider §46.407/50.54

<u>Reasonable opportunity</u>
to understand, prevent or
alleviate serious problem
affecting children's
health or welfare
(§46.407(a); 50.54(a))

Not a reasonable
opportunity
(§46.407(a);
50.54(a))
Disapprove

Understand or ameliorate
child's disorder or condition
(§46.406(c)/50.53(c))

No understanding or
amelioration of child's
disorder or condition
(§46.406(c)/50.53(c))
Disapprove or
Consider §46.407/50.54

Yield generalizable
knowledge of vital
importance
(§46.406(c)50.53 (c))
Approve

No generalizable knowledge
of vital importance
(§46.406(c)/50.53(c))
Disapprove

Conducted in accord
with sound ethical
principles
§46.407(b); 50.54(b)
Consider §46.407/50.54

Not conducted in
accord with sound
ethical principles
§46.407(b); 50.54(b)
Disapprove

If Considering Approval, Return to Section Three.

(to entice the individual into the study) will be lost. Still, such compensation
is an expression of respect and gratitude to the child.

On occasion, a child will suffer injury from his or her participation in a
study. Justice requires that parents and their child not become burdened with
the costs of medical care that results from an injury related to the research.
The investigators and the IRB should assume the financial responsibilities
related to injury during the study and cover all expenses.[9]

Payments offered to children and their families must be scrutinized carefully. Since children cannot legally protect their own interests, IRBs must ensure that there is no opportunity for a child to be exploited by financial incentives. Reimbursement for out-of-pocket costs is usually appropriate and eliminates financial barriers to participation in research. Inducement payments must be carefully examined for their ability to distort parental decision making.[29]

CONCLUSION

The 2004 vision statement of the American Academy of Pediatrics declares, "We believe in the inherent worth of all children. They are our enduring and vulnerable legacy."[31] Pediatric research ethics is based on respect for children and their best interests (Figure 5.1). The purpose of biomedical research is to contribute to knowledge, but this laudable goal may put children at risk of harm in clinical research, potentially stripping them of their rights and the respect they deserve. The research imperative even has the potential to overtake respect for a child and his family. Pediatric research ethics relies on this respect, sometimes at the expense of knowledge that could benefit society. Knowledge gained from research must be obtained in a way that recognizes the vulnerability of children and respects their best interests.

References

1. Emanuel EJ, Grady C, Crouch RA, Lie RK, Miller FG, Wendler D, eds. *The Oxford Textbook of Clinical Research Ethics.* New York: Oxford University Press; 2008.
2. Campbell AT. *State Regulation of Medical Research with Children and Adolescents: An Overview and Analysis.* Washington, DC: National Academy Press; 2004: 320–387.
3. Gordin MA, Alpert JJ. Children as participants in medical research. *Pediatr Clin North Am.* 1988;35:1389–1401.
4. Kodish E., ed. *Ethics and Research with Children.* New York: Oxford University Press; 2005:3–361.
5. Gaylin W. *Competence No Longer All or None.* In: Gaylin W, Macklin R, eds. New York: Plenum Press; 1982:27–54.
6. Levine RJ. *Ethics and Regulation of Clinical Research.* 2nd ed. New Haven, Conn: Yale University Press; 1988.
7. Coleman CH., ed. *The Ethics and Regulation of Research with Human Subjects.* LexisNexis; 2006.
8. United States Office of Human Subjects Research, National Institutes of Health. *Nuremberg Code.* Available at: http://ohsr.od.nih.gov/guidelines/nuremberg. html. Accessed June 26, 2008.
9. Alderson P. Competent children? Minors' consent to health care treatment and research. *Social Sci Med.* 2007;65:2272–2283.

10. Miller PB, Weijer C. Evaluating benefits and harms in research on healthy children. In: Kodish E, ed. *Ethics, and Research with Children*. Oxford: Oxford University Press; 2005:29–45.

11. Ramsey P. The enforcement of morals: nontherapeutic research on children. *Hastings Cent Rep.* 1976;6:21–30.

12. McCormick R. Proxy consent in the experimental situation. *Perspect Biol Med.* 1974;18:2–20.

13. Office of Human Subjects Research. *The Belmont Report: Ethical Principles and Guidelines for the Protection of Human Subjects of Research*. National Commission for the Protection of Human Subjects of Biomedical and Behavioral Research; April 1979. Available at: http://ohsr.od.nih.gov/guidelines/belmont.html.

14. Office for Human Research Protections. *Special Protections for Children as Research Subjects*. United States Department of Health & Human Services; November 2008. Available at: http://www.hhs.gov/ohrp/children/.

15. Ross LF. Informed consent in pediatric research. *Camb Q Healthcare Ethics.* 2004;13:346–358.

16. International Ethical Guidelines for Biomedical Research. Geneva: Council for International Organizations of Medical Sciences; 2002.

17. Wendler D. Protecting subjects who cannot give consent: toward a better standard for "minimal" risk. *Hastings Cent Rep.* 2005;35:37–43.

18. Bartholome WG. Ethical issues in pediatric research. In: Vanderpool HY, ed. *The Ethics of Research Involving Human Subjects: Facing the 21st Century*. Frederick, Md: University Group; 1996:356–361.

19. Collogan LK, Fleischman AR. Adolescent research and parental permission. In: Kodish E, ed. *Ethics and Research with Children*. Oxford: Oxford University Press; 2005:77–99.

20. Downie RS, Randall F. Parenting and the best interests of minors. *J Med Philos.* 1997;22: 219–231.

21. Sugarman J. Determining the appropriateness of including children in clinical research: how thick is the ice? *JAMA.* 2004;291: 494–496.

22. Kodish E, Eder M, Noll RB, et al. Communication of randomization in childhood leukemia trials. *JAMA.* 2004;291:470–475.

23. Dawson A, Spencer SA. Informing children and parents about research. *Arch Dis Child.* 2005;90:233–235.

24. Mastroianni AC, Kahn JP. Risk and responsibility: ethics, *Grimes v. Kennedy Krieger,* and public health research involving children. *Am J Pub Health.* 2002;7:1073–1076.

25. Glantz LH. Nontherapeutic research with children: *Grimes v. Kennedy Krieger Institute. Am J Pub Health.* 2002;7:1070–1073.

26. Piaget, J. The stages of the intellectual development of the child. *Bull Menninger Clin.* 1962;26:120–128.

27. Rogers AS, Schwartz DF, Weissman G, English A. A case study in adolescent participation in clinical research: eleven clinical sites, one common protocol, and eleven IRBs. *IRB.* 1999;2:6–10.

28. Weise KL, Smith ML, Maschke KJ, Copeland HL. National practices regarding payment to research subjects for participating in pediatric research. *Pediatrics.* 2002;110:577–582.

29. Diekema DS. Payments for participation of children in research. In: Kodish E, ed. *Ethics and Research with Children.* Oxford: Oxford University Press; 2005:143–160.

30. American Academy of Pediatrics, Committee on Drugs. Guidelines for the ethical conduct of studies to evaluate drugs in pediatric populations. *Pediatrics.* 1995;95:286–294.

31. American Academy of Pediatrics Core Vision Statement. July 27, 2004. Available at: http://www.aap.org/new/reachchild.pdf.

6

Truth Telling in Pediatrics

What They Don't Know Might Hurt Them

Christine Harrison

INTRODUCTION

Health care professionals are currently trained and practice in an environment where personal health information is considered to belong to the patient, and where honesty and truth telling are considered virtues foundational to the therapeutic relationship. Professional codes of ethics and position statements define practitioners' responsibilities with regard to honesty and disclosure of information, although these concepts require interpretation and contextualization in clinical encounters with patients and families. Truth telling is considered especially important in relationships with children, whose vulnerability creates in us a special obligation to protect and who are in the process of having their character shaped – at least in part – by the adults with whom they interact.[1]

The debate between those who support a consistent practice of telling the truth to children and those who believe this practice will cause them harm is not new. Pernick quotes Dr. Worthington Hooker, who in the 19th century argued that "[a] child can appreciate fair and honest treatment as well as an adult can, and he has as good a right to receive it."[2] Increasingly clear standards of practice in pediatrics are emerging. For example, the Canadian Paediatric Society holds that children

should be given developmentally appropriate information so that they may understand their situation. However, cultural norms or family values may underlie some parents' reluctance to discuss the child or adolescent's condition, diagnosis or prognosis in his or her presence. *While parents' views regarding disclosure are important, the child or adolescent's desire or need for information should remain paramount.*[3] (emphasis added)

An American Academy of Pediatrics (AAP) technical report, while advocating respect for family's wishes, values, and cultural perspectives in this matter, states that "[t]here is a moral and ethical obligation to discuss health and illness with the child patient."[4] This is consistent with an earlier AAP report's position that "[a]s children mature, they should be fully informed of the nature and consequences of their illness and encouraged to actively participate in their own medical care."[5] The British Medical Association maintains the position that "[o]n the whole, we are against the withholding of information if the child seems willing to know it, even where parents request secrecy."[6] Finally, when we read the United Nations Convention on the Rights of the Child statement that "[w]hen adults are making decisions that affect children, children have the right to say what they think should happen and have their opinions taken into account,"[7] we may surely infer that children also have the right to information necessary to form these opinions in a meaningful way.

In spite of these directives, there are still situations in which individual practitioners may disagree about the appropriateness of disclosing information to children, and sometimes even to their parents. A recurring ethical dilemma in pediatrics leading to requests for ethics consultation is the conflict between health care professionals' duty to disclose potentially distressing information to patients (in this case children) and their duty to respect parents' wishes to protect their children from harm. Another challenge is determining the nature and amount of information that should be given to parents and patients in situations of considerable medical uncertainty.

Three issues providing challenges in the area of truth telling in pediatrics will be explored. First, whether it is the duty of pediatric practitioners, regardless of their professional discipline, to disclose information to patients who are children or adolescents, and to the parents of their patients, is not absolute; in pediatrics there is also a duty to respect parents' role in shaping the context of care and information provision. Relevant contextual factors will be suggested to assist practitioners with decision making. Second, challenges associated with truth telling often arise because practitioners and family members have different cultural backgrounds, and one's cultural background affects the importance one places on truth telling in the health care context. Both the significance and limitations of this will be considered. Third, parents' desire to withhold information about their child's impending death from that child is especially challenging for the child's health care providers. Arguments supporting sensitive disclosure will be presented. Where there are differing perspectives as to what the child should be told, and no significant harm to the child is anticipated as a result of nondisclosure, parents' wishes should be respected, creating the need for careful and creative planning for providing the child's care and assisting team members with their moral distress.

I will make the following presumption, acknowledging that this may be arguable. Children and adolescents, and their parents, may ask professional caregivers direct questions. Once these questions have been clarified, they should be answered honestly and fairly, that is, sensitively and in a way that can be properly understood.

ISSUES OF TRUTH TELLING IN THE THERAPEUTIC RELATIONSHIP

Information is usually shared in the pediatric health care context so that the child's health condition can be understood, options can be identified and reflected upon, and decisions can be made. Ideally, pediatric practitioners would disclose diagnoses and test results to patients who were developmentally capable of understanding them, and then they would decide together how to proceed. Disclosure would be appropriately staged, in a way that was sensitive to the feelings and emotional state of the patient, and accompanied by compassion and support. Parents would be part of this process, unless for some reason the patient did not want to include them. If the patient was less mature and developmentally less able to process information and make decisions, the practitioner would speak with the patient and parents together or, when appropriate, with the parents first to enlist their assistance when talking to the child. Information in either context would be fully and truthfully communicated.

This ideal is often not realized in the pediatric context. Practitioners who have access to information that is likely to cause anxiety and is not necessary for decision making may be uncertain as to their duty to disclose. Parents may wish to withhold information from their child for a number of reasons, usually believing this will protect the child from being overwhelmed or highly distressed.[8] I will use three scenarios arising from clinical ethics consultations to help identify distinctions and general principles. One scenario involves the condition of sudden unexpected death in epilepsy (SUDEP). Currently there is a debate as to whether it is better for physicians to explain SUDEP to families or to withhold this information in the belief that it serves no useful purpose and may cause harm. The second scenario involves the disclosure of a diagnosis of HIV to a child. Parents have good reasons to delay the disclosure of this diagnosis to their child, and at the same time there are good reasons to believe that information and education may contribute to the child's well-being. The third scenario entails the infertility associated with Turner syndrome, which is sometimes not disclosed. This may lead to a sense of betrayal later in life and the development of a self-identity shadowed by false presumptions that might have been avoided.

Scenario 1: When Information May Harm and Not Help – SUDEP

Sudden unexplained death in epilepsy is the most common epilepsy-specific cause of death.[9] Persons with epilepsy die unexpectedly, often in their sleep, and the cause of their death is not known. Little is known about these otherwise unexplained deaths, and they are believed to occur rarely in children; on the basis of two studies, the incidence rate in children is estimated to be 1–2.7 deaths per 10,000 patient-years.[10] In cases where persons with epilepsy are receiving the best possible treatment and are following medical advice, it is believed that there is nothing more that might be done to decrease the risk of SUDEP.[11] It might reasonably be argued that telling parents (or children themselves) that this is a risk for their child, when there is nothing they can do with that information other than worry about it, is unnecessary. Indeed, it is possibly harmful in terms of the anxiety it causes parents[12] and potentially affects the parent–child relationship in negative ways. The argument that information about SUDEP need not be provided to families is that there must be a purpose or reason for disclosing information that might otherwise cause harm.

A problem with this argument, of course, is that in these situations it is the health care professional who decides whether or not there is a reason to disclose information, whether or not the reason is important, and that in fact the disclosure of *this* information to *this* person is likely to cause harm. Epilepsy support groups report the views of family members of persons who have died under these circumstances. They believe that, had they or the person who died known about the possibility of SUDEP, aspects of the person's life may have been handled differently and his or her death might have been avoided.

An approach that is more respectful of parents would be to take into account their information needs, views about truth telling, and communication preferences. As a general rule, when embarking on a relationship with patients and families, health care professionals should negotiate a consensus about how and what kind of information will be shared, and with whom, always presuming that when information is necessary for decision making it will be provided to the appropriate decision maker. Information about support groups should also be provided, and then families and patients may choose to consult these sources of information themselves.

The example of SUDEP reminds us that information may or may not be necessary for decision making, that it may have consequences that change relationships in negative and positive ways, and that parents may view any and all information about their child, or their child's condition generally, as something they have a right to be given. Health care practitioners may see these situations differently and may wish to protect families from what is perceived as unnecessary anxiety when these families are already caring for a child with serious health problems and the health care practitioner believes that the information is not needed for decision-making purposes.

Scenario 2: HIV and Family Secrets

Parents whose children have been diagnosed with HIV may wish to withhold this diagnosis from their child.[13] Three main reasons for this wish are summarized by Salter-Goldie et al. First, parents fear causing emotional harm to the child, especially when it is not the child him- or herself alone who is infected but other family members as well. Parents may feel guilty when they have some responsibility for being the cause of their child's illness, as when HIV is transmitted from parent to child. They worry that their child will blame them. Finally, parents are concerned that their child will tell others, and that the child and family may then be subject to discrimination and isolation.[14]

This is an example of a situation where it may be important to share information with the child about his or her condition in order to facilitate coping with a chronic illness and to win the child's trust and elicit the child's cooperation with treatment.[15] Pursuing a strategy of partial truth telling, which "involves building gradually on parts of the truth, without telling lies, until children have the full information about their own and their parents' HIV status,"[14] may help parents and health care practitioners achieve these goals. The actual term "HIV" or "AIDS" need not be used, and information would be developmentally appropriate. As the child entered adolescence and approached sexual maturity, discussions would have to be more explicit. Parents and the team could work together planning for this event, and as time would allow for trust to develop in many cases, conflict could be avoided.[16]

The partial-truth-telling model developed for information disclosure to children infected with HIV is one that would reasonably apply in other situations where children are diagnosed with a chronic illness at a young age. As children develop and mature – physically, emotionally, and cognitively – the emphasis should shift from honoring parents' wishes to withhold or filter information from the child to respecting the children's abilities and needs to be actively involved in their own care and thus the custodians of information about their heath condition and treatment plan.

Scenario 3: Knowledge of Self and Self-Identity – Turner Syndrome

Some children may be diagnosed at birth, or early on, with a condition that will in all likelihood affect the evolution of their self-identity. Turner syndrome, for example, is a chromosomal abnormality, usually diagnosed in utero or during childhood. Women with Turner syndrome are usually infertile. Historically they were not told of their diagnosis, or at least the implications for their ability to be a biological parent. This practice began to change in the 1970s and 1980s, although parents still sometimes withhold the diagnosis, or some parts of it (such as infertility).

Sutton and colleagues spoke with girls and women with Turner syndrome. One concern identified by some who did not know aspects of their diagnosis included the traumatic effects of learning of their infertility inadvertently. Another was the anger they felt when they discovered that this information had been kept secret from them. One individual explained to her mother, "I think it would have helped me to understand myself a little bit better." Another felt betrayed: "All I knew was that the people that I trusted forever were willing to betray me."[17]

Sutton and colleagues summarize a crucial point, one that is arguably generalizable beyond Turner syndrome, when they say that

[d]isclosing the diagnosis at a young age enables girls to incorporate TS [Turner syndrome] and its consequences for reproduction into their self-identity early in their development. By not telling young girls about their reproductive limitations, parents allow their daughters to create self-images that include biological motherhood.[17]

Disclosing information about the aspects of children's circumstances that might contribute to the development of their identity and self-esteem is also supported by literature promoting the disclosure of adoption status and by proponents of disclosure to those offspring of parents who used donor gametes.[18] Open and honest communication may positively affect family relationships and prevent the anger and sense of betrayal that may occur when disclosure either happens in an unplanned way or happens later on in life.

Lessons Learned. From these three scenarios we can garner some general recommendations:

- When establishing relationships with patients and families, health care practitioners should at the outset discuss their views about information disclosure and communication.
- In situations where children and adolescents are living with chronic illnesses, they benefit from receiving information and being educated about their condition, their role in their own care, and strategies for maximizing their own well-being.
- Parents may have good reasons for wishing to protect their children from information that may be distressing, overwhelming, or harmful to the child in other ways. Health care practitioners should collaborate with parents to plan disclosure strategies, such as that of partial truth telling.
- There are some aspects of one's own sense of self or personhood that are essential to one's identity and self-esteem. Secrets related to these may have a deleterious effect on family relationships.

CULTURAL CONTEXT OF TRUTH TELLING

Parents and families who raise children, as well as children's friends, teachers, and acquaintances, create the reality in which children live. Their use of language, including euphemisms and metaphors they may employ as placeholders or explanations for painful concepts such as death, and in potentially embarrassing conversations related to bodily functions and sexuality, and the stories they use to teach and communicate values and history may be well understood by the child and within the child's circle, but may be unfamiliar to the child's health care providers. Similarly, when the language a family uses to communicate with each other is different from that of their health care professionals, practitioners should take care that they do not use euphemisms or symbolic language that may be misunderstood.

The desire of family members to withhold potentially distressing information from a loved one is often ascribed to the cultural background and beliefs of the family. A recent UNESCO declaration describes culture "as the set of distinctive spiritual, material, intellectual and emotional features of society or a social group, and that it encompasses, in addition to art and literature, lifestyles, ways of living together, value systems, traditions and beliefs."[19] Culture is usually understood to be something that exists over time and is passed on through generations.

All patients, families, and health practitioners have culturally based beliefs that affect their understanding of health, disease, and illness, and that to some extent determine their child-raising practices.[20,21] Parents' wish to withhold information from their child may very well be culturally related. They may themselves be unwilling or unable to accept a diagnosis such as cancer or HIV infection, and they may believe that children are not able to handle such devastating news. Parents with certain cultural backgrounds (e.g., Japanese, Navajo, and Chinese) are likely to see it as their duty as parents to protect their child and that failing to do this may make the child's condition worse.[22,23]

Health care professionals who have been trained in the Western tradition are likely to place an almost absolute value on truth telling. In order to provide care that is respectful of the values of patients and families, they should understand the influence their own training and personal cultural beliefs have had on shaping their views. Forcing the view that has evolved relatively recently in the West onto a family from a different culture "ignore[s] the fact that the issue of truth telling in medicine is a function of a particular way of life."[22] While some individuals may do better when they participate actively in their own treatment, others may not. Children and families from Latin or Asian cultures, for example, may take a more passive approach to illness and not experience negative consequences because of this.[21] Families are likely to take comfort from familiar cultural practices. Health care practitioners should try to understand and support parents' wishes in these circumstances, to the extent possible given professional and legal constraints.[21,24]

While it is necessary that health care professionals understand cultural norms and practices in order to provide good patient care, they should focus on the individual patient and the individuals who make up that patient's family and support system. While these individuals may come from a particular cultural group, they do not necessarily follow any or all of the generally accepted practices of that group.[23,25] Children may have been influenced by others outside their cultural community and may hold somewhat different values than their parents. While it is essential to understand the influence that cultural values and beliefs have on parents' decisions and children's perspectives, stereotyping and judgmental attitudes should be avoided.

Lessons Learned

- Individuals' cultural backgrounds contribute to the value they place on truth telling as an ethical imperative.
- Health care practitioners who have been trained in the Western tradition are likely to consider truth telling to be one of the most highly ranked ethical principles. They should not presume that patients and families feel the same.
- Being familiar with cultural customs and traditions generally, and those practiced by patients and families specifically, allows for the provision of more respectful care.

TRUTH TELLING AND THE DYING CHILD

When children have a life-threatening illness or are dying, their vulnerability is great and the urge to protect them may be overwhelming. This may even include protecting them from the knowledge that death appears to be imminent and inevitable. Undoubtedly, telling a child that death is approaching – however sensitively this is done – will cause the child sadness, anxiety, and fear and will bring distress to the family and health care providers. This is not a case, however, where to hide the truth is to necessarily prevent harm. More harm may result from *not* telling the child, and so while the adults caring for the child may take comfort from the belief that they are protecting the child, it may actually be in the child's best interests that there be honesty and openness about his or her condition and likely future.

While parents may intuitively believe that "not telling" protects children from anxiety and fear, preserves their innocence (and ignorance), and relieves them from the unjustifiable burden of making impossible decisions, there is increasing evidence that this intuition is not supported generally in children (although it may be in the case of a particular child). When parents have processed the devastating news themselves, caregivers should share with them that research indicates the following:

- Most (almost all) children with cancer, when asked if they wanted to be told if they were not getting better and were likely to die, said yes.[26,27]
- Children who are terminally ill and dying typically know that this is so.[28-30]

- Children from whom information about a serious illness or impending death is withheld are more anxious and fearful than those who have the opportunity to discuss their feelings. They are often concerned about pain and abandonment, wonder how their families will cope, and have an awareness of death, which they might not explicitly express unless encouraged to talk about it.[13,31–33]
- Parents who discussed their child's impending death with the child did not regret doing so, while some parents who did not have those discussions regretted not doing so.[34]

Honoring parents' wish to "protect" may isolate children from supportive caregivers with whom they can discuss their fears and anxieties. "Deception does not succeed in keeping out the fears of sickness and death. It only succeeds in keeping out the loved ones, who could have helped them deal with the fears."[28] The arguments for offering opportunities to children to discuss their impending death are powerful.

There may be circumstances where, as uncomfortable as it might be for some members of the team, the parents' request that the child's impending death not be disclosed or discussed ought to be respected. Children who are aware of the seriousness of their condition may wish to go along with the pretense created by their parents. One practitioner relates an experience with a dying adolescent patient whose parents insisted that his impending death not be disclosed to or discussed with him. He himself made it clear that he did not want to speak about his death with either his professional caregivers or his family. His caregivers found this very difficult, but the author noted, "Truth-telling about dying is our principle, but it was not his."[35] Parents who are clearly motivated by love and concern, who know their child well, whose family ethos has always been to protect the child, and whose child does not give indications to the contrary might be correct in insisting that this is best for their child and that this is what the child would prefer. Members of the health care team are likely to experience moral distress in these situations, namely that they are not fulfilling their ethical and professional obligation to their patient.[33,36,37]

Constant pressure on parents to speak to the child, or to give the team permission to speak to the child, is likely to alienate parents and create a conflict-ridden environment that results in angry parents, frustrated team members, and a confused and anxious child. Professional caregivers should make parents aware of the potential consequences of nondisclosure, and even try to persuade them to discuss openly with the child his or her condition. Health care professionals' moral distress should be acknowledged. Case conferences, in-services, and ethics consultations may offer opportunities for decisions to be reviewed and caregivers to receive support from colleagues. The child's state of mind and awareness of his

or her condition should be constantly monitored. Children who ask direct
and explicit questions should have them answered truthfully.

Lessons Learned

- Children and adolescents who are terminally ill or who are dying are
  especially vulnerable, and the desire to protect them is heightened.
- A growing body of research suggests that attempts to preserve secrecy
  and withhold information from dying children may not be effective
  and may cause harm in the form of increased anxiety and isolation.
  The arguments for offering opportunities to children to discuss their
  impending death are powerful.
- In some exceptional situations, it may be ethically appropriate to support the parents' wish to refrain from speaking to their child about the
  seriousness of his or her condition.

CONCLUSION

The body of literature concerning challenges parents and children experience in communicating with health care practitioners, what information
they desire and how they want to receive it, and suggestions as to how to
improve practices of communicating complex and distressing information
continues to grow.[4,17,26,31,37–41]

Truth telling and transparency should be a presumed component of the
provision of health care to children and adolescents.

[I]f someone contemplates lying to a patient or concealing the truth, the burden
of proof must shift. It must rest, here, as with all deception, on those who advocate
it in any one instance. They must show why they fear a patient may be harmed or
how they know that another cannot cope with the truthful knowledge. A decision
to deceive must be seen as a very unusual step, to be talked over with colleagues
and others who participate in the care of the patient. Reasons must be set forth and
debated, alternatives weighted carefully. At all times, the correct information must
go to *someone* closely related to the patient.[1]

Desires and plans to withhold information from patients or their parents
should be carefully thought through and justified, as withholding information is contrary to our duty to respect persons.[42] Ongoing discussions with
parents may lead them to the realization that it is often less harmful for
children to know about their illness and that they may therefore, through
disclosure, better fulfill their duties of protection and care.

Truth Telling in Pediatrics – Recommendations and Summary

- Children and adolescents, and their parents, may ask professional caregivers direct questions. Once these questions have been clarified and

properly understood, they should be answered honestly and fairly, that is, sensitively and in a way that can be properly understood.

- When establishing relationships with patients and families, health care practitioners should at the outset discuss their views about information disclosure and communication.
- In situations where children and adolescents are living with chronic illnesses, they benefit from receiving information and being educated about their condition, their role in their own care, and strategies for maximizing their own well-being.
- Parents may have good reasons for wishing to protect their child from information that may be distressing, overwhelming, or harmful to the child in other ways. Health care practitioners should collaborate with parents to plan disclosure strategies, such as that of partial truth telling.
- There are some aspects of one's own sense of self or personhood that are essential to one's identity and self-esteem. Secrets related to these may have a deleterious effect on family relationships.
- Individuals' cultural backgrounds contribute to the value they place on truth telling as an ethical imperative.
- Health care practitioners who have been trained in the Western tradition are likely to consider truth telling to be one of the most highly ranked ethical principles. They should not presume that patients and families feel the same.
- Being familiar with cultural customs and traditions generally, and those practiced by patients and families specifically, allows for the provision of more respectful care.
- Children and adolescents who are terminally ill or who are dying are especially vulnerable, and the desire to protect them is heightened.
- A growing body of research suggests that attempts to preserve secrecy and withhold information from dying children may not be effective and may cause harm in the form of increased anxiety and isolation. The arguments for offering opportunities to children to discuss their impending death are powerful.
- In some exceptional situations, it may be ethically appropriate to support the parents' wish to refrain from speaking to their child about the seriousness of his or condition.

References

1. Bok S. *Lying: Moral Choice in Public and Private Life*. New York: Pantheon Books; 1978.
2. Pernick M. Childhood death and medical ethics: an historical perspective on truth-telling in pediatrics. In: Ganos D et al., eds. *Difficult Decisions in Medical Ethics: The Fourth Volume in a Series on Ethics, Humanism, and Medicine*. Proceedings of the Eighth and Ninth Conferences on Ethics, Humanism, and

Medicine, University of Michigan, Ann Arbor; 1981, 1982. New York: Alan R Liss; 1983:173–188.

3. Canadian Paediatric Society, Bioethics Committee. Treatment decisions regarding infants, children and adolescents. Canadian Paediatric Society Reference No. B04-01. *Paediatr Child Health.* 2004;9:99–103.

4. Levetown M. American Academy of Pediatrics Committee on Bioethics. Communicating with children and families: from everyday interactions to skill in conveying distressing information. *Pediatrics.* 2008;121:e1441–e1460.

5. American Academy of Pediatrics, Committee on Pediatric AIDS. Disclosure of illness status to children and adolescents with HIV infection. *Pediatrics.* 1999;103:164–166.

6. British Medical Association. *Consent, Rights and Choices in Health Care for Children and Young People.* London: BMJ Books; 2001.

7. United Nations. *Convention on the Rights of the Child.* 1989. Available at: http://www.unhchr.ch/html/menu3/b/k2crc.htm. Accessed October 29, 2008.

8. Claflin CJ, Barbarin OA. Does "telling" less protect more? Relationships among age, information disclosure, and what children with cancer see and feel. *J Pediatr Psychol.* 1991;16:169–191.

9. Beran RG. SUDEP: to discuss or not discuss – that is the question [comment]. *Lancet Neurol.* 2006;5:464–465.

10. So EL. Demystifying sudden unexplained death in epilepsy: are we close? *Epilepsia.* 2006;47(Suppl. 1):87–92.

11. Beran RG, Weber S, Sungaran R, et al. Review of the legal obligations of the doctor to discuss sudden unexplained death in epilepsy (SUDEP): a cohort controlled comparative cross-matched study in an outpatient epilepsy clinic. *Seizure.* 2004;13:523–528.

12. Morton B, Richardson A, Duncan S. Sudden unexpected death in epilepsy (SUDEP): don't ask, don't tell? *J Neurol Neurosurg Psychiatry.* 2006;77:199–202.

13. Kouyoumdjian FG, Meyers T, Mtshizana S, Meyers T, Mtshizana S. Barriers to disclosure to children with HIV. *J Trop Pediatr.* 2005;51:285–7.

14. Salter-Goldie R, King SM, Smith ML, et al. Disclosing HIV diagnosis to infected children: a health care team's approach. *Vulnerable Children and Youth Studies.* 2007;2:12–16.

15. Stewart KS, Dearmun AK. Adherence to health advice amongst young people with chronic illness. *J Child Health Care.* 2001;5:155–162.

16. Lipson M. What do you say to a child with AIDS? *Hastings Cent Rep.* 1993;23:6–12.

17. Sutton EJ, Young J, McInerney-Leo A, et al. Truth-telling and Turner syndrome: the importance of diagnostic disclosure. *J Pediatr.* 2006;148:102–107.

18. American Society for Reproductive Medicine, Ethics Committee. Informing offspring of their conception by gamete donation. *Fertil Steril.* 2004;82 (Suppl. 1):S212–S216.

19. United Nations Educational, Scientific,and Cultural Organization (UNESCO). Universal Declaration on Cultural Diversity; 2002. Available at: http://unesdoc.unesco.org/images/0012/001271/127160m.pdf. Accessed October 29, 2008.

20. Britton CV, American Academy of Pediatrics Committee on Pediatric Workforce. Ensuring culturally effective pediatric care: implications for education and health policy. *Pediatrics.* 2004;114:1677–1685.

21. De Trill M, Kovalcik R. The child with cancer: influence of culture on truth-telling and patient care. *Ann NY Acad Sci.* 1997;809:197–210.
22. Fan R, Li B. Truth telling in medicine: the Confucian view. *J Med Philos.* 2004;29:179–193.
23. Hurwitz Swota A. Cultural diversity in the clinical setting. In: Hester DM, ed. *Ethics by Committee: A Textbook on Consultation, Organization, and Education for Hospital Ethics Committees.* Lanham, Md: Rowman & Littlefield; 2008.
24. Crow K, Matheson L, Steed A. Informed consent and truth-telling: cultural directions for healthcare providers. *J Nurs Adm.* 2000;30:148–152.
25. Tse CY, Chong A, Fok SY, Chong A. Breaking bad news: a Chinese perspective. *Palliat Med.* 2003;17:339–343.
26. Ellis R, Leventhal B. Information needs and decision-making preferences of children with cancer. *Psycho-oncology.* 1993;2:277–284.
27. Wolfe L. Should parents speak with a dying child about impending death? [comment]. *N Engl J Med.* 2004;351:1251–1253.
28. Cassidy R. Tell all the truth? Shepherds, liberators, or educators. In: Cassidy R, Fleischman AR, eds. *Pediatric Ethics: From Principles to Practice.* Amsterdam: Harwood Academic; 1996:67–82.
29. Spinetta JJ, Rigler D, Karon M. Anxiety in the dying child. *Pediatrics.* 1973;52:841–845.
30. Wolfe J, Friebert S, Hilden J, Wolfe J, Friebert S, Hilden J. Caring for children with advanced cancer integrating palliative care. *Pediatr Clin North Am.* 2002;49:1043–1062.
31. Beale EA, Baile WF, Aaron J. Silence is not golden: communicating with children dying from cancer. *J Clin Oncol.* 2005;23:3629–3631.
32. Goldie J, Schwartz L, Morrison J. Whose information is it anyway? Informing a 12-year-old patient of her terminal prognosis. *J Med Ethics.* 2005;31:427–434.
33. Turkoski BB. A mother's orders about truth telling. *Home Healthcare Nurse.* 2003;21:81–83.
34. Kreicbergs U, Valdimarsdottir U, Onelov E, et al. Talking about death with children who have severe malignant disease [see comment]. *N Engl J Med.* 2004;351:1175–1186.
35. Hinds PS. Truth-telling with patients. *J Pediatr Oncol Nurs.* 1995;12:1.
36. Kendall S. Being asked not to tell: nurses' experiences of caring for cancer patients not told their diagnosis. *J Clin Nurs.* 2006;15:1149–1157.
37. Miles A. "Am I going to die?" … terminally ill child … has the right to know. *Am J Nurs.* 1994;94:20.
38. Krahn GL, Hallum A, Kime C. Are there good ways to give "bad news"? *Pediatrics.* 1993;91:578–582.
39. Levi RB, Marsick R, Drotar D, Kodish ED. Diagnosis, disclosure, and informed consent: learning from parents of children with cancer [see comment]. *J Pediatr Hematol Oncol.* 2000;22:3–12.
40. O'Connor P. Truth telling in pediatrics – in degrees. In: Ganos D et al, eds. *Difficult Decisions in Medical Ethics: The Fourth Volume in a Series on Ethics, Humanism, and Medicine.* Proceedings of the Eighth and Ninth Conferences on Ethics, Humanism, and Medicine, University of Michigan, Ann Arbor; 1981, 1982. New York: Alan R Liss; 1983.

41. Young B, Dixon-Woods M, Windridge KC, et al. Managing communication with young people who have a potentially life threatening chronic illness: qualitative study of patients and parents [see comment]. *BMJ.* 2003;326:305.

42. Sigman GS, Kraut J, La Puma J. Disclosure of a diagnosis to children and adolescents when parents object: a clinical ethics analysis. *Am J Dis Child.* 1993;147:764–768.

7

Pediatric Ethics Committees

Mark R. Mercurio

INTRODUCTION

Ethics committees have become nearly ubiquitous in American hospitals in the past quarter-century, and their use has been widely endorsed. The Universal Declaration on Bioethics and Human Rights recommends the use of independent, pluralistic, multidisciplinary ethics committees to provide advice on ethical problems in clinical settings and to establish educational forums for the discussion of issues in bioethics.[1] The Joint Commission on Accreditation of Healthcare Organizations has mandated that every health care organization in the United States have a mechanism in place to address ethical conflicts,[2] and for the majority of hospitals this requirement has been met by the creation of an ethics committee. The American Medical Association (AMA) and the American Academy of Pediatrics (AAP) have endorsed hospital ethics committees and have provided specific guidelines for their use.[3,4] The early proliferation of these committees occurred partially in response to landmark cases involving neurologically incapacitated adults, notably Karen Quinlan in 1976.[5] In 1983, the President's Commission for the Study of Ethical Problems in Medicine and Biomedical and Behavioral Research endorsed the creation and use of hospital ethics committees to promote effective decision making for incapacitated individuals. At that time fewer than 1% of all U.S. hospitals had such a committee.[6] In the years since then, ethics committees have become commonplace in U.S. hospitals, and more recently their use in European hospitals has grown as well.[7-9]

As the use of hospital ethics committees increased, it became apparent that many of the difficult issues confronted by these committees involved infants and children. Indeed, some of the early landmark cases that contributed to the spread of ethics committees involved newborns, such as the well-known 1982 "Baby Doe" case in Indiana, which involved the question of withholding lifesaving surgery from a child with trisomy 21.[5] Some hospital ethics committees, such as those in most general hospitals in the United States, are intended to deal with adult and pediatric cases. Some larger pediatric services and children's hospitals have a separate pediatric ethics committee (PEC), intended to deal exclusively with ethical issues related to the provision of medical care to pediatric patients.

This chapter is meant to provide the reader with an understanding of some ethical, social, and cultural issues at play in the operation of a PEC, as well as a practical guide to the formation and operation of such a committee. It is intended to be of use to those already well versed in the activities of an ethics committee, as well as to those for whom this is a new enterprise. Some suggestions are specific to PECs, but most of what is discussed is equally relevant to adult ethics committees. In no way, however, is it suggested that the approach outlined here is the only reasonable one. Experience has shown that there are many different ways to run a good ethics committee and consultation service.

ETHICS COMMITTEES: WHAT THEY ARE AND WHY THEY EXIST

Some problems faced in the delivery of medical care are so complex from an ethical standpoint that patients, families, and physicians are sometimes truly at a loss as to which of the options are morally permissible or preferable. Often family members will disagree among themselves or with hospital staff members. Furthermore, physicians and other health care providers are sometimes asked by parents to provide a course of treatment they feel is ethically unacceptable. There are those who maintain that physicians should generally follow the directives of parents and not seek to impose their own moral judgments on the plan. Everyone involved in the delivery of health care, however, is a moral agent, with responsibility for his or her actions. Thus, it is appropriate that members of the staff take the ethical component of their roles seriously and sometimes seek help when sorting out these difficult issues.

The purpose of the PEC is to provide guidance for each of these circumstances. It serves as a resource for patients, families, staff, and community. The purpose of the committee is not, however, to usurp the roles of patients, parents, or attending physicians in making therapeutic decisions. Indeed, PECs typically operate solely in an advisory capacity, with no authority to direct or dictate care.

The committee should be a group of individuals from various disciplines who come together to offer guidance, facilitate communication, and provide a framework for analysis in cases of ethical uncertainty. It should not, however, merely be a collection of intelligent, well-meaning individuals assembled to hear a case and render an opinion, based solely on their moral intuitions. Though there will be various levels of experience and formal training among members, the PEC should provide a level of expertise in such matters beyond that of most clinicians. All members should have some education in ethics, and one or more should have extensive training, ideally an advanced degree in this field. Also, at least some should have considerable experience in clinical ethics consultation. The ongoing training of PEC members is an obligation of the committee itself and the parent institution.

Skepticism among some hospital staff members about the inadequate expertise of PEC members ("What do these people know that we don't?") may sometimes be valid, and the committee and its ongoing educational programs should be designed with that concern in mind. That is, the membership and ongoing education of the committee should be such that the PEC does indeed have something to offer. Optimally, perhaps, most members of the PEC would have an advanced degree in ethics or a related field and/or extensive clinical ethics experience. For the majority of hospitals, however, this is not a realistic expectation. However, it must be recognized that PECs are sometimes called on to make recommendations with potentially very serious consequences, using whatever limited tools are at their disposal. The inability to optimize those tools does not relieve the committee or the parent institution of the obligation to provide them and to make ongoing efforts to sharpen them.

ETHICS COMMITTEES: WHAT THEY ARE NOT

It is important to be clear to patients, families, staff, and the PEC members themselves regarding what the committee is *not*. For example, the ethics committee is not a legal office or a court, and individuals seeking legal advice should be referred appropriately. With this in mind, members of the PEC consulting on a specific case should not become preoccupied with the legal "answer" to the question presented, but rather should seek to identify the ethical issues and work with the people involved to identify the morally preferable course of action. The question of whether that course of action is legal is, of course, an important one, but a separate one, often difficult to discern, and in any case is appropriately addressed in a different setting.

The PEC is not the institutional review board (IRB), whose domain includes the protection of human subjects of medical research. Questions involving clinical research protocols typically are referred to the IRB. It may occur that a PEC is presented with concerns about the care of an individual patient participating in such a protocol. In some such cases it may be reasonable for the PEC members to consult, but if so, they should work closely with the IRB.

Similarly, the PEC is not the chaplaincy. This mistaken impression may sometimes be held, particularly in hospitals with a religious affiliation. In such hospitals, if there are specific policies dictated by that affiliation, the PEC should be well versed in those policies. However, it is not the role of the

PEC to advise on or enforce a specific religious doctrine. In any hospital, questions about religious precepts, customs, or rituals should be referred to clergy of the appropriate faith.

The PEC is usually not responsible for organizational ethics. This important role, to provide guidance to (and monitoring of) the organization in areas such as business ethics, is typically carried out by a separate committee, commonly known as the compliance committee. Ethical concerns related to matters such as billing, employee contracts, and advertising activities should be referred to that group. There may be some potential for overlap, and it might be advantageous to have the chair of each committee serve on the other, so as to best determine which committee should become involved in referrals when this is not immediately clear. It should be noted, however, that in some hospitals the ethics committee does fill this role,[10] and if so, the committee should include individuals with the necessary expertise.

Finally, it is worth noting that the PEC is not a rubber stamp, put in place to provide pro forma approval of any plan. When the committee is asked to consider a situation, an appropriate sentiment of the request could be: "Help us to determine what the best course of action is," or "Help us to consider whether a proposed plan is ethically acceptable," or "Help us to reach an agreement with the family in this difficult decision." Occasionally, one gets the sense that what is really being asked is: "Tell us that our plan is acceptable and explain that to the family," or "We need you to confirm that we are right and the family is wrong, and to let them know." The credibility and the effectiveness of the PEC require that everyone involved, especially the members themselves, understand that the committee should not enter into any deliberation or consultation with its recommendation predetermined.

The American Society for Bioethics and Humanities (ASBH) Task Force for Bioethics Consultations have listed character traits associated with successful ethics consultations. Some are relatively obvious but nevertheless important, such as honesty, tolerance, and compassion. The most important, however, may well be integrity and courage.[11,12] Members of the PEC must be willing, when appropriate, to advise against a plan that has been strongly endorsed by powerful and respected members of the hospital's medical staff and/or administration. Such situations have occurred and will continue to occur.

HOW PEDIATRIC ETHICS COMMITTEES DIFFER FROM ADULT ETHICS COMMITTEES

Just as it is widely accepted that providing medical care for children is not akin to treating little adults, addressing the ethical issues that face children cannot be directly extrapolated from the approach applied in adult cases.[13]

While they have a great deal in common, there are fundamental differences between pediatric ethics and adult ethics, and thus in the questions the different committees are likely to confront. Adult medical ethics, and its application by ethics committees, commonly looks to the primacy of patient autonomy. The competent patient's right to refuse a recommended treatment, for example, is foundational. If the patient is unable to speak for him- or herself, autonomy is still somewhat respected by attempting to determine what the patient would have preferred (substituted judgment) and basing therapeutic decisions on that determination. Often, specific written instructions (advance directives) are available.

For the vast majority of pediatric cases (the possible exception being late adolescence), complete deference to patient autonomy is not an available option, as most questions brought to the PEC will concern patients who are not, and have never been, competent to make such decisions. The more complex notions of assent and the gradual increase in competence over the course of childhood must instead be considered. Patient autonomy is not usually at issue, but rather parental authority, which, while carrying considerable weight, is not as absolute as adult patient autonomy. Sometimes, as pediatricians know well, parental authority is most appropriately overruled by other considerations, most notably the patient's best interests. The PEC will usually work to craft a recommendation based on the patient's best interests, which is essentially a weighing of the anticipated benefits and burdens to the patient of a plan under consideration. It is often an extremely subjective judgment and a common source of disagreement between staff and families. The threshold at which patient's best interests, as perceived by the staff, should trump parental authority can be one of the most difficult ethical determinations in pediatrics.

If a surrogate decision maker is needed for an adult, there is usually one individual, such as the spouse, who fills that role. In some circumstances several relatives (e.g., grown sons and daughters) will be involved, but commonly one individual has the authority to speak on behalf of the patient. In most pediatric cases, on the other hand, there are usually two surrogate decision makers (the parents) with equal authority, who may disagree on their assessment of the child's best interests and/or on how they wish the medical team to proceed. Furthermore, it is not uncommon for one or both surrogate decision makers to be adolescents, who would not be considered adequate or appropriate surrogates for an adult patient, but with whom the pediatric staff and the PEC must work when trying to resolve an ethical question or conflict.[14]

Finally, a large percentage of questions brought to an ethics committee are related to end-of-life care. In the case of adults, this commonly involves elderly individuals, who regardless of the path chosen are very unlikely to survive for several more years. While some patients considered by the PEC will die soon regardless of the therapeutic path chosen, many could potentially survive another 70 or 80 years. For decisions such as the withdrawal of life-sustaining medical therapy from a severely impaired newborn, for example, a great deal more seems to be at stake.

STRUCTURE: PEDIATRIC ETHICS COMMITTEE MEMBERSHIP

The PEC, and in particular its consultation process, should be fair, efficient, and most of all helpful to the individuals it is meant to serve: the patients, families, and staff. The structure of the committee, and its processes, should be designed with those goals in mind. With that aim, let us now turn to the nuts and bolts of forming and operating a PEC, beginning with membership.

Although in the past some ethics committees were composed entirely of physicians, it is now widely recognized in the United States that membership should be multidisciplinary. As with any consultative service, if it is intended to serve as a resource to clinicians, then clearly the collective membership should have a fund of knowledge and/or a set of skills not generally possessed by most of those who consult the committee. Otherwise, it is difficult to see how the committee would be of any real use. That knowledge should be in a variety of areas relevant to ethics, consistent with ASBH recommendations discussed in more detail later, but should generally fall into two categories: ethical theory and landmark cases. This is knowledge that perhaps a few members of the PEC (e.g., those with advanced education in philosophy, law, theology, or bioethics) bring with them at the outset and that the others should be expected to acquire, at least to some degree, over their tenure on the committee.

The necessary expertise and experience take time to acquire. As such, the rapid rotation of members on and off the committee that is common to many hospital committees is not appropriate for the PEC. While permanent membership may be problematic, terms of membership should be longer than typical for other committees and should be clearly specified for those joining.

The specific process of membership selection is rarely discussed, but can be crucial to the effectiveness and fairness of the committee. The practices and policies considered by an ethics committee often involve issues that engender strong feelings on all sides, issues such as the withdrawal of life-sustaining treatment and the termination of pregnancy, among many others. It is best, therefore, that one individual (such as the committee chair) not be in a position to choose the majority of committee members, which could potentially result in PEC membership based on agreement on certain important questions. Even if the chair were not inclined to do so, the PEC must avoid even the appearance or potential of bias. The best way to achieve balance on the committee, and thus to maximize its credibility, is to delegate membership selection to several individuals. For example, the physicians on the committee could be appointed by the chair of the Pediatric Department, the nurses by the vice president of nursing, the clergy by religious leaders outside the hospital, the administrative representative by the hospital president, the community members by the PEC chair, and so on.

In addition, it is preferable that a majority of members not report to the same supervisor. The PEC may be called upon to provide advice on individual cases and on policies, which could be very controversial within the organization. As such, the committee should be able to operate with a significant degree of independence. Not having a majority of the committee answerable to one individual may be helpful in fostering that independence.

An ethics committee will be able to provide a much broader and richer fund of expertise as a result of its multidisciplinary nature. While the experience and perspectives of physicians and nurses are unique and essential to these discussions, they are greatly augmented by the perspectives provided by others from very different backgrounds. With that in mind, it is recommended that a PEC seek representation from the following disciplines.

Attending Physicians: At least four pediatricians should be on the committee, so that at least one will be available to participate in any given consultation. It would be best if these physicians were from disparate subspecialties – for example, intensive care, community-based general pediatrics, neonatology, or adolescent medicine – and not all employed by the hospital or university. It would also be valuable to have a surgeon and/or adult physician to provide the different perspectives that surgery and medicine often foster. It may be particularly helpful to include a pediatric neurologist or a specialist in neurodevelopmental outcome, as many of the questions will pertain to neurological prognosis. Individuals with any expertise in a subspecialty that are not represented on the committee, however, can be called upon to provide input on an ad hoc basis.

Resident Physicians: One or two members should be a resident or fellow. Though they will have to serve shorter terms, and thus generally be unable to acquire the same degree of expertise or experience as the other members, their perspective is often unique and helpful. In addition, their membership increases the visibility of the committee among the house staff, possibly augmenting utilization of the committee.

Nurses: At least three members should be pediatric nurses, preferably representing different units in the hospital. This also provides a different perspective and increases the visibility and utilization of the committee. It may also be helpful to have a nurse on the committee who is not employed by the hospital and is therefore less likely to be influenced by hospital political or administrative concerns.

Mental Health Professional: At least one member should have a background in mental health, ideally child psychiatry or psychology. Insight from such an individual can prove invaluable for understanding and resolving conflicts.

Social Workers: These members often bring unique insight into the family dynamics and/or conflicts being considered, but also typically have a very helpful understanding of the resources (both inside and outside the hospital) that could contribute to a practical solution.

Clergy: These individuals are often helpful not only for their expertise in specific faith traditions and how those may affect family thinking, but also for their experience and skill in working with families in times of crisis.

Individuals Trained in Philosophy and/or Bioethics: Clearly many hospitals do not have access to anyone with advanced training in these fields (recall that ethics is a branch of philosophy). However, many children's hospitals are part of a larger academic community, and thus there may be a faculty member who could contribute greatly, both to individual case discussions and to the education of the committee members and hospital community. Some clinicians may balk at the idea that an academic philosopher could be a valued member. After all, it might be argued, such philosophers usually do not have any real-world medical experience. It would be a mistake, however, to underestimate their analytical ability and their potential contribution to clinical ethics consultation. When included in the deliberations, they often provide valuable insight.

Attorney: As noted earlier, legal questions are not the purview of the PEC. Nevertheless, having an individual at the table with that expertise can often prove helpful as discussions unfold. When the attorney is a legal representative of the hospital, there is the potential for conflict between the interests of the hospital and those of the patient being discussed. While this concern does not outweigh the potential benefit of having an attorney on the committee, the attorney, the committee chair, and indeed all PEC members should be aware of this potential and how it could affect the discussion. One solution to this concern is to have an attorney from the community, with no ties to the hospital other than membership on the PEC.

Students: Members may wish to consider inviting one or two medical and/or nursing students to participate, both for the helpful perspective of younger individuals and because doing so would be consistent with the PEC's educational mission.

Administrator: It may be helpful to have an individual from the hospital administration to serve as a liaison to that group and to provide knowledge regarding policies and procedures. As with the attorney, however, there is clearly a risk of conflict of interest. With awareness of that risk, and given the right individual, a representative of administration can prove helpful to the functioning of the PEC and should be considered. In some cases, the hospital attorney might fill this role.

Other Hospital Staff Members: The PEC should ideally have representatives from each of the disciplines just listed, but additional hospital personnel may also prove valuable, such as those involved in child life, physical or occupational therapy, or other fields, including hospital staff members with no direct clinical exposure.

Community Representatives: Some of the individuals already discussed, such as clergy, will probably be unaffiliated with the hospital and could thus be considered community representatives. A balanced perspective and representation is further served by including additional community members unrelated to the hospital or to the health care professions. Possibilities include an individual who has worked closely with disabled individuals, a teacher in a local school, or a particularly mature young person, such as an undergraduate at a nearby college. There may also be value in having a culturally diverse committee. Though one or two individuals should not be thought to speak for all members of any group, their insights and their presence can often prove helpful.

Medical staff members may be reluctant to involve nonmedical individuals in ethics committee deliberations, perhaps in part because they are understandably perceived as being much less knowledgeable about the problem at hand. This is generally true for medical matters, but the objection can be overcome by the realization that the fundamental questions being addressed are usually not medical, in the sense that they are not physiological. Rather, the questions are more often moral ones, and once the relevant medical background has been presented in sufficient detail to consider the moral questions, non-clinicians are no less qualified than medical personnel to participate in the deliberation. The nonmedical participants may in fact be more qualified in some settings if they have more experience with such moral deliberations and/or have less emotional investment in a particular outcome.

Some hospital personnel have expressed concern about "airing their dirty laundry," including possible ethical breeches, to outsiders. To address this reasonable concern, committee members should be selected with care, and the chair should make every effort to ensure that all members understand and abide by strict rules of confidentiality. With that caution, however, the benefits of community representation most likely will outweigh the risks.

PEC Chair: The chair of the PEC need not be the individual on the committee with the most formal training in ethics, though that is one viable option, but should possess expertise and experience in this area. In particular, he or she should have significant experience in providing ethics consultations. Given the nature of many issues discussed, the chair should be receptive to the opinions of all, but also have the ability to keep meetings moving and focused on the issue at hand. He or she should have credibility with the medical staff and with the hospital community in general, or the PEC and its work are unlikely to be accepted.

One possible reason that a physician is commonly chosen as chair is that the multidisciplinary teams that provide patient care in the hospital are invariably led by an attending physician. Thus, physician leadership is part of hospital culture, at least on the patient-care level. Another reason may be the perception that the attending physician's responsibility in many of the difficult issues discussed is unique and best understood by another attending physician. In addition, a physician-chair may be more likely to appreciate the medical nuances of a case. Of course, it could also be argued that an ethicist-chair is more likely to appreciate the ethical nuances and that a chair with a nonclinical background would be more capable of providing a more objective viewpoint.

Perhaps the most practical reason for choosing a physician is to optimize acceptance of the committee by the attending medical staff. An understanding of the medical culture (i.e., its sometimes ill-advised reluctance to take advice from non-physicians) would suggest that this is most likely the case, and for this reason a physician with a strong background in ethics may be the best choice. Nevertheless, there are clearly some non-physicians who are capable of filling this role and who may be the best choice for a given hospital.

It is essential that the chair have the confidence of the medical staff and the hospital administration, and it is therefore recommended that both groups have input into his or her selection. One possibility is selection upon agreement between the hospital CEO and the chair of pediatrics. It is equally important that, once selected, the chair be permitted to direct the committee without undue influence or interference from either.

The PEC members should be selected to maximize effectiveness in carrying out the committee's three main functions: case consultations, education, and policy development. The execution of each of these functions will be considered next.

CASE CONSULTATION: ACCESS AND INDICATIONS

Access to the PEC for questions regarding the care of a patient within the hospital should be nearly universal. This includes all members of the clinical team regardless of status in the hierarchy, patients, members of the patient's family or broader support group, and other hospital employees. If someone from the housekeeping staff witnesses something he or she feels is an ethical problem, that person should have the same access to the PEC as would a nurse or physician. Every member of the staff, every parent, and (appropriate for age) every patient should be made aware of the PEC's existence, function, and how it can be accessed. Hospital employees should thus be able to immediately assist families wishing to speak with a representative of the committee. The staff should also clearly understand that initial contact of the PEC, whether by a patient, parent, or member of the staff, does not require anyone's permission.

The chair (or a designated PEC member) should be readily available for an initial telephone consultation, to determine whether the issue is appropriate for the committee or should be referred elsewhere. For example, if the problem is related to unprofessional behavior on the part of a staff member, the chair may choose to deal with the issue on an individual basis or refer the problem to the individual's supervisor. If the concern relates to the quality of medical care being provided by an individual physician, it may be more appropriate to refer to the physician's department chair, who will generally be better suited to determine the quality of the care and will have the responsibility of taking corrective action if needed. If there appears to be a miscommunication between two individuals, the PEC chair might attempt resolution simply by facilitating that communication.

It might sometimes take two or three conversations to determine whether the question is appropriate for the PEC. The chair should have those conversations in a timely fashion and generally be prepared to convene the PEC within 24–48 hours if necessary. As already noted, the attending physician's permission should not be required for an ethics consultation to be requested or to proceed, but the PEC chair should discuss the possibility of consultation with the attending physician before going forward.

Appropriate indications for PEC involvement include a request for help with a specific ethical question or decision concerning patient care (e.g., Should a certain therapy be offered, withheld, or withdrawn?) or a request for guidance with a more open-ended question (e.g., What should we do with this ethically complex situation?). It is also appropriate for the PEC to become involved if there is concern that a specific ethical breech in patient care has occurred or is ongoing.

There are other situations wherein it may or may not be appropriate to involve the PEC, depending on the culture of the committee and the organization. The PEC is sometimes consulted to assist with conflict resolution, usually involving a family's resistance to the staff's recommended approach, but occasionally involving disagreements among staff members themselves. Some PECs choose not to become involved in such disputes, but only in cases where there is a clear ethical question to be resolved. Others, however, see conflict resolution as a valuable service they can sometimes provide. Similarly, a PEC meeting sometimes serves as a forum for the clinical team to air its frustrations, even if no specific ethical question is articulated. This may have therapeutic value for the team and may also help bring forth new ideas and approaches not previously considered. Here again, some PECs may avoid such discussions if there is no specific ethical question, while others may elect to offer this service to clinicians.

CASE CONSULTATION: THREE MODELS

Once the chair has decided that the PEC should be involved, it must next be determined how the consultation will be carried out. There are generally three models for case consultation: consultation with an individual, consultation with the entire committee, or consultation with a small team.[15] While some committees have chosen one particular model they feel works best, it seems preferable to allow the chair some flexibility in choosing which is best for the case at hand. For example, if he or she receives a call from a physician requiring input on a difficult decision within the hour, an individual consultation, or perhaps recruiting one or two additional members, seems most feasible. Also, if the situation calls for mediation of a disagreement, working with a single consultant may sometimes be the best approach. Clearly, if the single-consultant model is used, the individual should have considerable experience and expertise in ethics consultation. The biggest advantage of this model is the ability to respond quickly, or even immediately, to a request for help. The biggest disadvantage is that the judgment of only a single individual is provided. When there is an ethical question to be addressed, it is preferable, even on very short notice, to assemble at least a small subset of the PEC if at all possible and to give the question the consideration and deliberation it warrants.

The entire PEC, or a large subset, will offer a much wider and richer fund of knowledge and experience than a single consultant. It will, however, take longer to assemble the group. Also, it may be intimidating to the patient and/or parents, if they are present, to meet with such a large group, along with several members of the clinical team, particularly if the issue is one of conflict. For most consultations, the advantages of both approaches can usually be achieved by including a moderate-sized subgroup of the PEC. The consultation group would consist of a minimum of four and up to eight members. Ideally, at least two should be physicians. With a committee consisting of 15–20 members, a group of this size can nearly always be available for a meeting within one or two days.

This small-group approach is recommended for most clinical case consultations, particularly when the patient and/or family will be present. However, if no family members will be at the meeting, it may prove helpful to have more members of the PEC contributing to the discussion, and there is less need to limit attendance. One should keep in mind, however, that using a group (small or large) to determine a recommendation risks the phenomenon known as "groupthink," wherein a collection of people can reach an ill-advised conclusion that none would have made as individuals. Put simply, I may have serious reservations about the plan, but do not voice them and agree to move forward because you appear to endorse it and I trust you. You endorse it, at least in part, because I do. Our trust in the perceived collective wisdom of the group may exceed our trust in ourselves. History is replete with unfortunate examples of groupthink.[16] The best way to avert this problem is to create an environment wherein members feel comfortable voicing any concerns, they are encouraged to do so, and counterarguments to the prevailing opinion are actively sought and considered.

CASE CONSULTATION: WHOM TO INVITE

Once it is determined that a PEC consultation should take place, a time (optimally within 48 hours) should be set. This will be based in part on the availability of individuals essential to the process, such as the attending physician, the individual(s) requesting the consult, and the parents. The chair should determine the optimal size of the PEC consultation team based on considerations described in the preceding section. Specifically who is chosen may sometimes depend on the specific circumstances of the case, and nearly always on who is available. Any member of the PEC who offers to attend but will need to arrive late should be discouraged from attending. Given the gravity of the recommendations sometimes reached, everyone contributing to those recommendations should have been witness to the entire deliberation.

In addition to the attending physician, other physicians (e.g., consultants, the primary care pediatrician, and/or residents involved in the care) may prove helpful to the discussion. The same is true for nurses, social workers, and/or a hospital chaplain if they have been involved in the case. Each of these individuals often have information and insights about the patient and/or family that the physicians do not, and their participation may also help achieve buy-in to the recommendation reached. If the patient or family will not be at the meeting, it may be reasonable to open it up to as many members of the care team as wish to attend, to maximize the available information, as well as to expose as many of the staff members as possible to the deliberations that led to the recommendation. If family will be there, the number of staff members present should be limited, but nurses should nearly always be there, as should social workers and/or a chaplain, if they have been involved with the case.

A central question in planning the meeting is whether to invite the patient and/or parents. For cases brought before the PEC, the presence of the patient at the meeting is usually not at issue. In the majority of cases, however, parents should be invited to participate. If the purpose of the PEC meeting is to help resolve a conflict between parents and staff, it seems both counterproductive and unfair to exclude one party. If the purpose is to facilitate deliberations regarding a difficult ethical question, it will be valuable for the parents to observe the process and important for everyone else to hear their thoughts on the question. In a survey of physicians after ethics consultations, it was specifically noted that one benefit of these meetings was that they helped bring the parents' perspective into focus.[17] Furthermore, the ethical questions considered are often laden with value judgments. In such cases the values of the family, while not always determinative, must be central to the discussion and recommendation.[18] For all of these reasons, parents should generally be invited to attend.

There may be some situations wherein parental attendance is not advisable – for example, if the purpose of the meeting is to mediate a dispute between clinicians. Also, the clinical team sometimes seeks the PEC's help in deciding what to offer a family or how to deal with a difficult family and might specifically request that the family not be included. Such a request should be honored, but the chair might in some cases encourage the clinical team to invite the parents, by explaining the advantages of their presence. In the end, whenever it remains the choice of the clinical team to meet in the absence of the parents, that request should be honored, with two important qualifications. First, in most such cases the parents deserve to know that the meeting has occurred and to be given the opportunity to meet with the PEC, with or without the clinicians present. Second, the PEC (or anyone, for that matter) should be very cautious about making a recommendation regarding a conflict between two parties without having first heard from both, or at the very least having offered the opportunity to both.

Parents should be given the opportunity to invite anyone they choose and should often be encouraged to bring persons who will provide some support, such as relatives, friends, or clergy, and who might put them more at ease. In addition, these individuals sometimes help articulate the parents' position and sometimes help the parents understand the situation more clearly or realistically. It may be especially helpful, when the PEC is working with very young parents, to strongly encourage them to include the grandparents.

CASE CONSULTATION: THE MEETING

Before the meeting takes place, it is often helpful for the PEC chair to have briefly discussed both the purpose of the meeting and the specifics of what will take place with the relevant clinician(s) and the parents. At the beginning of the meeting, the chair should introduce him- or herself and very briefly explain the purpose of the meeting, how it will transpire, and how long it will last. It should be stated that the PEC has no authority to make or enforce decisions, but rather is there to facilitate the discussion and decision-making process and often to make a specific recommendation. It should also be made clear that the PEC does not serve as a legal adviser. If the chair anticipates that the meeting will be followed by an executive session of the PEC before a recommendation is made (which is generally advisable), the entire group present should be so informed at the outset and told when to expect the recommendation.

All those present should introduce themselves, and in one sentence state their relation to the case. The patient's attending or resident physician should present a brief clinical summary, providing data relevant to the ethical question, in language that everyone in the room (many or most being non-physicians) can understand. Other members of the clinical team should be invited to add anything they feel is relevant. Everyone present should then be invited to ask for clarification of the clinical information. The parents should then be asked if they have anything to add. If the parents requested the meeting, they should be invited to speak before the clinical presentation, to state their concerns at the outset of the meeting.

After the initial presentations, the chair should summarize and articulate in straightforward terms the specific ethical question being brought before the group. It is essential, for example, that distinct questions not be conflated. For example, the question "Which of these options is the ethically preferable one?" should not be confused with "Which of these options would be ethically permissible?" One might be determined to be preferable, yet both to be permissible. This should be made clear at the outset, and if both questions are to be considered, they must be addressed separately in the discussion and in the final recommendation.

Once there is agreement on the question, open discussion should begin, with all present invited to participate. Different PECs will have different ideas as to how these meetings are approached. One possibility is a "facilitation approach," in which the committee does not so much seek to make a specific recommendation at the end of the meeting as to use the deliberations to educate those involved in the case about the ethical issues, get them to share their thoughts on those issues, and help them to reach their own judgment and agreement about what the best answer would be.[19] Other committees may aim to make their own specific recommendation at the end of the session and in that way be somewhat more directive. In either case, the PEC's role should include exploring, with all of those present, the ethical issues and principles at play.

The conversation should include practical matters, such as the patient's prognosis and the reliability of the prognostic data, treatments, and support services available, and details of the family's situation. It should also include consideration of specific ethical approaches, such as an application of the patient's best-interests standard, and thus an attempt to identify the potential types of benefit and harm of a proposed course of action. PECs may choose to discuss and employ various other ethical models and considerations as well, such as the fundamental principles of autonomy, beneficence, nonmaleficence, and justice,[20] prior cases (casuistry), effects on relationships, and the relative importance of the family's interests. The patient's best interests, however, should remain prominent in all of these considerations.

A meeting length of 60–90 minutes is generally sufficient for adequate discussion, without being onerous to those asked to attend. Near the end, the chair should bring the discussion to a close by summarizing where things stand and invite anyone to make a final brief comment before the session is adjourned. In some cases the issue will have been clearly resolved to the satisfaction to all present, and it should be so stated. Often, however, the PEC has been asked for a specific recommendation, which is usually made only after discussion in executive session. If so, at the close of the meeting the PEC members should remain for that discussion.

Executive sessions, wherein the members of a committee meet in private, are controversial but may sometimes prove helpful. Though such sessions seem contrary to the goal of a transparent process, there may be circumstances wherein a member of the committee has something important to share with other members but is reluctant to do so in the presence of the clinical team and family. It may relate, for example, to a perception of credibility or motives. Executive sessions give members the opportunity to speak openly and to air all concerns before a recommendation is reached. Often, the gravity of the recommendation will justify this extra step.

The chair, if possible with another member of the committee, should then communicate with the attending physician, as well as other relevant parties (e.g., parents and nurses), regarding the recommendations. It should be stated whether the recommendations reached were unanimous or represented a majority of the committee with some dissent. If no consensus could be reached by the PEC, that, too, may be helpful information to a clinician or family struggling with a difficult decision. The chair should write a brief note in the medical record stating the committee's recommendation. A longer report should subsequently be generated for the PEC's records and should include the names of those present, the questions raised, a brief description of the case, the recommendations reached, and the ethical rationale for those recommendations.

CHAIRING A CASE CONSULTATION

In addition to the points made in the preceding section, there are some specific suggestions for chairing the meeting that may prove helpful. It is permissible to choose certain PEC members to participate depending on the specifics of the case, but not to "stack" the meeting to achieve an answer the chair prefers. At the meeting, the chair should set a tone of open, frank, and respectful dialogue. It is important that everyone who wishes to speak be given the opportunity to do so, and thus no one be permitted to dominate the discussion to the exclusion of others. It is the role of the chair to keep the conversation focused on the issue at hand, which can sometimes be surprisingly difficult.

One reason that it may be helpful to have a physician serve as the chair, and that it is essential that physician members of the PEC at least be involved, is that any flaws in the medical information presented are more likely to be appreciated. The chair (with the help of the other members) will need to decide if the medical "facts" presented should be accepted at face value or warrant further investigation. This concern refers not so much to the specifics of the case as to prognostic data that may be out-of-date or otherwise incorrect. In general, the chair (and thus the PEC) will be able to rely on the clinical team's presentation, but that may not always be the case, and they should be alert to the possibility of inaccurate data. Sound ethical reasoning applied to bad data can, and has, led to poor recommendations. For example, the decision reached in the classic Baby Doe case, mentioned at the outset of the chapter, was based in part on the dubious prognostic information presented, that children with trisomy 21 have no chance at any quality of life.

In the executive session, the chair should question each PEC member present for his or her opinion, being clear that it is permissible to "pass." He or she should also consider the possibility that a second meeting of the PEC, perhaps after a brief time for data acquisition or further reflection, should occur before a recommendation is made. The feasibility of this may, of course, depend on the urgency of the question. Finally, the chair should avoid inappropriately influencing or limiting the discussion, either in the general meeting or in the executive session, by stating his or her opinion early in the process. It is best to appear objective, questioning any argument given and providing the counterargument for consideration. In the executive session, for example, when soliciting the opinion of each member, the chair should generally be the last to weigh in and should also discourage others who may have excessive influence (e.g., the department chair, hospital attorney, or hospital CEO) from voicing a definitive judgment early in the process, thus closing off what could be valuable dialogue.

CONSULTATION FOLLOW-UP AND EVALUATION

As with every other service in health care, ethics consultations should be subject to review and quality improvement.[21–23] Every consultation, including the ethical reasoning applied, should be reviewed retrospectively by the entire committee. This will serve as a quality check and as a way to maximize the educational value of each case. Most consultations should also be followed up by contacting relevant parties (e.g., the parents and person who requested the consultation) to determine the outcome, to decide whether any further PEC involvement would be helpful, and to solicit suggestions for improving the process. Periodic retrospective reviews of consultations should also be carried out and presented to the committee and to those to whom the committee is responsible (e.g., the department chair or medical board), to assess utilization of the committee, look for trends, and identify potential areas of improvement.

While the effectiveness of a service such as this is difficult to quantify, studies have shown that most physicians and families are satisfied with the process. In addition, randomized prospective studies have shown that ethics consultation in the intensive care setting, while having no effect on overall mortality, is associated with a reduction in hospital days and in the use of life-sustaining treatments, among patients who failed to survive to discharge.[24,25] This suggests that the discussions fostered by the PEC may facilitate an understanding and acceptance of the outcome sooner than would otherwise be the case, thus reducing the tendency to continue invasive, expensive, or inappropriate treatments at the end of life. Though an individual PEC may lack the resources or case volume to do a study of this nature, every committee should make a good-faith effort to ensure that it is providing a helpful, accessible, and efficient service based on sound ethical reasoning and a fair process.

EDUCATION

The second of the PEC's three main functions is the provision of educational support within the organization, and perhaps to the community as well. Before considering either, however, the PEC must first and foremost see to the education of its own members. As stated previously, the usefulness of this service requires note only that it be available, but also that those who provide it bring some measure of expertise. The ASBH has made it clear that ethics committees must be educated on a large range of topics, and their curriculum is available for use by those wishing to establish or maintain such a committee.[12] While the list of potential topics is extensive, a suggested basic curriculum for PEC members can be outlined as follows:

The structure and function of the PEC
Fundamentals of ethical theories
Landmark cases relevant to pediatric ethics
Surrogate decision making
Conflict resolution
Parental rights
Informed consent and assent
End-of-life decisions
Approach to parent–physician conflict
Adolescent rights
Ethical issues related to reproduction
Ethical issues specific to newborn medicine
Religion and medical decisions

Withholding and withdrawing life-sustaining medical treatment, including (but not limited to) mechanical ventilation and artificial nutrition and hydration

Conflicts of interest

Many other topics would surely be relevant as well, but this list represents a solid foundation. A monthly seminar series covering these topics could be an ideal format. In addition, PEC members should be familiar with the relevant policies of their hospital and those of the AAP Committee on Bioethics. A review of the AAP policies on bioethical questions, with brief commentaries and useful references, is available.[26-29] Perhaps most importantly, the committee should be considered a work in progress, and therefore its efforts at self-education should be ongoing.

The educational activities of the PEC should be extended to include all members of the staff involved in the care of children, including physicians, nurses, therapists, social workers, chaplains, and others. It is also appropriate, and has been beneficial, to offer a session on the basics of medical ethics to members of the hospital administration. This provides them with a better understanding of the issues at stake and the methods applied to their resolution, while also increasing the visibility of the PEC within that group.

POLICY DEVELOPMENT

The experience and expertise of the committee should be utilized not just on a case-by-case basis, but in the overall approach to patient care. Thus, PECs should play an active role in the development of hospital policies related to ethical concerns in the care of pediatric patients. This is not to suggest that all such policies need to be primarily generated by the PEC (though in some cases that may be appropriate), but the committee should provide input as they are developed. Examples include resuscitation policies and end-of-life care policies. The AAP and the AMA have provided many guidelines and policies that can serve as a resource or framework for those being developed by a PEC.[3,27]

INTERNAL SUPPORT FOR THE PEDIATRIC ETHICS COMMITTEE

In order for the PEC to function adequately within the hospital, it must be supported by the administration and the medical leadership. The committee should appear on the hospital's organizational chart, be included in the institution's bylaws, and be openly recognized as an essential part of the hospital. An appropriate space should be provided for meetings and consultations. Membership on the committee should be seen as an important service to the organization, and thus members who are hospital employees should be allotted sufficient time to participate. Secretarial support and funding for educational endeavors, including the education of the PEC members and hospital staff, should be provided as regular budget items. In addition, given the time and availability usually required of the chair, the hospital should provide at least partial salary support for that individual. The institution should also provide liability coverage for all PEC members for work carried out in that role.

Most importantly, there must be a culture within the organization that recognizes the seriousness and value of the PEC's work. Hospitals should seek to establish a recognition that everyone, regardless of level of experience, could sometimes benefit from outside help. Once that is understood, to occasionally seek such input would not be seen as a sign of weakness or failure, as might sometimes be the perception, particularly among physicians. Rather, to seek input would be seen as evidence of maturity and self-confidence. As one senior attending physician noted in a survey study, seeking a view from outside the immediate clinical team is a sign of professional strength.[18]

The PEC members should also be aware of its natural partners within the organization, such as the institutional review board (sometimes called the human investigations committee), the palliative care committee, the compliance committee (also known as the organizational ethics committee), and the chaplaincy, among others. Each of these groups will share common interests and goals with the PEC and be a potential source of information and expertise.

EXTERNAL SUPPORT AND RESOURCES FOR THE PEDIATRIC ETHICS COMMITTEE

External support includes several professional organizations, such as the AAP Section on Bioethics (whose main function is education), the AAP Committee on Bioethics (whose main function is policy and guideline development), the AMA Council on Ethical and Judicial Affairs, and the ASBH, all of which have generated many helpful documents and guidelines. Within the ASBH there is a Pediatric Ethics Affinity Group devoted to the discussion of ethical issues related to pediatrics. Also, there is an informal coalition or listserve of professionals with an interest in pediatrics called the Pediatrics Ethics Consortium, where helpful ideas about PECs are frequently exchanged.[30] Anyone with an interest in pediatric ethics should be encouraged to participate in one or more of these groups and to occasionally attend one of the national meetings where matters of mutual interest are discussed.

Finally, resources sometimes overlooked include the adult ethics committee at the same or an affiliated institution and ethics committees at other hospitals. Committees could benefit from combining educational programs and also on occasion from soliciting the opinion of the committee of a nearby (or faraway) ethics committee regarding a difficult case. Sometimes a more objective viewpoint from a colleague (e.g., another PEC chair) with no personal loyalties to consider can be very helpful.

CONCLUSION

The pediatric ethics committee can be an important part of a pediatric service or children's hospital, but its value will depend on forming and maintaining an educated committee and on developing an accessible and helpful service that is valued by the hospital staff and administration.

References

1. United Nations Educational, Scientific, and Cultural Organization (UNESCO). Universal Declaration on Bioethics and Human Rights; 2005. Available at: http://portal.unesco.org/shs/en/ev.php URL_ID=1883&URL_DO=DO_ TOPIC&URL_SECTION=201.html. Accessed October 23, 2008.
2. Joint Commission on Accreditation of Healthcare Organizations. *Comprehensive Accreditation Manual for Hospitals: Update 1*. Oakbrook Terrace, Ill; 1999:R1–R11.
3. American Medical Association, Council on Ethical and Judicial Affairs. *Code of Medical Ethics*. Chicago: American Medical Association; 2006.
4. American Academy of Pediatrics, Committee on Bioethics. Institutional ethics committees. *Pediatrics*. 2001;107:205–209.
5. Pence, G. *Classic Cases in Medical Ethics*. 4th ed. Chicago: McGraw-Hill; 2004.
6. Deciding to forgo life-sustaining treatment: a report on the ethical, medical, and legal issues in treatment decisions. *President's Commission for the Study of Ethical Problems in Medicine and Biomedical Behavioral Research*; 1983:160–170. Available at: http://www.bioethics.gov/reports/past_commissions/index. html. Accessed October 23, 2008.
7. Pedersen R, Akre V, Forde R. Barriers and challenges in clinical ethics consultations: the experiences of nine clinical ethics committees. *Bioethics*. 2008. Available at: http://lib.bioinfo.pl/auid:5046596. Accessed October 23, 2008.
8. Williamson L, McLean S, Connell J. Clinical ethics committees in the United Kingdom: towards evaluation. *Med Law Int*. 2007;8:221–237.
9. Mino J, Copel L, Zucker J. *A French perspective on hospital ethics committees. Camb Q Healthcare Ethics*. 2008;17:300–307.
10. Blustein J, Post L, Dubler N. *Ethics for Healthcare Organizations: Theory, Case Studies, and Tools*. New York: United Hospital Fund of New York; 2008.
11. Society for Health and Human Values/Society for Bioethics Consultation, Task Force on Standards for Bioethics Consultation. *Core Competencies for Health Care Ethics Consultation: The Report of the American Society for Bioethics and Humanities*. Glenview, Ill: American Society for Bioethics and Humanities; 1998:21–22.
12. Aulisio M, Arnold R, Younger S. *Ethics Consultations: From Theory to Practice*. Baltimore: Johns Hopkins University Press; 2003:39.

13. Lyren A, Ford P. Special considerations for clinical ethics consultations in pediatrics: pediatric care provider as advocate. *Clin Pediatr.* 2007;9:771–776.
14. Ladd RE, Mercurio MR. Deciding for neonates: whose authority, whose interests? *Sem Perinatol.* 2003;27:488–494.
15. Smith ML, Kempfer AJ, Adams B, Candelair TG, Blackburn RK. Criteria for determining the appropriate method for an ethics consultation. *HEC Forum.* 2004;16:95–112.
16. Janis, IL. *Victims of Groupthink.* Boston: Houghton Mifflin; 1972.
17. Forde R, Pedersen, Akre A. Clinicians' evaluation of clinical ethics consultations in Norway: a qualitative study. *Med Health Care Philos.* 2008;11:17–25.
18. American Academy of Pediatrics, Committee on Bioethics. Guidelines on forgoing life-sustaining medical treatment. *Pediatrics.* 1994;93:532–536.
19. Shelton W, Bjarnadottir D. Ethics consultation and the committee. In: Hester DM, ed. *Ethics by Committee.* Lanham, Md: Rowman & Littlefield; 2008:49–78.
20. Beauchamp TL, Childress JF. *Principles of Biomedical Ethics.* 5th ed. Oxford: Oxford University Press; 2001.
21. Lo, B. Behind closed doors: promises and pitfalls of ethics committees. *N Engl J Med.* 1987;317:46–50.
22. Craig JM, May T. Evaluating the outcomes of ethics consultation. *J Clin Ethics.* 2006;17:168–180.
23. Williamson L. Empirical assessments of clinical ethics services: implications for clinical ethics committees. *Clin Ethics.* 2007;2:187–192.
24. Schneiderman LJ, Gilmer T, Teetzel HD. Impact of ethics consultations in the intensive care setting: a randomized, controlled trial. *Crit Care Med.* 2000;28:3920–3924.
25. Schneiderman LJ, Gilmer T, Teetzel HD, et al. Effect of ethics consultations on nonbeneficial life-sustaining treatments in the intensive care setting. *JAMA.* 2003;290:1166–1172.
26. American Academy of Pediatrics Policy Web site. Available at: http://aappolicy.aappublications.org/. Accessed October 23, 2008.
27. Mercurio MR, Adam MB, Forman EN, Ladd RF, Ross LF, Silber TJ. American Academy of Pediatrics policy statements on bioethics: summaries and commentaries, part 1. *Pediatr Rev.* 2008;29(January):e1–e8.
28. Mercurio, MR, Maxwell MA, Mears BJ, Ross LF, Silber TJ. American Academy of Pediatrics policy statements on bioethics: summaries and commentaries, part 2. *Pediatr Rev.* 2008;29(March):e15–e22.
29. Mercurio MR, Forman EN, Ladd RE, Maxwell MA, Ross LF, Silber TJ. American Academy of Pediatrics policy statements on bioethics: summaries and commentaries, part 3. *Pediatr Rev.* 2008;29(May):e28–e34.
30. Pediatrics Ethics Consortium Web site. Available at: http://www.pediatricethics.org/. Accessed October 23, 2008.

B

GENETICS AND THE NEWBORN

8

Newborn Screening

Lainie Friedman Ross

INTRODUCTION

Today, newborn screening is a rite of passage. The practice began in the United States in 1957 when California initiated screening for phenylketonuria (PKU) by testing urine in infants' diapers for phenylpyruvic acid.[1] Objections to urine sample collection were raised by both parents and physicians, and testing was not routinely performed. In the 1960s, the ability to measure phenylalanine from blood spots collected on filter paper (Guthrie cards) made large-scale newborn screening possible. In 2008, that small amount of dried blood was collected from virtually every infant born in the United States and tested for a number of conditions. But there is wide state variability in (1) the number of conditions; (2) how testing is done (different methodologies and different cutoff points leading to different rates of false positives and false negatives); (3) when testing is done (before discharge and whether a second screen is offered or mandated); (4) what follow-up screening services are offered by the states (many of the conditions require special formulas that are expensive; only some are state-subsidized); and (5) whether the cards are stored and are made accessible to researchers.

A major technological revolution in newborn screening is the use of tandem mass spectrometry (MS/MS). Mass spectrometry was developed more than 100 years ago, but the use of mass spectrometers in series (tandem) was not applied to newborn screening until the 1990s.[2] MS/MS allows newborns to be screened for a large number of inherited metabolic conditions simultaneously at an incrementally small price for each additional condition included.[3] Whereas the number of conditions in state newborn screening (NBS) panels in the 1980s varied from 3 to 10, today

Dr. Ross's research on newborn screening was funded by an R01 grant from the National Institute of Child Health and Human Development, "Newborn Genetic Screening: For Whose Benefit?"

the distribution ranges from 4 to more than 40. However, not all of the conditions identified by MS/MS are well understood or have available treatments, 2 of 10 criteria enumerated in the World Health Organization (WHO) guidelines to justify population screening.[4] Some supporters of expanded NBS argue that the multiplex platform provided by MS/MS makes some of the WHO criteria obsolete,[5,6] but no consensus exists nationally or internationally.

Despite calls for a rational evidence-based approach to expanding NBS,[7,8] the main variability in state NBS panels is political. Parent advocacy groups were integral to passage of the PKU legislation in the 1960s and 1970s, and in the expansion of NBS to include MS/MS in the 1990s and 2000s.[9] Parent advocacy groups also deserve significant credit for the passage of the Newborn Screening Saves Lives legislation passed in April 2008. Other political factors that have been important in influencing the number of conditions on the state NBS panels are (1) the fact that each states has unique NBS legislation that can either facilitate or discourage additions and eliminations; (2) differences in state funding of public health departments; and (3) the priority given to NBS programs within each public health department.

The expansion of NBS is tempting. It is tempting because the newborn period is the most efficient time to screen an entire cohort of individuals; tempting because newborns are already tested for a variety of conditions and so additional testing using the same Guthrie card samples can be incorporated easily into standard practice; tempting because we can study these children longitudinally and learn the natural history of these conditions, their prevalence, and what factors either exacerbate or minimize their expression; and tempting because we can, period.

And yet there are reasons to "proceed with caution."[10] We do not know much about how families will react to abnormal genetic screens, even if follow-up studies are normal or if the condition is mild.[11] We do not know much about how these children, once labeled, will be treated by outside institutions, including insurers, schools, and future employers. Given the familial implications of genetic tests, we must understand their impact on the extended family that may be labeled by blood ties. Often, we will not know whether the therapies we offer are necessary or effective, in part because we do not know how many children with these conditions would have remained asymptomatic or done well regardless – particularly for conditions that do not express themselves in the newborn period.[12]

I began this chapter with a short discussion of the controversies surrounding the passage of mandatory PKU screening. Whereas PKU represents the paradigmatic case of a public health program in which early screening prevents serious morbidity and mortality, there is great interest in expanding NBS beyond the public health emergency paradigm. The paradigm shift from public health emergency to public health service[13] would allow for the inclusion of conditions for which there is no known effective therapy and for the inclusion of conditions that present later in childhood. I will use the case of NBS for Duchenne muscular dystrophy as a case study. I will then examine one of the unintended consequences of NBS: the identification of carriers. Most conditions included in traditional NBS panels are autosomal-recessive (an abnormal gene must be inherited from both parents), but some of our screening tests identify those who are "carriers" (they have only one abnormal gene), and sometimes carriers are identified during confirmatory testing. Next, I will consider how public health programs must consider the potential disparities created by different screening methodologies. I will subsequently discuss issues about the storage of Guthrie cards and their use for research. Finally, I will examine the issue of informed consent for NBS and how this may be affected by whether the appropriate paradigm for NBS is a public health emergency or a public health service, whether screening identifies and discloses genetic carrier information, and whether samples can be used for nonclinical purposes.

Although the focus of this chapter is newborn genetic screening, NBS is not limited to genetic conditions. Testing newborns for hypothyroidism is universal in the United States and has successfully prevented significant morbidity.[14] There is also widespread support for newborn hearing screening using audiometric tests that identify both genetic and nongenetic causes of deafness,[15] and there is limited but growing support for NBS for infectious diseases.[16–18]

PKU: THE PARADIGMATIC PUBLIC HEALTH EMERGENCY PROGRAM

Phyenylketonuria is an autosomal-recessive enzyme deficiency that leads to the accumulation of phenylalanine and causes several forms of mental retardation and seizures. The development of universal screening for PKU is a story of successful advocacy.[19] By 1961, Guthrie had developed both the bacterial inhibition assay to detect excess phenylalanine and the filter paper on which to collect blood samples to make large-scale testing feasible. To expedite the adoption of PKU screening universally, the National Association of Retarded Children (NARC, now known as the Association of Retarded Citizens, or ARC) encouraged Guthrie to circumvent the usual channels of peer review and to publish his methods as a letter to the editor[20] rather than as a journal article. The journal article would appear two years later;[21] meanwhile, Guthrie and the NARC lobbied for mandatory state screening, despite opposition from the Institute of Medicine and the American Academy of Pediatrics, which argued that not enough was known about the natural history of the disease and the efficacy of screening.[7,22]

Guthrie and the NARC won. In 1963, Massachusetts adopted a mandatory screening program, and by 1967, 37 states had passed PKU screening laws.[9] These laws were passed even though a collaborative project to study the effects of dietary restriction on the physical, cognitive, and psychosocial development of affected children did not begin until 1967.[23] The studies would show that there were children with elevated levels of phenylalanine who would not respond to a phenylalanine-restricted diet and that there were some benign causes of elevated levels of phenylalanine that did not require treatment.[7,24] The result was that some healthy children were placed on diets that led to iatrogenic retardation, and in some cases the treatment itself caused severe malnutrition and death.[24] Today, much more is known, but there are still many unknowns.[25] All states test for PKU, although various methods are used with various degrees of sensitivity and specificity. The diagnosis and treatment of a child with PKU prevents severe mental retardation and allows a child to live a healthy life. However, the treatment is a strict diet, and this may cause serious familial tension, particularly if there are other children in the family who do not have PKU and need to be on a less restrictive diet. While virtually everyone would agree that the benefits of preventing mental retardation outweigh the costs and harm of doing so, these should not be trivialized.[26] As the historian Diane Paul explains, "The ultimate success of screening for PKU has sometimes obscured the fact that these were reasonable concerns reflecting what in some cases turned out to be very real problems."[19]

CASE STUDY: NBS FOR DUCHENNE MUSCULAR DYSTROPHY

Duchenne muscular dystrophy (DMD) is an X-linked condition, a progressive untreatable neuromuscular condition that presents in boys around 4–6 years of age and leads to serious disability and death in young adulthood. One potential benefit of early diagnosis is that family planning decisions – both logistical (e.g., the need to have a house without stairs) and reproductive – can be made. Early diagnosis also prevents diagnostic delays,[27,28] but this benefit could accrue even if screening occurred later in infancy. One reason to delay screening until later in infancy is to avoid the confusion created by bundling conditions that meet the traditional WHO guidelines for population screening and have a high medical benefit–risk ratio versus those conditions for which it is reasonable for parents to elect not to test because the benefit–risk ratio is more dependent on personal assessment of psychosocial risks and benefits. A second reason to delay screening is to avoid labeling an asymptomatic newborn with a lethal genetic condition because of the potential to interfere with parent–child bonding and child rearing.[8,29,30]

Many of the psychosocial implications of NBS for DMD come from data from Wales. The screening test for DMD measures creatinine phosphokinase

(CPK), a chemical normally found in muscle fibers, which is elevated in children with muscular dystrophy. Confirmatory testing usually involves a muscle biopsy to distinguish different types of muscular dystrophies. In Wales, more than 94% of parents consent to have their sons screened, and most of the families are quite positive about the program.[31] Still, one wonders whether a 94% uptake is too high. Consider that in Germany, where screening is offered in the offices of the primary care provider for a small fee, the uptake is 5%.[32]

One of the principal investigators in Wales concerned about the high uptake suggested requiring more active parental involvement (e.g., requiring parents to mail the blood spot for the DMD screening): "To suggest that a lower uptake rate for a screening test would be preferable, that we should set a threshold of motivation so that infants are not screened unless their parents actively choose it, is certainly unusual but is perfectly appropriate in the context of an untreatable disease."[33] In a pilot project in the United Kingdom, parents were required to mail the blood spot, and the result was that consent decreased to 78%.[33]

Interestingly, the program in Wales screens only boys. While it is true that most girls who carry the abnormal dystrophin gene are asymptomatic carriers, this is not always so. There are cases, albeit rarely, of affected girls.[34,35] It is also true that being a carrier is not as benign a situation as we have traditionally believed it to be. Twenty percent of female carriers of an abnormal dystrophin gene develop cardiomyopathies in young adulthood.[36] In addition, if a benefit of NBS is to provide reproductive knowledge to parents, then diagnosing carrier girls would be quite informative to parents who otherwise may be unaware until an affected son is born. From a cost–benefit analysis, it may also make sense to screen all infants, because otherwise one must consider the cost of separating the blood spots by gender. Early programs in France and Germany screened girls and boys, as did a supplemental DMD screening program provided by NeoGen (now Pediatrix) in some hospitals in Pennsylvania, Puerto Rico, Texas, and New York.[32]

In 2005, the Centers for Disease Control and Prevention (CDC) in the United States funded two pilot programs for DMD screening of boys – one in the newborn period (Ohio) and one later in infancy (Georgia). The pilot programs were feasibility studies in measuring CPK and in procuring consent. As in Wales, uptake in Ohio exceeded 90%, although follow-up on the few positive families has not been reported.[37] Uptake in Georgia was much lower[37] and similar to that in Germany. The main practical obstacle to screening at a later date is the need for a second blood collection. Uptake may also be lower because parents have more time to think about the risks and benefits of diagnosing an asymptomatic child. In focus groups in Illinois in which parents were asked to think about whether they would want to be offered NBS for DMD, the participants were evenly divided about whether they would want to have this information.[38] Parents expressed concerns about its impact on child rearing and their preference to wait until the child had symptoms. Those who supported testing spoke about planning and about activities that they would do with their child at a younger age. No one expressed concern about being unable to care for a child with a positive screen.[38]

How the CDC pilot studies will inform future policies is unknown. However, the studies show that the issue of whether to screen is only the first question. If it is answered affirmatively, the debate must include the question of when to screen. Given that no therapies are needed presymptomatically, some have argued for screening later in infancy. The advantage of this is that it avoids labeling affected children during the vulnerable newborn period, and the disadvantage is that the infrastructure exists for NBS but not for population screening at a later point in childhood. It is also the case that, in affected boys, the CPK level is abnormal in both the newborn period and later in infancy. Carrier girls frequently have an abnormal CPK level at birth, but this often reverts to the normal range later in infancy. Thus, the debate about timing cannot be solved independent of the debate about whether to screen only boys or both boys and girls. If one wants to identify female carriers using CPK, one needs to screen in the newborn period.

CASE STUDY: THE IDENTIFICATION OF SICKLE CELL TRAIT AND CYSTIC FIBROSIS CARRIERS

Although the issue of carrier identification in X-linked conditions like DMD is a gendered issue, most conditions included in the NBS programs are autosomal-recessive, and the detection of carriers affects boys and girls equally, although its meaning may differ by gender.

The identification of carriers in NBS programs has been a concern since 1973, when Norm Fost and Michael Kaback wrote an article for the journal *Pediatrics* entitled "Why Do Sickle Screening in Children? The Trait Is the Issue."[39] Sickle cell disease (SCD) is an autosomal-recessive condition characterized by anemia, pain crises, increased risk of infections in young children, and increased risk of stroke. The article criticized sickle cell screening programs of school-age children because they used sickle cell screening as a primary screening tool. The authors argued that hematological screening of children should focus on identifying children with anemia and that only children with anemia should undergo sickle cell testing. The reason for this two-tiered approach was twofold. First was the concern that there would be confusion about SCD and sickle cell carriers (known as sickle cell trait), as was common at the time the article was written.[7,22] Second was the concern that there was no need to identify children with sickle trait because that was reproductive information for adults. Thus, if we tested only those with anemia, we could identify those with SCD who might benefit from diagnosis and would reduce the number of sickle cell carriers identified in childhood.

With the discovery in 1986 that penicillin prophylaxis could prevent serious morbidity and even mortality in infants and young children with SCD,[40] there was a rapid increase in support for NBS for sickle cell disease and other hemoglobinopathies. The problem of identifying sickle cell carriers in NBS programs was accepted as a foreseen but unintended consequence. However, what to do with the information was not at all settled. An entire issue of *Pediatrics,* in May 1989, discussed NBS for SCD.[41] Different attitudes were expressed about what to do with the identification of carriers. Some public health programs reported the information to the parents as the fiduciaries of their children, other programs reported the results to the physicians to ensure that the information was given with appropriate counseling, and others decided not to disclose the information on the grounds that it was "incidental."[41] National recommendations in favor of routine disclosure to parents would not be developed until 1994.[8]

The issue of carrier identification of newborns for autosomal-recessive conditions reemerged in the United States in the early 1990s following the 1989 cloning of the cystic fibrosis gene. Cystic fibrosis (CF) is an autosomal-recessive condition characterized by pulmonary and gastrointestinal problems. At the time of the gene's discovery, NBS for CF was being piloted in a few states by measuring immunoreactive trypsinogen (IRT),[42,43] but this method required two samples followed by confirmatory sweat testing. With the identification of the $\Delta F508$ mutation, a two-tiered screening IRT/DNA protocol was developed.[44] Samples were tested for elevated levels of IRT, and those with levels above a certain threshold were then tested for the $\Delta F508$ mutation to reduce the number of children who had to undergo confirmatory sweat testing. Today, more than 1,300 CF mutations have been identified, and different NBS programs include different mutations and different numbers of mutations in their panel. The more mutations that are included, the larger is the number of carriers identified. However, none of the programs seeks to maximize the identification of carriers, which could be done by screening for mutations as a first-tier screening protocol. That is, carrier identification and reproductive knowledge are "incidental" and not primary to the screening activity.

When the Wisconsin study changed from IRT/IRT to IRT/DNA, the researchers revised their protocol to include genetic counseling for parents whose children were diagnosed as carriers but had a negative sweat test.[44] Today, the practice of reporting carrier results discovered incidentally in NBS is standard and is supported by professional guidelines.[8,30,45]

THE IMPACT OF METHODOLOGY ON NBS PUBLIC
HEALTH PROGRAMS

The goals of public health programs are to reduce disease, premature
death, and disability in human populations. The emphasis is at the population level, and in this regard, the concept of social justice is integral to its
structure and function.[46] Consider, then, how the different methodologies
for NBS for CF affect different ethnic communities.[47]

Consider first the IRT/IRT method. On average, African American children have higher IRT levels than do Caucasian children, even though they
have a much lower risk for CF.[48] Using an IRT/IRT methodology means
that false positives, which create anxiety and misunderstanding,[49] will be
more common in African Americans. Methods that include genetic testing
(IRT/DNA) can be done using a single sample; however, these methods
raise questions about the appropriate number of mutations to include in
the genetic test. The answer depends in part on the heterogeneity of the
population. The most common CF mutation is ΔF508. It is found in 72%
of the U.S. non-Hispanic Caucasian CF population, but in much lower
percentages of patients with CF of other ethnicities (Hispanic Caucasian,
54%; African American, 44%; Asian American, 39%; Ashekenazi Jewish,
31%).[50] In 2001, the American College of Medical Genetics Cystic Fibrosis
Carrier Screening Working Group recommended a panel of 25 mutations,
which would account for more than 80% of CF alleles in the pan-ethnic
U.S. population with CF.[51] This panel was updated in 2004 on the basis of a
larger, more pan-ethnic CF database that now finds 6 additional mutations
with a frequency of greater than 0.10% and another 14 that occurred at
slightly lower frequency (0.09–0.01%) but would be useful for specific ethnic minority communities.[50] Adding mutations will improve sensitivity but
decrease specificity. And yet fewer mutations in a screening panel may lead
to an increased number of false negative newborn screens in minorities.

The selection of mutation panels, then, is not a simple medical decision. The IRT/IRT methodology will identify more African Americans
as false positives, but the IRT/DNA method will yield a disproportionate
number of false negatives in minorities. False negatives in minorities may
be of greater concern for a condition like CF, which has historically been
perceived as a "white child's illness." The frequency of CF is much higher
in non-Hispanic Caucasians than in any other ethnic community. The
decreased frequency of CF in ethnic communities means that the diagnosis of CF may be delayed in these individuals both when no screening program exists[52] and when an infant screens negative,[53] because physicians
may seek other diagnoses to explain the clinical symptoms. A concern,
then, is that screening will lead to complacency in physicians who will
not work up a child with failure to thrive for CF because that diagnosis
was "ruled out" in the newborn screen. If the introduction of a screening

program leads to a delay in diagnosis mainly for minority children, the methodology may cause more disproportionate harm than realized. Thus, in the United States, justice concerns may lead one to support the use of the IRT/IRT method despite the fact that (1) the frequency of the disease is lower in minority communities, and (2) the need for two samples is more cumbersome.[47]

RESEARCH USING GUTHRIE CARDS

Approximately 4 million Guthrie cards are collected annually in the United States, which could lead to the world's largest biobank. Biobanks are repositories of stored tissue or blood samples. Their research potential could be incalculable, particularly if the samples are linked to medical records and information about environmental exposures, dietary habits, and other factors that influence health. The National Children's Study is one such effort and plans to enroll more than 100,000 children across the United States, following them from before birth until age 21.

Currently all states store Guthrie cards for a period of time; some states do so indefinitely,[54] despite questions regarding the cards' stability (and therefore utility) over time.[54,55] If stored properly, Guthrie cards could serve as a national biobank![56] But the use of these cards for research raises serious ethical questions. Consent is a major concern, particularly with respect to the use of NBS samples, which were almost always procured without consent. Ideally, samples stored today could be reused for years to come, for research that is not yet even imagined, but this raises many ethical issues, including how one consents to such research participation and how a surrogate consents to such research. While a competent adult may choose to "sign a blank check" and permit research on his or her samples for any and all purposes for an indefinite period of time, it is not so clear that a surrogate has such wide discretion. It is not clear that a surrogate can or should authorize his or her proxy's participation when the researchers cannot describe the goals or the methods of the research. It also raises the question of whether and how to address the issue of re-consent when the minor becomes an adult. What if the individual cannot be located? What if the individual has died?

THE ROLE OF CONSENT IN NEWBORN SCREENING

Let us examine the practice of performing NBS without informed consent. In 48 of the 50 states, NBS is mandatory. The major benefit of mandatory screening is that it ensures that all children are screened so that those who are affected (true positives) can be treated quickly and accurately and those who do not have the disease (true negatives) can be reassured. The main arguments against requiring parental consent for NBS are that the process is time-consuming and that, even when consent is sought, the consent is perfunctory and not informed.[57] That consent is perfunctory does not argue against the need for consent, but rather is a criticism of the professionals who are not fulfilling their role in the consent process.[58] Another argument against consent is that it is unnecessary because to refuse such clearly beneficial tests would constitute neglect. And in fact the Nebraska Supreme Court has removed children from parental custody in order to perform NBS on a child whose parents refused NBS.[59] In contrast, most states have religious and some even have philosophical exemptions that permit parents to refuse screening.[45]

The main argument in support of the practice of seeking parental consent for NBS is that consent is the hallmark of all patient–physician interactions. When the patient cannot consent for him- or herself, a surrogate is chosen. When the patient is a child, the parents are presumed to be the surrogate. Thus, seeking parental consent is consistent with the authority and responsibility accorded to parents in all other aspects of their children's health care.[60]

There are several reasons for taking parental consent seriously. First, informed consent is a basic principle of all medical care. Consent serves as a symbol of respect for the patient and family, which is important given that families are the primary source of child rearing and given that families, and not the state, will bear the greatest costs if an affected child is not screened and diagnosis is delayed.[58]

Second, procuring parental consent serves a valuable educational role. If consent is meaningful, it must be informed, which requires education – about both the purpose and the limitations of screening. This education may increase the likelihood that parents will follow up on abnormal screening results. Knowledge of negative test results also may be reassuring to parents, particularly those with personal knowledge of the conditions being tested.[58]

Third, as we move from NBS as a public health emergency to NBS as a public health service that includes conditions that do not meet the WHO criteria for a public health screening program, the justification for mandatory screening become less compelling.

Fourth, the need for consent is further supported by the identification and disclosure of carrier status of newborns. The usual practice of genetic testing involves a very extensive informed-consent process that includes pre- and post-test counseling. However, when NBS identifies a newborn as a carrier, it also identifies a parent as a carrier despite the fact that the parents did not consent to genetic testing. In fact, often parents are unaware that the testing was being done![61]

Fifth, the potential value of Guthrie cards for research may be a catalyst for reform, as the first principle of research is the essential role of informed consent.[62] Thus, ethical issues related to the evolving scope of clinical care and research in NBS are all converging to make consent reform imperative.

CONCLUSION

Despite its controversial beginnings, newborn screening is now an integral component of public health and pediatric practice. And yet it was and remains the only test that is routinely performed without consent. Although the Institute of Medicine[8] and the American Academy of Pediatrics[45] have guidelines that recommend the practice of seeking parental permission for NBS, few states have heeded these recommendations. With the expansion of NBS to include the identification of carriers, conditions that have a later onset, and conditions that are not treatable, one must acknowledge that there may be families who will not want to know some or all of this information. These and other factors demand a reevaluation and transformation of the current practice of mandatory NBS to require a voluntary informed-consent process that will engage parents in clinical decisions regarding the health and well-being of their children and in research decisions regarding the health of the broader pediatric population.

References

1. Pass KA. Lessons learned from newborn screening for phenylketonuria. In: Khoury MJ, Burke W, Thomson EJ, eds. *Genetics and Public Health in the 21st Century.* New York: Oxford University Press; 2000:385–404.
2. Millington DS, Kodo N, Norwood DL, Roe CR. Tandem mass spectrometry: a new method for acylcarnitine profiling with potential for neonatal screening for inborn errors of metabolism. *J Inherited Metabol Dis.* 1990;13:321–324.
3. Report of a workgroup: using tandem mass spectrometry for metabolic disease screening among newborns. *MMWR: Morbidity and Mortality Weekly Report.* 2001;50(RR03):1–22.
4. Wilson JM, Jungner G. Principles and practice of screening for disease. Geneva: World Health Organization; 1968. Public Health Papers, No. 34.
5. Pollitt RJ. Principles and performance: assessing the evidence. *Acta Paediatr Suppl.* 1989;432:110–114.
6. Alexander D, van Dyck PC. A vision of the future of newborn screening. *Pediatrics.* 2006;117(5 Pt. 2):S350–S354.
7. National Research Council, Committee for the Study of Inborn Errors of Metabolism. *Genetic Screening: Programs, Principles, and Research.* Washington, DC: National Academy of Sciences; 1975.
8. Andrews L, Fullarton J, Holtzman N, Motulsky G, eds. for the Institute of Medicine. *Assessing Genetic Risks: Implications for Health and Social Policy.* Washington, DC: National Academy Press; 1994.
9. Paul DB. Patient advocacy in newborn screening: continuities and discontinuities. *Am J Med Genet. Part C.* 2008;148C:8–14.

10. Holtzman NA. *Proceed with Caution.* Baltimore: Johns Hopkins University Press; 1989.

11. Green JM, Hewison J, Bekker HL, Bryant LD, Cuckle HS. Psychosocial aspects of genetic screening of pregnant women and newborns: a systematic review. *Health Technol Assess.* 2004;8(33).

12. Wilcken B, Wiley V, Hammond J, Carpenter K. Screening newborns for inborn errors of metabolism by tandem mass spectrometry. *N Engl J Med.* 2003;348:2304–2312.

13. Grosse SD, Boyle CA, Kenneson A, Khoury MJ, Wilfond BS. From public health emergency to public health service: the implications of evolving criteria for newborn screening panels. *Pediatrics.* 2006;117:923–929.

14. Hunter MK, Mandel SH, Sesser DE, et al. Follow-up of newborns with low thyroxine and nonelevated thyroid-stimulating hormone-screening concentrations: results of the 20-year experience in the Northwest Regional Newborn Screening Program. *J Pediatr.* 1998;132:70–74.

15. Davis A, Bamford J, Wilson I, Rankalawan T, Forshaw M, Wright S. A critical review of the role of neonatal hearing screening in the detection of congenital hearing impairment. *Health Technol Assess.* 1997;1(10).

16. Cameron T. Mandatory HIV testing of newborns in New York State: what are the implications? *J Health Social Pol.* 2002;14(3):59–78.

17. Anonymous. Connecticut will test newborns if mother isn't tested first. *AIDS Policy & Law.* 1999;14(13):7.

18. Hsu HW, Grady GF, Maguire JH, Weiblen BJ, Hoff R. Newborn screening for congenital toxoplasmosis infection: five years experience in Massachusetts USA. *Scand J Infect Dis. Suppl.* 1992;84:59–64.

19. Paul DB. The history of newborn phenylketonuria screening in the U.S. In: Holtzman NA, Watson MS, eds. *Promoting Safe and Effective Genetic Testing in the United States: Final Report of the Task Force on Genetic Testing.* Baltimore: Johns Hopkins University Press; 1998:137–160.

20. Guthrie R. Blood screening for phenylketonuria. *JAMA.* 1961;178:863.

21. Guthrie R, Susi A. A simple phenylalanine method for detecting phenylketonuria in large populations of newborn infants. *Pediatrics.* 1963;32: 338–343.

22. Reilly P. *Genetics, Law and Social Policy.* Cambridge, Mass: Harvard University Press; 1977.

23. American Academy of Pediatrics, Committee on Genetics. New issues in newborn screening for phenylketonuria and congenital hypothyroidism. *Pediatrics.* 1982;69:104106.

24. Holtzman N. Dietary treatment of inborn errors of metabolism. *Annu Rev Med.* 1970;21:335–356.

25. National Institutes of Health Consensus Development Panel. National Institutes of Health Consensus Development Conference Statement: Phenylketonuria: Screening and Management, October 16–18, 2000. *Pediatrics.* 2001;108:972–982.

26. Unger I, Awiszus D. Coping with PKU: results of narrative interviews with parents. *Eur J Pediatr.* 1990;149(Suppl. 1):S45–S51.

27. Bushby KMD, Hill A, Steele JG. Failure of early diagnosis in symptomatic Duchenne muscular dystrophy. *Lancet.* 1999;353:557–558.

28. Mohamed K, Appleton R, Nicolaides P. Delayed diagnosis of Duchenne muscular dystrophy. *Eur J Paediatr Neurol.* 2000;4;219–223.
29. Clayton EW. Issues in state newborn screening programs. *Pediatrics.* 1992; 90:641–646.
30. American Society of Human Genetics/American College of Medical Genetics. Points to consider: ethical, legal, and psychosocial implications of genetic testing in children and adolescents. *Am J Hum Genet.* 1995;57:1233–1241.
31. Bradley DM, Parsons EP, Clarke AJ. Experience with screening newborns for Duchenne muscular dystrophy in Wales. *BMJ.* 1993;306:357–360.
32. Conference: Newborn Screening for Duchenne Muscular Dystrophy. Sponsored by the Centers for Disease Control and Prevention, Atlanta; March 12, 2004.
33. Clarke AJ. Newborn screening. In: Harper PS, Clarke AJ, eds. *Genetics, Society and Clinical Practice.* Oxford: Bios Scientific; 1997:107–117.
34. Lesca G, Demarquay G, Llense S, et al. Symptomatic carriers of dystrophinopathy with chromosome X inactivation bias [in French]. *Rev Neurol.* 2003;159(8–9):775–780.
35. Tachi N, Sasaki K, Yamada T, Imamura S, Mike T. Mosaic pattern of dystrophins in Duchenne muscular dystrophy. *Pediatr Neurol.* 1990;6(1):54–56.
36. Grain L, Cortina-Borja C, Hilton-Jones D, Hopkin J, Burch M. Cardiac abnormalities and skeletal muscle weakness in carriers of Duchenne and Becker muscular dystrophies and controls. *Neuromuscular Disorders.* 2001; 11:186–191.
37. Conference: Screening for Duchenne Muscular Dystrophy: What's the Best Age? American College of Medical Genetics 15th Annual Meeting. Phoenix, Ariz; March 13, 2008.
38. Campbell E, Ross LF. Parental attitudes regarding newborn screening of PKU and DMD. *Am J Med Genet.* 2003;120A:209–214.
39. Fost N, Kaback MM. Why do sickle cell screening in children? The trait is the issue. *Pediatrics.* 1973;51:742.
40. Gaston MH, Verter JI, Woods G, et al. Prophylaxis with oral penicillin in children with sickle cell anemia: A randomized trial. *N Engl J Med.* 1986; 314(25):1593–1599.
41. Newborn screening for sickle cell disease and other hemoglobinopathies. *Pediatrics.* 1989;83:813–914.
42. Anonymous. Newborn screening for cystic fibrosis. Proceedings from the Fourth International Conference, Denver; October 8–9, 1990. *Pediatr Pulmonol Suppl.* 1991;7:1–92.
43. Farrell PM, Mischler EH. Newborn screening for cystic fibrosis: the Cystic Fibrosis Neonatal Screening Study Group. *Advan Pediatr.* 1992;39:35–70.
44. Farrell PM, Aronson RA, Hoffman G, Laessig RH. Newborn screening for cystic fibrosis in Wisconsin: first application of population-based molecular genetics testing. *Wis Med J.* 1994;93(8):415–421.
45. American Academy of Pediatrics, Committee on Bioethics. Ethical issues with genetic testing in pediatrics. *Pediatrics.* 2001;107:1451–1455.
46. Dabrock P. Public health genetics and social justice. *Commun Genet.* 2006;9:34–39.
47. Ross LF. Newborn screening for cystic fibrosis: a lesson in public health disparities. *J Pediatr.* 2008;153:308–313.

48. Rock MJ, Mischler EH, Farrell PM, Bruns WT, Hassemer DJ, Laessig RH. Immunoreactive trypsinogen screening for cystic fibrosis: characterization of infants with a false-positive screening test. *Pediatr Pulmonol.* 1989;6:42–48.
49. Baroni MA, Anderson YE, Mischler E. Cystic fibrosis newborn screening: impact of early screening results on parenting stress. *Pediatr Nurs.* 1997;23:143–151.
50. Watson MS, Cutting GR, Desnick RJ, et al. Cystic fibrosis population carrier screening: 2004 revision of American College of Medical Genetics mutation panel. *Genet Med.* 2004;6:387–391.
51. Grody WW, Cutting GR, Klinger KW, Richards CS, Watson MS, Desnick RJ. Laboratory standards and guidelines for population-based cystic fibrosis carrier screening. *Genet Med.* 2001;3:149–154.
52. Spencer DA, Venkataraman M, Weller PH. Delayed diagnosis of cystic fibrosis in children from ethnic minorities. *Lancet.* 1998;342:238.
53. Wagener JS, Sontag MK, Sagel SD, Accurso FJ. Update on newborn screening for cystic fibrosis. *Current Opinion in Pulmonary Medicine.* 2004;10:500–504.
54. Clayton EW, Steinberg KK, Khoury MJ, et al. Informed consent for genetic research on stored tissue samples. *JAMA.* 1995;274:1786–1792.
55. American College of Medical Genetics, Storage of Genetics Materials Committee. ACMG statement on storage and use of genetic materials. *Am J Hum Genet.* 1995;57:1499–1500.
56. McEwen JE, Reilly PR. Stored Guthrie cards as DNA "banks." *Am J Hum Genet.* 1994;55:196–200.
57. Statham H, Green J, Snowdon C. Mother's consent to screening newborn babies for disease. *BMJ.* 1993;306:858–859.
58. Ross LF, Fost N. Ethical issues in pediatric genetics. In: Miller SM, McDaniel SH, Rolland JS, Feetham SL, eds. *Individuals, Families, and the New Era of Genetics.* New York: WW Norton; 2006:486–505.
59. *Douglas County v. Anaya No. S-03-1446*, SUPREME COURT OF NEBRASKA, 269 Neb. 552; 694 N.W.2d 601; 2005 Neb. LEXIS 61, March 25, 2005, Filed, US Supreme Court certiorari denied 546 U.S. 826; 126 S. Ct. 365; 163 L. Ed. 2d 71; 2005 U.S. LEXIS 6097; 74 U.S.L.W. 3202, October 3, 2005.
60. Ross LF. *Children, Families, and Health Care Decision Making.* Oxford: Oxford University Press; 1998.
61. Campbell E, Ross LF. Incorporating newborn screening into prenatal care. *Am J Obstet Gynecol.* 2004;190(4):876–877.
62. Nuremberg Code. See *Trials of War Criminals Before the Nuremberg Military Tribunals under Control Council Law*, No. 10, Vol. II. Washington, DC: US Government Printing Office; 1948.

9

Presymptomatic Genetic Testing in Children

Kimberly A. Quaid

Isn't ignorance the same as hope?

Jean Barema, *The Test*[1]

As the fruits of the Human Genome Project transition into clinical care, the number of genetic conditions that medical professionals can test for is increasing rapidly. DNA-based tests are being developed to diagnose genetic disease, to determine predisposition to genetically based disorders, and to identify carrier status. Genetic testing may offer considerable benefit, but it is not without some peril. Because our ability to identify those at high risk for genetic conditions far outpaces our ability to treat or cure such conditions, many of those at risk are choosing not to be tested.

The genetic testing of children may have numerous diagnostic and prognostic applications for those who already have symptoms or who may develop them in the future. However, genetic testing in childhood for disorders that do not manifest until adult life is an area of particular sensitivity. Parental requests for the genetic testing of unaffected children and adolescents have raised a number of ethical issues and have led to several statements by professional organizations. The boards of directors of the American Society of Human Genetics (ASHG, 1995), the American College of Medical Genetics[2] (ACMG 1995), the Council on Ethical and Judicial Affairs of the American Medical Association[3] (AMA 1995), and National Society of Genetic Counselors[4] (NSGC 1995) have all published statements on this issue.

The most ethically worrisome situations involve the testing of asymptomatic children for (1) genes for a late-onset disorder when there is no medical benefit to the child in the near future and (2) carrier status for a recessive or X-linked disorder when the information is not immediately useful for the child's reproductive decision making. The aforementioned organizations have all expressed caution regarding the testing of minors in these two situations, especially if the request is made by the parents rather than the child. Authors in both the United States and the United Kingdom have recommended that testing be performed only if there is clear benefit for the minor.[5-7]

A systematic review of the ethical and clinical guidelines and position papers from 1991 to 2005 concerning the presymptomatic and predictive genetic testing of minors led to the conclusion that the main justification for such testing is direct benefit for the minor either through medical intervention or preventive measures. If there are no urgent medical reasons, all guidelines recommend postponing testing until the child can consent to testing as a competent adolescent or as an adult.[8] Borry and his colleagues recently conducted a survey of the practices and attitudes of geneticists in Europe with regard to presymptomatic and predictive genetic testing of minors. In particular, they were interested in whether the clinical geneticists supported the rule of earliest onset, which states that genetic testing "should be permitted no earlier than the first possible onset of the disease."[9] They found that there is strongest support for testing young children when it provides clear medical benefit. Most clinical geneticists were unwilling to perform presymptomatic or predictive tests for adult-onset diseases, unless they would be of medical benefit.[10] To summarize, to date, there has been a nearly universal presumption that immature minor children should not be tested for late-onset disease. Testing of "mature" minors is somewhat less controversial.[11] However, all guidelines recommend a default position whereby even mature minors should not be tested unless there is a strong justification for doing so.

Despite this presumption, requests for the presymptomatic and carrier testing of children are likely to increase. One U.S. survey of genetics service providers indicated that 44% had received requests to test children for adult-onset disorders.[12] A survey of the general public showed that 53% thought that parents should "[b]e able to have their children under the age of 18 tested for a genetic condition that may appear much later in life," even if the condition was "neither preventable nor treatable."[12] One study of the attitudes of pediatric residents indicated that 39% would order testing for Huntington disease (HD) for a 10-year-old at his parents' request.[13] A survey of individuals at risk for HD who had themselves chosen not to be tested indicated that when asked, "Do you believe that a child younger than 18 years of age should be tested at their parents' request?" fully 78.6% replied yes. When asked, "Do you believe that a child younger than 18 years of age should be tested at their own request?" 74% said yes. Interestingly, when asked, "What is the youngest age at which a child at risk should be able to request genetic testing for HD for him- or herself?" the answer was 18.63 years (S.D. = 4.84).[14]

There has been a spate of articles advocating the genetic testing of children for late-onset disease at their parents' request. In 2005, in discussing a case from my own book[15] involving the testing of minors, and citing Lainie

Ross's model of constrained parental autonomy,[16] Sevick and colleagues argued that the family must be empowered to make the best choices given the circumstances of the child and the values of the family.[17] Mary Kay Pelias, a lawyer, argues that the role of parents as decision makers for their minor children has been reinforced by four seminal holdings of the United States Supreme Court. She rejects arguments about protecting the future autonomy of children and argues that parents have a right, perhaps even a duty, to exercise their own vested autonomy in making decisions that they believe are in the best interests of their families.[18] Most recently, Malpas examined two types of psychological harm that are posited to possibly result from testing minors: a limited future and damage to the child's self-esteem. He concluded that parents generally want what is best for their children and are as likely to overindulge children with positive test results as they are to deprive them of opportunities. However, geneticists responding to surveys regarding the genetic testing of minors have reported that parents requested testing of children for HD in order to decide whether or not to save money for the child's education. If the child had the gene, the parents would not "waste" family resources.[19] He further concluded that children in families who are treated with respect, are accepted, and are the recipients of affection and support are less likely to experience damage to their self-esteem "because they are situated in a strongly supportive and caring environment where confidence in their abilities is nurtured."[20]

As genetic testing becomes an integral part of clinical practice, the issue of the genetic testing of minors for late-onset disease is likely to once again be a subject of considerable debate. In this chapter, I will examine the arguments for and against predictive genetic testing of minors for late-onset disease for which there is no treatment or cure and will draw my conclusions on the basis of the evidence that we have to date coupled with my 22 years of experience in providing genetic testing for HD. But first, I will offer a little background.

Huntington disease is the most commonly inherited neurological disorder, with a prevalence ranging from 4.1 to 7.5 cases per 1,000,000 in Caucasians.[21] It is inherited in an autosomal-dominant pattern such that each child of a parent affected with the disorder has a 50% chance of inheriting the HD mutation. Penetrance is close to 100%, and most people who inherit the mutation that causes HD begin to show the classic symptoms of the disease in their late 30s or early 40s. These symptoms include abnormal involuntary movements, accompanied by intellectual impairment and a variety of psychiatric disturbances, most commonly depression.[22] Death normally occurs 10–17 years after onset.[23] There is no treatment and no cure.

In 1983, HD became the first disease to be mapped to a previously unknown location on chromosome 4 through the use of restriction enzymes, which cleave DNA at sequence-specific sites.[24] Inherited variations of these DNA sequences, also known as restriction fragment-length polymorphisms, or RFLPs, can be used as genetic markers to map diseases on chromosomes as well as to trace the inheritance of disease within families. The discovery of polymorphic markers linked to HD was a significant advance in HD research. Not only did it provide a possible clue to finding the gene and to understanding the mechanism by which the gene caused brain cells to die, it also meant that presymptomatic or predictive testing for those at risk was possible. In 1993, the discovery of an expanded CAG trinucleotide repeat as the underlying mutation that causes HD led to the availability of direct predictive testing.[25] CAG repeats greater than or equal to 40 are indicative of HD and can either confirm a diagnosis of HD in a symptomatic individual or confer increased risk with a virtually 100% chance of those who are asymptomatic developing symptoms at some point in time. While direct gene testing made testing cheaper, faster, and less complicated, it did not change the underlying psychological effects of testing.

In light of the initial discovery of linked markers, and in concert with HD patients and families, Milton Wexler, head of the Hereditary Disease Foundation, convened a meeting of geneticists, genetic counselors, bioethicists, and other health care professionals to establish guidelines for offering genetic testing for HD. The guiding principle at the time was "First do no harm." This was necessary for several reasons. First, there was no treatment or cure for HD; therefore, there was no medical benefit to be derived from testing. Second, the suicide rate for those with or at risk for HD was four times the national average, suggesting that this was a vulnerable population for which this information could potentially be devastating.[26] Third, this type of predictive testing had not been possible before, and a cautious approach was deemed appropriate. The workshop, convened in 1985, developed preliminary guidelines for testing protocols, including a neurological examination before testing, psychiatric screening, extensive pre-test counseling, and post-test follow-up.

Also in 1985, a committee of representatives of the International Huntington Association (IHA) and the World Federation of Neurology (WFN) Research Group on Huntington's chorea was established specifically to produce recommendations for the use of the predictive test for HD. The IHA–WFN guidelines published in 1990 and in 1994 recommend specifically that children under the age of 18 not be tested.[27,28] In 1989, the Huntington Disease Society of America (HDSA) published *Guidelines for Predictive Testing in Huntington's Disease.*[29] Crafted by a similar group of patients, at-risk family members, scientists, and health care professionals with extensive experience in caring for families with HD, these guidelines included mandatory counseling, the assumption of informed choice about testing on the part of the test taker, and the restriction of testing to those 18 years of age or older, except when a pregnancy was involved.

Most studies on the effects of predictive testing have focused on adults. The majority of evidence to date suggests that non-carriers and carriers differ significantly in terms of short- but not long-term psychological distress. How carriers adjust to the test result tends to depend more on their psychological adjustment before testing than on the test result itself.[30,31] One criticism of several of these studies is that the most distressed carriers were often lost to follow-up,[32] leading to an underestimation of distress following testing. A study of the long-term effects of testing indicate that, while carriers and their partners were more distressed immediately after testing, their outlook improved somewhat in the two- to three-year post-test period. As they approached the expected age of onset, carriers became more pessimistic.[33]

Calls for caution continue to be made. There are indications that both carriers and non-carriers have problems coping with, and adjusting to, their new knowledge of their genetic status.[34-36] In most studies, the effects of genetic testing for HD on psychological health have been assessed mainly in terms of depression and well-being.[32,37,38] When other psychiatric symptoms are assessed, presymptomatic carriers complain more about sadness, low self-esteem, aggressive behavior, and compulsions than do non-carriers.[39] A double-blind longitudinal follow-up study showed increasing irritability and cynical hostility among presymptomatic carriers compared with non-carriers.[40] A study focusing on depression and suicidal ideation found that depression scores and the frequency of suicidal thoughts increased for carriers after testing compared with non-carriers.[41] The study based on the largest sample measured hopelessness and found that differences between carriers and non-carriers may persist in the long term.[42] This finding is particularly disturbing given that hopelessness has been identified as a predictor of suicide, a particular cause of concern in this population.[43] The point must also be made that the majority of those tested in these studies went through fairly rigorous testing protocols that included neurological exams, psychiatric screening, pretest counseling, and follow-up, a situation unlikely to be the case when a minor is tested.

In addition to the types of harm experienced by adults, children may face other risks. Potential types of harm that might be caused by the genetic testing of a minor for late-onset conditions include the loss of future decision-making capacity and confidentiality; damage to the child's self-esteem; discrimination in education, insurance, or employment; and adverse effects on the child's ability to form future relationships.[44] Some of the potential harm that may occur as a result of testing may affect the entire family. For young children, harm may include changes in the family dynamic, alterations in parent–child bonding, survivor guilt, heightened anxiety and impaired comprehension, and risk for misunderstanding.[45] For the adolescent, harm may include interference with successful resolution of the major psychosocial tasks that must be mastered during adolescence, including seeking freedom from parental figures, establishing a personal identity, handling sexual energies and interpersonal intimacy, and remodeling former idealizations of others and self.[45] Stigmatization and discrimination, especially in employment and insurance, are also possible.[46,47]

The advantages of such testing have been considered to be relief from anxiety about possible early signs, a reduction in family uncertainty about the future, more accurate genetic counseling, more responsible attitudes toward reproduction, alteration of parental expectations, and more practical planning for education, housing, and family finances.[48] Further advantages are that the child has an opportunity to adapt to his or her circumstances and openness is fostered within the family.[49] And yet few of these advantages accrue specifically to the child, while the disadvantages most surely do.

There are three key arguments against predictive testing in young people. These are that (1) testing fails to protect the future autonomy of the young person, (2) testing young people is a breach of confidentiality, and (3) testing may cause psychosocial harm.[7] There is little empirical evidence on the effects of genetic testing of minors for late-onset disease, despite the fact that this debate surfaced soon after the introduction of testing in the late 1980s.[50] Duncan and Delatycki postulate four possible reasons for this state of affairs: (1) such tests are rarely performed, (2) such tests are usually the exception in a clinical setting and therefore are not assessed in the same way that they would be as part of a research study, (3) clinicians involved in the provision of such tests to young people are placed in a potentially vulnerable situation, and (4) there is an absence of a single, leading group to coordinate such research.[51] Given the number of guidelines advocating against such testing, it is also unlikely that any institutional review board would approve of research of this type.

An international survey of clinical geneticists in the United States, Canada, the United Kingdom, Australia, and New Zealand indicated that children had been tested for nonmedical reasons a total of 49 times.[52] The most common condition tested for was Huntington disease, and in 22 (45%) of those cases the young person tested was immature, defined as under the age of 14 years. The most common reason cited for testing was that the parents wanted to know. Results were disclosed to only two immature minors, and in three cases the parents experienced clinically significant anxiety related to how they would pass on the information to their gene-positive child. There were no reports of adverse events with immature young persons tested, but only two were reported as having been informed of the result. In 27 (55%) cases the young person tested was mature. Ten (37%) of the requests for testing were made by the young person alone, and 13 (48%) were made by the young person and his or her parents. Four (15%) requests were made by the parents alone. Results were disclosed to 26 mature minors, and it was reported that two individuals experienced an adverse event. One adverse event following an increased-risk result for HD in a 17-year-old male was described as "[i]nitial depression and rebellion, but eventual acceptance." Another adverse event followed a decreased-risk result for HD in a 17-year-old female described as follows: "[n]o psychological disturbance but worry and responsibility for affected mother and untested brothers." There were nine reports of beneficial effects. Six followed decreased-risk results, with one example given as follows: "Enabled him to focus on school etc. and parents say behavior improved and he deals with difficulties in a more mature way." Three followed increased-risk results, with an example given as follows: "So far she is doing fine and seems to have integrated this information into her thoughts about her future in a healthy way."

A second study presented qualitative interviews with eight young people who had undergone predictive genetic testing for HD.[53] The participants were four males and four females, who ranged in age from 17 to 25 at the time of testing. Two had received a gene-positive result. Three major themes arose in these interviews: (1) living as though gene-positive, (2) risky behaviors, and (3) complex pasts. The authors concluded that predictive genetic testing not only may have the potential to create harm and benefit for young people at risk for HD, but may have the potential to alleviate preexisting harm. Some of those interviewed felt that uncertainty about their genetic status was a barrier in their lives that prevented them from moving forward.

The same eight interviews were used in a later study of the experience of genetic testing for HD and for familial adenomatous polyposis (FAP). In this study, the kinds of harm associated with a gene-positive result included knowledge of future illness, witnessing distress in parents, identifying with other gene-positive family members, experiencing a range of negative emotions, feeling that the knowledge resurfaced at difficult times in life, feeling distanced from family members, friendships being affected by negative mood, feeling let down by the reactions of others, experiencing anxiety about other people gossiping, experiencing concern about implications for employment, and feeling regret about having the knowledge. The kinds of harm associated with a gene-negative test result included experiencing unexpected negative emotions, worrying about the implications for siblings, feeling guilty, and feeling distanced from family members. The types of harm associated with the testing process in general included having to confront the issue, experiencing the stress placed on the family, experiencing irritability, feeling anxious while waiting for the test results, interference with school, feeling a lack of control about the testing process, and experiencing anxiety about the needle used for the blood test. The benefits experienced from a gene-positive test included experiencing relief from uncertainty, feeling able to move forward with life, bonding with other gene-positive family members, strengthened friendships, experiencing clarity about what is important in life, and feeling a sense of control about managing the condition (FAP only). The benefits associated with a gene-negative result included finding out that the genetic condition will not develop, witnessing relief in parents, feeling able to plan for the future, experiencing relief from uncertainty, feeling able to move forward, and feeling generally more positive about life. The benefits associated with the testing process in general included feeling empowered, developing awareness of the support that is available, improved family relationships, and undergoing counseling.[54]

The authors drew three major conclusions. First, the range of effects described by young people far exceeds the range of effects that have been empirically assessed to date. Second, the distribution of harm and benefit is not fundamentally intuitive in that harm and benefit result from both gene-negative and gene-positive results. Third, the testing process itself can create a range of harm and benefit, distinct from the results of the test itself. The small number of interviews and the qualitative nature of this study make it difficult to generalize. The authors concluded, somewhat arbitrarily in my view, that "in order to support a stance in which young people are not able to access tests in the same way that adults are, evidence is required that the effects for young people are worse than those for adults."[54]

These studies focused on the psychosocial implications of testing, as opposed to the other two key objections to testing: concern about future autonomy and confidentiality. Arguments based on the ethical principle of autonomy hold that it is unethical for minors to undergo testing, especially at the request of their parents, as they lose the opportunity to make that same decision as an autonomous adult.[55-57] These arguments are buttressed by the fact that the majority of adults at risk for HD have not decided to take the predictive test[58,59] and consider their autonomy to make the decision whether or not to be tested "sacred."[60] Since the advent of predictive testing for HD, only about 20% of those at risk have had testing.[61] This is, I believe, a powerful argument against childhood testing for late-onset disease. In a study of qualitative interviews, many individuals at risk stated that the uncertainty about their at-risk status was what gave them hope and allowed them to lead a relatively normal life.[62]

Other arguments against testing appeal to the notion of a child's right to an open future.[63] Feinberg distinguishes certain rights, called "C-rights," that are generally characteristic of children and possessed by adults only in unusual or abnormal circumstances. He divides these C-rights into two subclasses: dependency rights (rights deriving from a child's dependence on others for the basic instrumental good of life – food, shelter, and protection) and rights in trust (rights that the child is not yet capable of exercising but that must be preserved for exercise by the adult that the child is expected to become). According to Feinberg, conduct that would count as violating a C-right-in-trust is conduct that guarantees now that, when a child is an adult, certain key options will already be closed.[64] In ethics, rights and duties are correlative in that, when someone has a right, someone else has a duty. In the context of genetic testing, if one accepts a child's right to an open future, one can posit that the parental duty imposed by this right is the duty not to request testing in order to preserve the child's ability to decide for him- or herself whether or not to be tested.

Proponents of testing advance three main arguments. The first is that some young people are mature enough to be involved in making such decisions and that not to allow them to begin making choices about their life as they mature is, in fact, detrimental to the development of their autonomy. This response applies only to more mature young people and is not relevant to the testing of younger, less mature persons.[65] In general, I would support the argument that mature minors who request testing should have their requests assessed on a case-by-case basis.[11] Parental requests for testing are often disguised requests for more information or for the opportunity to express anxiety and concern for their children. The possibility of coercion makes me hesitant to wholeheartedly support requests even by mature minors and their parents without extensive counseling.[66] Testing even a mature minor because of his or her parents' need to know is, I believe, unsupportable.

The second argument is that testing young people does no more to reduce their future autonomy than does not testing them. This is because the untested child loses the opportunity to grow up with the genetic knowledge and adapt to it during his or her formative years. This response is applicable to immature young people.[67] However, the thought of growing up with genetic risk may, in fact, make one less likely to choose testing. In one study comparing individuals who chose to be tested with those who declined testing, those who declined were more likely to have learned about their at-risk status in adolescence rather than adulthood.[68] The authors suggest that, during adolescence, the individual is challenged to become psychologically independent from his or her parents. In adolescents at risk for HD, this process of individuation and separation may be influenced and burdened by the fearsome idea of an HD-doomed adulthood and the expected loyalty toward an affected parent. They further suggest that guilt, anxiety, and anger may increase pessimistic expectations with regard to the future, which makes minors less likely to choose testing as an adult. There is also some evidence that when minors are tested, the information is not shared with them,[52] thus completely negating this potential benefit. Individuals at risk report great difficulty in speaking with their children about their risk,[62] much less a positive test result, and there is some evidence that some parents experience great anxiety when thinking about how to share information about a positive test with their child.[52] I would add that, all too often, the child's adaptation to knowledge about the risk for HD leads to depression and an increase in suicidal thoughts.[41] Advocates of testing appear not to appreciate the likely dynamic of a parent with HD whose symptoms are worsening and a gene-positive adolescent struggling with both the illness and impending death of his or her parent and the certain knowledge of his or her own fate.

The third argument, also applicable to "immature" young people, is that parents have the right to make a decision about testing on behalf of their child, as they know the child best and have primary responsibility.[69] Although this may be legally correct, as Pelias states,[18] there is a growing tendency to afford children more say in their health care decisions.[70] Huntington disease clearly has effects on the family as a whole.[71] Sensitivity to the impact of illness within the family must be taken into account. While most families handle HD with grace and dignity, some are quite chaotic, sometimes violent, not necessarily providing the best environment for coming to terms with potentially devastating information. In addition, as with surrogate decision making in general, there is always a chance that the surrogate will be unduly influenced by conflicts of interests and will make decisions that serve the interests of the surrogate rather than the best interests of the child.

It is also argued that the testing of young people is a breach of their confidentiality, as their parents or guardians are also aware of the test result.[72] One response to this is to offer mature young persons complete confidentiality of their test results.[65] This suggestion does not negate the problem of breaching the confidentiality of younger children. Proponents of testing argue that parents are privy to all sorts of sensitive information about their children. The difference here is that most of that information is in real time and usually relevant to medical and other decisions that need to be made at the moment. Comparing information about a genetic test result for a disease that is unlikely to manifest for several decades to other sensitive information about the child is, I would argue, like comparing apples to oranges. This response also fails to take into consideration the fact that genetic test results are likely to become part of the permanent medical record and thus may lead to stigma and potential discrimination.[46,47]

A recent qualitative study looked at perceptions of genetic stigmatization and discrimination among adults who had completed genetic testing for HD and provides some insight into the impact of a positive result. Participants reported perceptions of genetic discrimination following disclosure of genetic test results in three areas: employment, insurance, and social relationships. While the majority of employed participants initially had a low level of concern about employment discrimination and revealed their test results to their employer, eight out of nine said they would not disclose this information when seeking new employment. Participants reported feeling stuck in their current position because of their gene test results due to uncertainty about being hired, receiving benefits, making a long-term commitment, or passing performance evaluations. Two individuals experienced specific discrimination involving termination. Concerns about insurance discrimination were initially high, and though few instances of insurance discrimination were found, subjects went to great lengths to keep their genetic results from insurers by, for example, paying out of pocket or using false names on the paperwork. With the passage of the Genetic Information Non-discrimination Act in 2008, we will see whether these fears diminish. Interestingly, the social impact of testing was the dominant concern of these subjects. All participants reported perceptions of differential treatment after having shared their test results. Nearly all (93%) reported at least one negative impact on family relationships. Additional social consequences included finding it difficult to convey health information while dating, concern for the implications of a positive result for other at-risk family members, increased concern about reproductive decisions, and an increase in depression and greater anxiety about their children's and grandchildren's lives. Nearly half expressed concern that others would monitor their behavior in order to identify disease symptoms. These social costs cannot be legislated away and provide some evidence that the predicted effects on family relationships do occur.[47]

There is one last ethical and social complexity associated with the testing of minors. This is a concern for the "genetic eligibility" for marriage or partnership and, ultimately, reproduction associated with the prediction of future, particularly untreatable, disease. Some individuals at risk feel that the availability of a genetic test generates a moral imperative that it be used for responsible reproductive decision making and that to knowingly abstain from doing so could result in future guilt, self-censure, or broader social censure.[60] Individuals who have been tested report that one of the social consequences of testing is having to decide if and when to share this information with a prospective partner.[47] Honesty would dictate that this information be shared at some point in the relationship, but the risk of rejection would be very real.[71] As marriage comes to be more like a contract with a growing number of conditions, and as dating often involves Googling a prospective partner in order to check out his or her eligibility, can checking out a partner's genes be far behind? There is a vast difference between undergoing genetic testing as an adult, when one may have been in a stable relationship for many years, and finding out this information about an acquaintance in whom one is not heavily invested.

CONCLUSION

For scientists, it is always preferable to rely on data. The fact of the matter is that, for the question of whether to perform genetic testing of minors for late-onset disorders, there are few data on which to base a decision.

What we do know is the following: The suicide rate for those with or at risk for HD is four times the national average. The majority of adults at risk for HD have chosen not to be tested. The majority of parents at risk for HD believe that it is their right to request such testing even when they themselves have chosen not to be tested. They also believe that the youngest age at which such testing should be done is past the age of majority, at 18.63 years. As time goes on, some adults who have received positive genetic test results experience increased depression and suicidal thoughts. In the few cases where such testing has been done on minors, few have been informed of their results, and some parents experience significant anxiety when thinking about how to give their children this information. Those who test negative as well as those who test positive experience both benefit and harm, and the testing process itself may have harmful effects on those at risk. Those who have tested gene-positive have experienced what they perceive as genetic discrimination related to their positive gene status and have reported a significant negative impact on their social relationships. To me, the very real burdens to individuals outweigh the often theoretical potential benefits. Although parents may have the legal right to request testing of minor children, they ought not to do so. Parents should preserve the autonomy of their children to decide for themselves as adults whether they wish to be tested.

References

1. Barema J. *The Test: Living in the Shadow of Huntington's Disease.* New York: Franklin Square Press; 2005:49.
2. American Society of Human Genetics Board of Directors and American College of Medical Genetics Board of Directors. Points to consider: ethical, legal, and psychosocial implications of genetic testing in children and adolescents. *Am J Hum Genet.* 1995;57:1233.
3. American Medical Association Council on Ethical and Judicial Affairs. Testing Children for Genetic Status. Chicago: *American Medical Association;* 1995. Code of Medical Ethics, Report No. 66.
4. National Society of Genetic Counselors. Prenatal and childhood testing for adult onset disorders. *Perspect Genet Couns.* 1995;17:5.
5. Harper PS, Clarke A. Should we test children for "adult" genetic diseases? *Lancet.* 1990;342:1205–1206.
6. Institute of Medicine, Committee on Assessing Genetic Risks. *Assessing Genetic Risks.* Washington, DC: National Academy Press; 1994.
7. Clarke A, Flinter F. The genetic testing of children: a clinical perspective. In: Marteau T, Richards M, eds. *The Troubled Helix: Social and Psychological Implications of the New Human Genetics.* Cambridge: Cambridge University Press; 1996:164–176.
8. Borry P, Stultiens L, Nys H, et al. Presymptomatic and predictive genetic testing in minors: a systematic review of guidelines and position papers. *Clin Genet.* 2006;70:374–381.

9. Kodish ED. Testing children for cancer genes: the rule of earliest onset. *J Pediatr.* 1999;135:390–395.

10. Borry P, Goffin T, Nys H, et al. Attitudes regarding predictive genetic testing in minors: a survey of European clinical geneticists. *Am J Med Genet, Part C (Sem Med Genet).* 2008;148C:78–83.

11. Binedell J, Soldan JR, Scourfield, et al. Huntington's disease predictive testing: the case for an assessment approach to requests from adolescents. *J Med Genet.* 1996;33:912–918.

12. Wertz DC, Reilly PR. Laboratory policies and practices for the genetic testing of children: a survey of the Helix network. *Am J Hum Genet.* 1997;61:1163–1168.

13. Rosen A, Wallenstien S, McGovern MM. Attitudes of pediatric residents toward ethical issues associated with genetic testing in children. *Pediatrics.* 2002;110:360–363.

14. Quaid KA, PHAROS Investigators and Coordinators. Attitudes towards genetic testing for Huntington's disease in PHAROS participants. *J Neurol Neurosurg Psychiatry.* 2005;76(Suppl. 4):A53.

15. Smith DH, Quaid KA, Dworkin RB, et al. *Early Warning: Cases and Ethical Guidance for Presymptomatic Testing in Genetic Diseases.* Indianapolis: Indiana University Press; 1998.

16. Ross LF. Predictive genetic testing for conditions that present in childhood. *Kennedy Inst Ethics J.* 2002;12:225–244.

17. Sevick MA, Nativio DG, McConnel T. Genetic testing of children for late onset disease. *Camb Q Healthcare Ethics.* 2005;14:47–56.

18. Pelias MK. Genetic testing of children for adult-onset diseases: is testing in the child's best interest? *Mt. Sinai J Med.* 2006;73:605–608.

19. Wertz DC. International perspectives. In: Clarke AJ, ed. *The Genetic Testing of Children.* Oxford: BiosScientific; 1998;271–287.

20. Malpus PJ. Predictive genetic testing of children for adult-onset diseases and psychological harm. *J Med Ethics.* 2008;34:275–278.

21. Folstein SE. *Huntington's Disease: A Disorder of Families.* Baltimore: Johns Hopkins University Press; 1989.

22. Conneally PM. Huntington disease: genetics and epidemiology. *Am J Hum Genet.* 1984;36:506–536.

23. Harper P. "The natural history of Huntington disease." In: Harper PS, ed. *Huntington's Disease.* London: WB Saunders; 1991:4–21.

24. Gusella JF, Wexler NS, Conneally PM, et al. A polymorphic DNA marker genetically linked to Huntington's disease. *Nature.* 1983;306:234–238.

25. Huntington's Disease Collaborative Research Group. A novel gene containing a trinucleotide repeat that is expanded and unstable on Huntington's disease chromosomes. *Cell.* 1993;74:971–983.

26. Farrer L. Suicide and attempted suicide in Huntington's disease: implications for preclinical testing of persons at risk. *Am J Med Genet.* 1986;24:305–311.

27. The International Huntington Association and the World Federation of Neurology Research Group on Huntington's Chorea. Ethical issues policy statement on Huntington's disease molecular genetics test. *J Med Genet.* 1990;27:34–38.

28. The International Huntington Association and the World Federation of Neurology Research Group on Huntington's Chorea. Guidelines for the

molecular genetics predictive test in Huntington disease. *J Med Genet.* 1994;31:555–559.

29. Huntington Disease Society of America. *Guidelines for Predictive Testing in Huntington's Disease.* New York: Huntington Disease Society of America; 1989.

30. Meisser B, Dunn S. Psychological impact of genetic testing for Huntington disease: an update on the literature. *J Neurol Neurosurg Psychiatry.* 2000; 69:574–578.

31. Duisterhof M, Trijsburg RW, Niermeijer MF, et al. Psychological studies in Huntington disease: making up the balance. *J Med Genet.* 2002;38:852–861.

32. Tibben A, Timman R, Bannink EC, et al. Three-year follow-up after presymptomatic testing for Huntington's disease in tested individuals and partners. *Health Psychol.* 1997;16:20–35.

33. Timman R, Roos R, Maat-Kievet A, Tibben A. Adverse effects of predictive testing for Huntington disease underestimated: long term effects 7–10 years after the test. *Health Psychol.* 2004;23:189–197.

34. Bloch M, Adam S, Wiggins S, et al. Predictive testing for Huntington disease in Canada: the experience of those receiving an increased risk. *Am J Med Genet. Part A.* 1992;42A:499–507.

35. Huggins M, Bloch M, Wiggins S, et al. Predictive testing for Huntington's disease in Canada: adverse effects and unexpected results in those receiving a decreased risk. *Am J Med Genet. Part A.* 1992;42A:508–515.

36. Robins Wahlin TB, Lundin A, Backman L, et al. Reactions to predictive testing in Huntington disease: case reports of coping with a new genetic status. *Acta Neurol Scand.* 2000;102:150–161.

37. Decruyenaere M, Evers-Kiebooms G, Cloostermans T, et al. Psychological distress in the 5-year period after predictive testing for Huntington's disease. *Eur J Hum Genet.* 2003;11:30–38.

38. Timman R, Roos R, Maat-Kievit A, et al. Adverse effects of predictive testing for Huntington disease underestimated: long terms effects 7–10 years after the test. *Health Psychol.* 2004;2:189–197.

39. Witjes-Ane M, Zwinderman AH, Tibben, et al. Behavioral complaints in participants who underwent predictive testing for Huntington disease. *J Med Genet.* 2002;39:857–862.

40. Close Kirkwood S, Siemers E, Viken J, et al. Evaluation of psychological symptoms among presymptomatic HD gene carriers as measured by selected MMPI scales. *J Psychiatr Res.* 2002;36: 377–382.

41. Larsson M, Luszcz MA, Bui TH, et al. Depression and suicidal ideation after predictive testing for Huntington disease: a two-year follow-up study. *J Genet Couns.* 2006;15:361–374.

42. Codori AM, Hanson R, Brandt J. Psychological costs and benefits of predictive testing for Huntington's disease. *Am J Med Genet. Part B (Neuropsychiatr Genet).* 1994;54B:167–173.

43. Beck A, Brown G, Berchick RJ, et al. Relationship between hopelessness and ultimate suicide: a replication with psychiatric outpatients. *Am J Psychiatry* 1990;147:190–195.

44. The genetic testing of children: report of a working party of the Clinical Genetics Society. March 1994. Available at: http://www.clingensoc.org/Docs/Testing_of_Children1994.pdf.

45. Fanos JH. Developmental tasks of childhood and adolescence: implications for genetic testing. *Am J Med Genet Part A.* 1997;71A:22–28.

46. Bombard Y, Penziner E, Decolongon J, et al. Managing genetic discrimination: strategies used by individuals found to have the Huntington disease mutation. *Clin Genet.* 2007;71:220–231.

47. Penziner E, Williams JK, Erwin C, et al. Perceptions of discrimination among persons who have undergone predictive testing for Huntington disease. *Am J Med Genet. Part B (Neuropsychiatr Genet).* 2008;147B:320–325.

48. Clarke A. Genetic testing of children: Working Party of the Clinical Genetics Society (U.K.). *J Med Genet.* 1994;31:785–797.

49. Dalby S. Genetics Interest Group response to the UK Clinical Genetics Society report "The genetic testing of children." *J Med Genet.* 1995;32:490–491.

50. Sharpe NF. Presymptomatic testing for Huntington disease: is there a duty to test those under the age of eighteen years? *Am J Med Genet.* 1993;46:250–253.

51. Duncan RE, Dalatycki MB. Predictive genetic testing in young people for adult-onset conditions: where is the empirical evidence? *Clin Genet.* 2006; 69:8–16.

52. Duncan RE, Savulescu J, Gilliam L, et al. An international survey of predictive genetic testing in children for adult onset condition. *Genet Med.* 2005; 7:390–396.

53. Duncan RE, Gilliam L, Savulescu J, et al. "Holding your breath": interviews with young people who have undergone predictive genetic testing for Huntington disease. *Am J Med Genet. Part A.* 2007;143A:1984–1989.

54. Duncan RE, Gilliam L, Savulescu J, et al. "You're one of us now": young people describe their experiences of predictive genetic testing for Huntington disease (HD) and familial adenomatous polyposis (FAP). *Am J Med Genet. Part C (Sem Med Genet).* 2008;148C:47–55.

55. Bloch M, Hayden M. Opinion – predictive testing for Huntington disease in childhood: challenges and implications. *Am J Hum Genet.* 1990;46:1–4.

56. Davis D. Genetic dilemmas and the child's right to an open future. *Rutgers Law J.* 1997;28:549–592.

57. Holland J. Should parents be permitted to authorize genetic testing for their children. *Fam Law Q.* 1997;31:321–353.

58. Nance M, Myers RH. The US Huntington Disease Testing Group: trends in predictive and prenatal testing for Huntington's disease, 1993–1999 [abstract]. *Am J Med Genet.* 1999;65A:406.

59. Tibben A. Genetic counseling and presymptomatic testing. In: Bates G, Harper P, Jones L, eds. *Huntington Disease.* 3rd ed. New York: Oxford University Press; 2002:198–248.

60. Taylor S. Predictive genetic test decisions for Huntington disease: context, appraisal and new moral imperatives. *Social Sci Med.* 2004;58:137–149.

61. Binedell J, Soldan JR, Harper PS. Predictive testing for Huntington's disease: predictors of uptake in South Wales. Clin Genet. 1998;54:477–488.

62. Quaid KA, Sims SL, Swenson MM, et al. Living at risk: concealing risk and preserving hope in Huntington disease. *J Genet Couns.* 2008;17:117–128.

63. Feinberg J. The child's right to an open future. In: Aiken W, La Follette H, eds. *Whose Child? Children's Rights, Parental Authority and State Power.* Totowa, NJ: Rowman & Littlefield; 1980:124–153.

64. Lotz M. Feinberg, Mills, and the child's right to an open future. *J Social Philos.* 2006;37:537–551.

65. Duncan RE. Predictive genetic testing in young people: when is it appropriate? *J Paediatr Child Health.* 2004;40:593–595.

66. Gaff CL, Lynch E, Spencer L. Predictive testing of eighteen year olds. *J Genet Couns.* 2006;15:245–251.

67. Robertson S, Sevulescu J. Is there a case in favor of predictive genetic testing in young children? *Bioethics.* 2001;15:2.

68. Van der Steenstraten IM, Tibben A, Roos RAC, et al. Predictive testing for Huntington's disease: non-participants compared with participants in the Dutch program. *Am J Hum Genet.* 1994;55:618–625.

69. Clayton EW. Genetic testing in children. *J Med Philos.* 1997;22:233–251.

70. Ambuel B, Rapaport J. Developmental trends in adolescents' psychological and legal competence to consent to abortion. *Law Hum Behav.* 1992;16:129–154.

71. Sobel SK, Cowan DB. Impact of genetic testing for Huntington disease on the family system. *Am J Med. Genet.* 2000;90:49–59.

72. Fryer A. Genetic testing of children. *Arch Dis Child.* 1995;73:97–99.

10

Extreme Prematurity

Truth and Justice

Geoffrey Miller

In this chapter I will consider some of the ethical issues that surround the management of the extremely preterm infant (EPTI). Such infants are characterized by a gestational age (GA) of less than 28 weeks. However, in practice, within this group, those who give rise to the most ethical concern are the ones who are born at less than 26 weeks. The issues raised by this group are discussed in several chapters in this book and include, in particular, parental rights and responsibilities; the forgoing of life-sustaining treatment; and the usefulness or otherwise of such words as "best interests," "benefits," "burdens," and "futility," which, incorrectly used, can both cloud and taint a coherent moral approach. I will not repeat these topics, but rather I will highlight the lack of use, misuse, and misinterpretation of empirical data to shape and drive ethical and medical management. This will include perceptions concerning prognosis, delivery room resuscitation, and justice, both distributive and personal.

There is an ongoing concern that continuing to care for and save the lives of EPTIs comes at the inevitable expense – to some babies, families, and society – of disability, emotional trauma, and financial cost. Because mortality and morbidity increase with decreasing GA and weight, it is argued that a line should be drawn on the basis of these measures, such that the provision of active care to a baby born at less than 25 weeks or 600 g should be optional. But not only is there uncertainty about the outcome for the individual child, there is also poor understanding of the types of disability that may occur and the accuracy of predicting GA and weight. The estimation of GA is not reliably accurate to within one week using the dates of the last menstrual period, obstetric estimates, or postnatal clinical methods.[1,2] Similarly, estimates of fetal weight can be inaccurate by 15–20%.[3] Furthermore, not all preterm infants are at the same developmental level after delivery because of differing genetic and environmental influences.[4] Despite this, the American Academy of Pediatrics, in 2002, wrote that it was appropriate to not initiate resuscitation at 23 weeks gestation while acknowledging the inaccuracies of GA estimation and the various factors that affect outcome.[5] Previously, in 1994, the Canadian Paediatric Society and the Society of Obstetricians and Gynecologists of Canada published guidelines for the management of an infant of extremely low GA.[6] They did not acknowledge the inaccuracies of GA estimation and recommended that, because the outcomes for infants with a GA of 23–24 completed weeks vary greatly, careful consideration should be given to the limited benefits for the infant and potential harm of cesarean section as well as to the expected results of resuscitation at birth. I will comment later on what these expected results of resuscitation are. It is disturbing that such influential bodies should issue such incoherent statements. However, similar conclusions were reached in other parts of the world. An Australian consensus work group recommended management practice according to the week of GA. Neither how this was estimated nor its accuracy was reported. The work group stated that at 26 weeks the obligation to treat was very high, but at 23–25 weeks it was acceptable not to resuscitate if the parents so wished.[7] In the United Kingdom the Nuffield Council on Bioethics came to conclusions very similar to those of the Australians based on the same tainted evidence.[8]

At this point in the chapter it is important to acknowledge that I do not want, or tolerate easily, the occurrence of children with conditions that hamper their opportunities for a full life, nor do I belittle the economic and emotional stresses that accrue from this. However, I am arguing not for a preference, the alternative to which I very much would want to prevent, but rather, given the circumstances, for what ought to be permissible. This permissibility is affected not only by the validity of clinical data but also by the manner in which it is presented. For example, in 2005, Marlow and his colleagues published an influential paper on the outcome rates of the EPIcure study. This was a prospective observational study of all births in Britain from 20 to 25 weeks gestation during 1995.[9] Leaving aside the inaccuracies of GA estimation and the effects of different types of management before and at birth, I would like to address the interpretation of the neurodevelopmental outcomes and what the words "severe," "moderate," or "mild disability" mean to parents and health professionals if these words are not defined during counseling. Clearly if the parents are informed that there is considerable risk of a severe disability, the perception of the outcome may be much worse than it is actually likely to be. In the EPIcure study, severe disability occurs in less than a quarter of infants and is defined as highly dependent on caregivers (e.g., if the child is unable to walk or has an I.Q. of less than 55, which may be comparable to Down syndrome). Within this group of severely disabled individuals, however, the majority are sentient, interactive, and loving. Emphasizing this information may well influence what is ethically permissible, rather than preferable. Also of note in this study is that the percentage of those who were classified as severely disabled varied little between the groups of 23, 24, and 25 weeks gestation and was greatest at 24 weeks gestation. However, perceptions of outcome are changing. Advances in management are leading to increased survival and a decrease in the incidence of severe neurodevelopmental disabilities.[10-12] This is not only because of treatment factors such as antenatal steroids and exogenous surfactant, but also because of a willingness to treat an EPTI intensively.[13-15] For example, in a 2004 study from Sweden,[16] the authors reported that a proactive management, rather than a selective treatment strategy, more than doubled survival for infants of 22–25 weeks gestation without an increase in long-term morbidity. The conclusion is that the interpretation of outcome studies requires knowledge of the management strategies, which themselves may lead to self-fulfilling prophesies and ethical decisions that are not fully informed.

The dangers of making false assumptions concerning outcome can also be seen when one examines the efficacy of active resuscitation of an EPTI in the delivery room. In 1996 Rennie wrote that the outcome after cardiopulmonary resuscitation (CPR) following delivery of a very preterm infant was "appalling."[17] This opinion was based on a small number of infants in case reports from the 1980s and early 1990s.[18-20] In sharp contrast to these reports are later ones suggesting that the condition at birth of an EPTI may not be a good indicator of viability or later outcome.[21] Jankov, Asztalos, and Skidmore evaluated whether vigorous resuscitation of EPTI infants at birth improved survival or increased the chances of major neurodevelopmental disability. The infants in their study received CPR in the delivery room. The majority survived and were free of major neurodevelopmental disability at follow-up,[22] and similar findings have been reported by others.[23,24] In practice, most neonatologists would want to resuscitate an infant of 25 or more weeks gestation and an estimated weight of more than 650 g, given the relatively good outcome of doing so. For that very small number of infants with an estimated GA of 23–24 weeks and less than 650 g, the prediction of outcome in the delivery room is not accurate, given individual variations in maturity and response to extreme prematurity, even if GA and birth weight could be estimated more accurately.[25] But despite this, there are still many U.S. neonatologists who base their decisions on whether to resuscitate the smallest of EPTIs on their condition in the delivery room. In 2007 Singh et al. asked more than 600 U.S. neonatologists how they would manage a group of infants of 500–600 g and GAs of 23–24 weeks whom the authors had cared for previously in Chicago and Cleveland. The majority of those questioned reported that they would decide whether to actively resuscitate the babies in the delivery room on the basis of their appearance. However, this appearance, based on Apgar scores and heart rates at one and five minutes, was neither sensitive nor predictive of death before discharge, survival with a neurological abnormality, or intact survival.[26] This misperception also exists among neonatal and obstetric resident physicians and delivery room nurses, who are often the first health professionals to see a mother in premature labor after she arrives at a hospital. Janvier et al. conducted a study to compare the attitudes of 172 neonatal and obstetric residents and 136 neonatal and delivery room nurses toward resuscitation of an EPTI if they are told only the GA or if they are given only prognostic information for infants at that GA.[27] They were asked whether they would resuscitate a depressed 24-week-gestation baby at birth and whether they would resuscitate a depressed preterm infant with a 50% chance of survival, knowing that, of those who survived, 50% would develop normally, 20–25% would have a serious handicap, and 40% might have behavioral or specific learning difficulties. In response to the first question, entailing only GA, 21% reported that they would resuscitate, but in response to the second question, entailing only prognosis, 51% reported that they would resuscitate. The authors concluded that the relative unwillingness to resuscitate the 24-week baby was surprising because modern outcomes for such babies are the same as or better than the outcome data that were given without specifying GA. The authors' explanations for this were that the respondents had irrational negative associations with low GAs or that they were unaware of the actual outcomes.

Are many of us unjust to EPTIs? Distributive justice refers to a fair and equitable distribution of resources. Some might argue that the costs of neonatal intensive care for an EPTI, and the costs and burdens to society of providing for disabled children, are not justified because they threaten the overall welfare of society. If one observes a modern neonatal intensive care unit (NICU), the impression is that of a labor-intensive environment filled with highly trained staff members managing the precarious existence of the smallest and most fragile of patients with the aid of frighteningly invasive procedures and expensive, technologically sophisticated equipment. It is not surprising that the question arises as to whether all of this is just, or worth it, in terms of economic, societal, and personal outcomes. Indeed, when the figures for resource use by NICUs are examined in relation to EPTIs, they appear daunting. For example, in a study of 17 Canadian NICUs,[28] the authors reported that, although EPTIs constituted only 4% of admissions, they accounted for 22% of deaths, 31% of severe intraventricular hemorrhage, 22% of chronic lung disease, 59% of severe retinopathy of prematurity, and 20% of necrotizing enterocolitis. They consumed 11% of NICU days, 20% of mechanical ventilator use, 35% of transfusions, 21% of surgically inserted central venous catheters, and 8% of major surgical procedures. But the cost of such care should be examined in relation to how much and the manner in which society spends on other aspects of health care and the proportion of this that is generated by the population in question. Neonatal intensive care cost per life-year gained is considerably less than that for adults given intensive care.[29] The vast majority of NICU expenditure is consumed by infants who survive and go home without major disability.[30,31] The longer an EPTI stays in the NICU, the more likely it is that the infant will survive, which is not necessarily the case in the adult ICU. In Japan, Nishida calculated the economic costs of providing for EPTIs, including lifelong costs, and concluded that there was a net financial benefit, which was generated by normal survivors.[32,33] Certainly it can be argued that the relatively favorable outcome for an EPTI generates more lifelong beneficence than that gained from resource allocation to the very elderly. As Buchh and colleagues write,[34] "[T]here are no credible distributive justice arguments to NICU care for ELBW infants now, when survival is good. But, surprisingly, even when NICU survival was much worse there have never been credible distributive justice arguments against NICU care for infants with birth weights <1000g."

In general, the principle of justice concerns fairness and rights and dictates that an EPTI be treated in the same way as other infants with treatable conditions. Personal experience and the literature would suggest that this is not always the case. EPTIs are systematically devalued, in comparison with older patients whose outcomes are the same or worse.[35] Much is written about the aspects of treatment of an EPTI based on outcomes. But the same considerations are not made for other infants whose treatments may lead to similar or worse adverse outcomes. For example, Janvier and colleagues write that the initiation of treatment for a 2-month-old baby with pyogenic bacterial meningitis is considered obligatory, but maybe considered optional for a 700 g 24-week infant who requires resuscitation at birth to survive.[36] The 2-month-old baby probably has a worse long-term prognosis than the EPTI. This, the authors suggest, may be because they are viewed in a morally different fashion than are older children and adults, and this bias is supported by unquestioned positive attitudes toward the treatment of very serious disorders in adults whose outcomes may be similar to or worse than that of a small EPTI. Some reasons given for this are that EPTIs may be viewed as non-persons or "less of a person"[13] or that in the "broad scheme of things" they are replaceable – what Janvier et al. term the "better luck next time approach."[36] There are many examples of this skewed approach. Parenchymal intracranial hemorrhage in an EPTI may be the stimulus for considering less active management, even though the severity of outcome may be unknown, but in an older child aggressive management is continued if there is a chance of a tolerable outcome. Hypoplastic left heart syndrome is another example. For those who are listed for transplant, there is a survival rate of 54% at five years.[37] With respect to the three-staged surgical repair, the survival rate after Stage 1 ranges from 48% to 71%.[38,39] Neurodevelopmental disability is common following hypoplastic left heart syndrome repair, with one study reporting mental retardation in 18% of survivors.[40,41] The survival and morbidity rates for EPTIs compare quite favorably with the hypoplastic left heart syndrome figures.[39] However, it is very unlikely, at least in North America, that operative intervention for hypoplastic left heart syndrome would be viewed as optional.

It is difficult to understand the reasons for this unjust prejudice against EPTIs. I can speculate that compromised babies are viewed as morally different and are owed less than older children and that their relationship with their caregivers, in particular health professionals, is not as well established. Conversely, the perceived harm inflicted on such small, vulnerable premature infants might trigger a response that is directed toward the removal of that stress. Also in the realm of speculation is the existence of an instinctual sense, perhaps teleological or evolutionary, that a disabled infant may be a burden and a threat to the community, tribe, or family. Although these are speculations, it is important to emphasize that biases in our approach to the management of the EPTI should be recognized and appreciated.

References

1. Mongelli T, Wilcox M, Gardosi J. Estimating the date of confinement: ultrasonographic biometry versus certain menstrual dates: *Am J Obstet Gynecol.* 1996;174:278–281.
2. Lynch CP, Zhang J. The research implications of the selection of a gestational age estimation method. *Paediatr Perinatol Epidemiol.* 2007;21(Suppl. 2):86–96.
3. Vavasseur C, Foran A, Murphy JFA. Consensus statements on the borderlands of neonatal viability: from uncertainty to grey areas. *Irish Med J.* 2007;100:561–564.
4. Leviton A, Blair E, Damman O, Allied E. The wealth of information conveyed by gestational age. *J Pediatr.* 2005;146:123–127.
5. American Academy of Pediatrics, Committee on Fetus and Newborn. Perinatal care at the threshold of viability. *Pediatrics.* 2002;110:1024–1027.
6. Fetus and Newborn Committee, Canadian Paediatric Society; Maternal–Fetal Medicine Committee, Society of Obstetricians and Gynecologists of Canada. Management of the woman with threatened birth of an infant of extremely low gestational age. *Can Med Assoc J.* 1994;151:547–553.
7. Lui K, Bajuk B, Foster K, et al. Perinatal care at the borderlines of viability: a consensus statement based on a NSW and ACT consensus workshop. *Med J Austral.* 2006;185:477–478.
8. Nuffield Council on Bioethics. *Critical Care Decisions in Fetal and Neonatal Medicine: Ethical Issues.* London: NCB; 2006.
9. Marlow N, Wolke D, Bracewell MA, Samara M. EPIcure Study Group: neurologic and developmental disability at six years of age after extremely preterm birth. *N Engl J Med.* 2005;352:9–19.
10. Platt MJ, Johnson A, Surman G, Topp M, Torriol MG, Krageloh-Mann I. Trends in cerebral palsy among infants of very low birth weight (<1500g) or born prematurely (<32 weeks) in 16 European centres: a database study. *Lancet.* 2007;369:45–50.
11. Wilson-Costello D, Freidman H, Minich H, Faneroff A, Hack M. Improved survival rates with increased neurodevelopmental disability for extremely low birth weight infants in the 1990s. *Pediatrics.* 2005;115:997–1003.

12. Wilson-Costello D, Friedman H, Minich N, et al. Improved neurodevelopmental outcomes for extremely low birth weights in 2000–2002. *Pediatrics.* 2007;119:37–45.

13. Miller G. *Extreme Prematurity: Practices, Bioethics, and the Law.* Cambridge: Cambridge University Press; 2007.

14. Riley K, Roth S, Sellwood M, Wyatt JS. Survival and neurodevelopmental morbidity at 1 year of age following extremely preterm delivery over a 20 year period: a single centre cohort study. *Acta Paediatrica.* 2008;97:159–165.

15. Steinmacher J, Pohlandt F, Bode H, Sander S, Kron M, Franz AR. Neurodevelopmental follow up of very preterm infants after proactive treatment at a gestational age of ≥23 weeks. *J Pediatr.* 2008;152:771–776.

16. Hakansson S, Farooqi A, Holmgren PA, Serenius F, Hagberg U. Proactive management promotes outcome in extremely preterm infants: a population-based comparison of two perinatal management strategies. *Pediatrics.* 2004; 114:58–64.

17. Rennie JM. Perinatal management at the margin of viability. *Arch Dis Child Fetal Neonatal Ed.* 1996;74:214–218.

18. Sims DG, Heal CA, Bartle SM. Use of adrenaline and atropine in neonatal resuscitation. *Arch Dis Child Fetal Neonatal Ed.* 1994;70:3–9.

19. Sond S, Glacois P. Cardiopulmonary resuscitation in very low birth weight infants. *Am J Perinatol.* 1992;9:130–133.

20. Davis DJ. How aggressive should delivery room CPR be for ELBW neonates? *Pediatrics.* 1993;92:447–450.

21. MacFarlane PI, Wood S, Bennett J. Non-viable delivery at 20–23 weeks gestation: observations and signs of life after birth. *Arch Dis Child Fetal Neonatal Ed.* 2003;83:199–202.

22. Jankov RP, Asztalos EV, Skidmore MB. Favourable neurological outcomes following delivery room cardiopulmonary resuscitation of infants <750gs at birth. *J Paediatr Child Health.* 2000;36:19–22.

23. Doron MW, Veness-Meehan KA, Margolis LH, et al. Delivery room resuscitation decisions for extremely premature infants. *Pediatrics.* 1998;102: 574–582.

24. Finer NN, Tarim T, Vaucher YE, Barrington K, Bajar R. Intact survival in extremely low birth weight infants after delivery room resuscitation. *Pediatrics.* 1999;104:40–44.

25. Meadow W. 500-Gram infants – and 800 pound gorillas – in the delivery room. *Pediatrics.* 2006;117:2276.

26. Singh J, Fanaroff J, Andrews B, et al. Resuscitation in the "gray zone" of viability: determining physician preferences and predicting infant outcomes. *Pediatrics.* 2007;120:519–526.

27. Janvier A, Lantos J, Dechenes M, Couture M, Nadeau S, Barrington KJ. Caregivers' attitudes for very premature infants: what if they knew? *Acta Paediatrica.* 2008;97:276–279.

28. Chan K, Ohlsson A, Synnes A, Lee DS, Chien L, Lee SK. Survival, morbidity, and resource use of infants of 25 weeks gestational age or less. *Am J Obstet Gynecol.* 2001;185:220–226.

29. Tyson JE, Younes N, Verter J, Wright LL. Viability, morbidity, and resource use among newborns 501–800g birth weight. *JAMA.* 1996;276:1645–1651.

30. Meadow WL, Lantos J. Epidemiology and ethics in the neonatal intensive care unit. *Qual Manage Health Care.* 1999;7:21–31.
31. Meadow WL, Lee G, Liu K, Lantos JD. Changes in mortality for ELBW infants in the 1990s: implications for treatment decisions and resource use. *Pediatrics.* 2004;113:1223–1229.
32. Nishida H. Perinatal care in Japan. *J Perinatol.* 1997;17:70–74.
33. Nishida H, Oishi M. Survival and disability in extremely tiny babies less than 600g birth weight. *Sem Neonatalol.* 1996;1:251–256.
34. Buchh B, Graham N, Harris B, et al. Neonatology has always been a bargain – even when we weren't very good at it! *Acta Paediatrica.* 2007;96:659–663.
35. Janvier A, LeBlanc I, Barrington KJ. The best-interest standard is not applied for neonatal resuscitation decisions. *Pediatrics.* 2008;121:963–969.
36. Janvier A, Bauer KL, Lantos JD. Are newborns morally different from older children? *Theoret Med Bioethics.* 2007;28:413–425.
37. Chrisant MRK, Naftel DC, Drummond-Webb J, et al. Fate of infants with hypoplastic left heart syndrome listed for cardiac transplantation: a multicenter study. *J Heart Lung Transplant.* 2005;24:576–582.
38. Checchia PA, McCollegan J, Daher N, Kolornos N, Levy F, Markovitz B. The effect of surgical case volume on outcome after Norwood procedure. *J Thorac Cardiovasc Soc.* 2005;129:754–759.
39. Mercurio MR, Peterec SM, Weeks B. Hypoplastic left heart syndrome, extreme prematurity, comfort care only, and the principle of justice. *Pediatrics.* 2008;122:186–189.
40. Mahle WT, Clancy RR, Moss EM, Gerdes M, Jobes DR, Wernovsky AG. Neurodevelopmental outcome and lifestyle assessment in school-aged and adolescent children with hypoplastic left heart syndrome. *Pediatrics.* 2000;105:1082–1089.
41. Tabutt S, Nord AJ, Jarvik GP, et al. Neurodevelopmental outcomes after staged palliation for hypoplastic left heart syndrome. *Pediatrics.* 2008;121:476–483.

11

Disorders of Sex Development

Alice D. Dreger and David Sandberg

In this chapter, we explore ethical issues in the treatment of children who have disorders of sex development. This term, "disorders of sex development" (DSD), has recently been adopted by medical professionals as a replacement for irregularly employed umbrella terms for congenital sex anomalies, including "intersex" and "(pseudo)hermaphroditism." The term covers "congenital conditions in which development of chromosomal, gonadal, or anatomical sex is atypical."[1] Thus, it includes such conditions as Klinefelter syndrome, Turner syndrome, androgen insensitivity syndrome (AIS), gonadal dysgenesis, and various manifestations of atypical genital development, to name just a few. Some types of DSD are diagnosed prenatally or at birth; some involve external (i.e., visible) sex atypicality; some involve an increased likelihood that children will grow up to feel a gender identity different from the gender assigned at birth. Despite this heterogeneity in diagnosis and clinical presentation, all types of DSD raise concerns among clinicians and parents about gender, fertility, and sexual function and hold the potential for producing disabling shame and secrecy. These concerns are ultimately both clinical and ethical matters, as we show here.

We begin this chapter with this discussion of terminology not only to clarify which conditions are under consideration here, but also because, in DSD clinical care, nomenclature implicates ethical considerations.[2] Unlike outdated, shame-inducing terms like those based on the root "hermaphrodite," the term "disorders of sex development" seems to predispose clinicians to openly disclose to their patients the true nature of their conditions, which we take to be an ethical good. Avoiding vague, imprecise terms (and concepts) like "pseudo-hermaphrodite" and "intersex" encourages a focus on precise medical diagnoses and evidence-based medical care for individual patients. Employing unhelpful terms that signify a special identity – some of which (e.g., "intersex") have been politicized well past the point where they can be beneficial to medical science or to families coping with what can be complex, even life-threatening, medical conditions – unnecessarily clouds discussions, investigations, and decision making.[3] It seems self-evident that care that produces more clarity and less shame is better care. Thus, nomenclature, in the context of DSD, becomes an ethical issue.

For the past half-century, much of the medical literature on the treatment of children with DSD has focused on gender, including patient gender identity, gender role, and sexual orientation.[4] ("Gender identity" refers to a sense of oneself as boy/man or girl/woman; "gender role" refers to behaviors or traits that exhibit sex-related variation in a culture at one point in time; "sexual orientation" refers to sexual arousal to individuals of the same sex [homosexual], opposite sex [heterosexual], or both sexes [bisexual].) Historically, in the pediatric care of children diagnosed with DSD, modern medical approaches have focused on attempting to produce an individual who is gender-typical in terms of physical appearance, self-identity, and behavior, including sexual orientation. Beginning in the 1950s, the standard of care as it emerged primarily out of Johns Hopkins University assumed that making a child's body look gender-typical would facilitate consistent rearing of a child in the assigned gender.[5] As this system spread beyond Hopkins to become a standard of care, some advocated withholding personal medical histories and other important medical information from patients so as not to potentially challenge the sense of gendered self.[5,6]

The heavy clinical focus on gender identity, gender role, and sexual orientation (i.e., psychosexual differentiation) reflected the weight of interest coming from sexologically oriented researchers like psychologist John Money. This clinical work represented a natural extension of animal experimental research demonstrating that early sex hormone exposure during sensitive periods of brain development has permanent (i.e., "organizational") effects on brain structure and physiology. Persons with DSD were accordingly seen by some researchers as "experiments of nature," natural models for the study of the roles of sex chromosomes and hormones in the sexual differentiation of human brain and behavior. What few longitudinal studies existed therefore tended to focus on gender-related outcomes to the exclusion of patients' quality of life. Thus, psychological outcome studies considered whether patients identified as girls/women or boys/men were attracted to males or females (or both), but not whether they experienced emotional equanimity or satisfying peer and romantic relations, or how they functioned in various roles across the life span. Surgical follow-up considered whether neo-vaginas had stenosed, not whether patients were experiencing satisfying sex lives. This left many patients feeling embittered enough that, once the Internet made finding others with DSD possible, an effective patients' rights movement prospered, forcing clinicians to reexamine the system.[5]

To date, the most obvious outcome of this reexamination has been the production of an important consensus statement, in 2006, by the

Lawson Wilkins Pediatric Endocrine Society and the European Society for Paediatric Endocrinology.[1] We will here refer to this as the DSD consensus statement, because therein the two societies argued for the substitution of the terminology of "DSD" and associated nosology. The DSD consensus statement is a critical document with which anyone treating DSD must be familiar, as it represents what experts in the field see as the fundamental principles of DSD care. Although the DSD consensus statement suggests a highly integrated team-management style of care that, arguably, is not yet available as described, it amounts to a road map that clinicians must follow if they are to understand that they are aiming for what is considered high-quality care for patients with DSD and their families. That the document has been accepted as a policy statement of the American Academy of Pediatrics (AAP) reflects the degree to which clinicians ought to understand it as a statement of what is today considered appropriate pediatric care for persons with DSD. One might then ask why we do not simply reprint the DSD consensus statement here. The answer is that, although the statement is clearly a response to a decade of strong ethical critique of the standard of care for children with DSD, it lacks any overt discussion of the ethical issues.

One of the most important insights contained in the DSD consensus statement regards the issue of gender. Substantial evidence now challenges the idea that one can simply "make" a child ultimately feel or behave like a girl or a boy by means of surgery and postnatal hormones. Nor can one easily predict – for example, from prenatal androgen levels – what gender identity a person will ultimately grow to have, or whether a gender identity will remain stable across a person's life span. Particular gender identities are certainly associated with particular biological conditions; for example, the vast majority of typical females end up self-identifying as women, as do the vast majority of – if not all – girls with XY chromosomes and complete androgen insensitivity syndrome (CAIS).[7] But for any given child, it is impossible to know or to engineer with certainty his or her ultimate gender identity.

Perhaps, then, more important than the insight that gender is not exclusively a product of nurture is the insight that a narrow clinical focus on gender obscures what ought to be the real goal in the treatment of DSD, namely, better health-related quality of life for patients than they would have without health care provided by an integrated interdisciplinary team as envisioned in the DSD consensus statement. Whether a patient ultimately changes gender assignment is not a good surrogate measurement for whether she or he has ultimately benefited from health care. Former patients have indicated that primary clinical outcome goals should include an emphasis on good health and sexual function (physical and psychological), positive social relationships, including those with family and romantic/sexual partners, and the promotion of patients' sense of being fully

educated and empowered rather than confused and ashamed by the care
they received from health professionals and their own parents.[8] To be clear,
former patients rarely complain that they got the wrong gender assignment. What some complain of is having lost functional tissue, being made
to feel isolated and ashamed of themselves and their bodies, and having
been misled about their own medical histories.[9]

The multidisciplinary team as envisioned in the DSD consensus statement includes specialists in pediatric endocrinology, pediatric surgery or
urology (or both), psychology and/or psychiatry, gynecology, genetics, neonatology, and (if possible) social work, nursing, and medical ethics. We
suggest that every major hospital have available social workers, nurses, and
medical ethicists who can be recruited to help these patients and their
families; that is, developing a team requires finding, educating, and training people who can provide the truly integrated care these families need
to deal, in the long term, with the issues before them. In lieu of bringing
together the necessary health care resources, the institution is ethically
bound to advocate on behalf of the patient and family to receive these
services at a center where they are available. To allow such children to be
treated only by, say, pediatric endocrinologists or urologists is to practice
in a way that is ethically questionable. This is because DSDs are universally
understood to necessarily involve psychosocial issues, and thus it is critical that professionals trained to deal with psychosocial issues (e.g., behavioral health experts) be intimately involved in the care from the time of
diagnosis.[8]

A well-functioning multidisciplinary team meets regularly to discuss
patients under their care and presents to the family a unified vision of how
to promote the long-term physical and psychological health of the children
they seek to help. Behavioral health experts on the team, such as psychologists and social workers, are critical for ensuring that the team does not
overemphasize lab results or procedures to the neglect, for example, of the
parents' and child's psychological health. Behavioral health professionals
can also ensure that the team attends to the family's understanding of the
medical facts, familial struggles with misattributed guilt, shame, and anger,
and contextual variables, like the family's religious beliefs, cultural values,
and socioeconomic realities. A recommendation for early surgery to make
a clitoris smaller may potentially be motivated by a desire to alleviate parental distress. The behavioral health member of the team can assist in determining whether, in fact, there exists parental distress over the anatomic
differences and, if so, why. Does the parental concern mirror health care
professionals' initial negative reactions (in awkward medical explanations
or more subtle facial expressions) that DSDs carry stigma (i.e., iatrogeni-
cally engendered distress)? The behavioral health team member not only
educates patients and parents, but also models for other DSD team members a style of interaction that communicates to the family that DSD does

not necessarily place limitations on ultimate quality of life. The inclusion of mental health professionals on DSD management teams also increases the likelihood that longitudinal studies will focus on the ultimate goal – positive health-related quality of life – rather than inadequate surrogates like sexual orientation or appearance of the genitals.

Medical centers today lack the integrated multidisciplinary care for DSD that is described in the DSD consensus statement, not only because of the perception that trained specialists are unavailable, but also because the systems do not adequately reimburse members of the management team or provide time to coordinate care as recommended by the DSD consensus statement. We would argue that the failure of health care systems to financially and institutionally support optimal care is in and of itself an ethical issue. It does not do simply to blame insurers and leave it at that, as we know that hospitals frequently find ways to absorb the costs of unreimbursed or under-reimbursed care. One option is for medical institutions to contract with insurers in a way that requires reimbursement of multidisciplinary teams for DSD, in the way many have for children with cleft lip and palate, diabetes, or cystic fibrosis.[10] "Standard of care" implies a diagnostic and treatment process that clinicians should adhere to for a certain type of patient, illness, or clinical circumstance regardless of the patient's health care coverage. Given the AAP's endorsement of the DSD consensus statement, it would seem that clinicians have an ethical duty to see that their institutions provide the care built on this model. If the psychosocial component of care for DSD and the coordination of multidisciplinary team interactions with the family are understood to be fundamental and indispensable, as they are, institutions must work toward these goals.

The existence of an integrated multidisciplinary team care would not, of course, lead to the resolution of all ethical questions in the pediatric care of DSD. We turn now to two of the thorniest ethical issues in this realm, namely medical history disclosure to patients and the use of surgical "normalization" procedures on children too young to consent for themselves.

As already noted, a few clinicians have advocated or participated in the withholding of medical histories from patients with DSD, ostensibly out of the belief that full disclosure would harm patients. Some have even employed peculiar euphemisms to try to manage nondisclosure, such as telling a woman with AIS she was born with "an X chromosome with a short arm" (when what she really has is a Y chromosome) and referring to the removal of her "gonads" instead of her "testes."[8] Clinicians' reluctance to disclose is sometimes motivated by their own discomfort in discussing sex and especially sex anomalies. This again reflects the importance of clinicians' working with behavioral health professionals specifically trained to manage issues like fear, shame, and sexuality.

Regarding disclosure, the DSD consensus statement indicates that "the process of disclosure concerning facts about karyotype, gonadal status, and prospects for future fertility is a collaborative ongoing action which requires a flexible individual based approach."[1] We cannot stress enough the importance of disclosing clear, accurate information from a medical standpoint; DSDs and the ways they are treated often come with attendant medical issues (such as a need for lifelong hormone replacement therapy [HRT], after gonadectomy, to prevent osteoporosis), and patients simply cannot fully understand and manage their own medical needs if they do not know their diagnoses and medical histories. Notably, many adults with DSD have reported feeling relieved upon finding out the truth about their medical histories, in part because it allowed them to obtain more medical information and to find others with the same conditions.[11]

Although we do not have specific data on the benefits of disclosure in pediatric DSD cases, there is persuasive evidence that disclosure of difficult pediatric issues often benefits children as well as parents. For example, regarding children infected with HIV, "[s]tudies suggest that children who know their HIV status have higher self-esteem than children who are not explicitly informed. Parents who have disclosed the status to their children experience less depression than those who do not."[12] A study of the communication of cancer diagnoses to pediatric patients also supports the idea that disclosure translates into better mental health for both children and parents: "[E]arly knowledge of the cancer diagnosis is related to good psychosocial adjustment among long-term survivors of childhood malignancies. ... Many of those parents who did not initially share the diagnosis with their child identified this lack of candor as a source of stress or other difficulty both during and after the treatment period." The authors of this study might have been describing DSD when they wrote about cancer that "honesty and openness with these children can be advocated out of a practical concern about the mental health of those patients who will ultimately survive the disease, as well as out of a humanitarian concern about the feelings of isolation, guilty fantasies, and unexpressed fears that have been found among seriously ill children."[13] Studies of adoption also indicate that disclosure improves the psychosocial adaptation of adoptees.[1]

Thus, developing a model that incorporates a deliberative approach to educating patients with DSD about their own bodies as they grow is not just ethical in and of itself; it is ethical in that it is likely to improve patient outcomes. We think it self-evident that practicing, without very good reason, in a way that is incompatible with the evidence is unethical. The DSD consensus statement recommends that disclosure "should be planned with the parents from the time of diagnosis." Again, we emphasize that behavioral health clinicians have training in this kind of counseling and that clinical services are available, far in excess of those enjoyed by medical and surgical subspecialists, and the benefits of such an approach can accrue to these families. The aforementioned study of cancer survivors suggests that, in having mental health professionals to help families be open about difficult issues related to cancer, the professionals have an opportunity to model communication and coping styles that will apply to other circumstances.[13]

Even if a multidisciplinary team has a commitment to and a plan for educating pediatric DSD patients as they grow, parents may sometimes ask that their children not be told the truth about their conditions and medical histories. Parents who ask for nondisclosure are typically dealing with their own shame and fear, and sometimes also their own guilt about the situation; thus, clinicians should regard parents' requests for nondisclosure as a form of asking for help. Parents may need help in understanding that their children will ultimately have the right to know – and most likely *will* know – what has happened and that they will develop more trust in their parents and health care professionals if they are treated with honesty early and often.

Obviously health care professionals find themselves in an ethical bind when parents seek medical treatment for children with DSD who are old enough to be educated about their conditions but whose parents have refused disclosure. For example, a parent may request that a 10-year-old child who was born 46,XX with congenital adrenal hyperplasia and raised male be given a puberty-delaying hormone to prevent the onset of menstruation, but not be told why he is being given the drug or what it will do to his body. Clinicians do not want to antagonize parents while trying to provide care; antagonizing parents, in and of itself, isn't in a child's best interests. At the same time, in such instances the parents' unwillingness to disclose may interfere with the patient's well-being. If parents cannot at this point be convinced that disclosure – ideally facilitated by behavioral health professionals in cooperation with the parents – is in the child's (and, indeed, the family's) best interests given the evidence and ethical reasoning, clinicians should ask for an ethics consultation and express their concern to the ethics consultants about participating in a deception that may harm the patient (at least psychologically and possibly also physically) in the long run. Pediatricians have a professional obligation to act as advocates for their patients. They can do this most effectively by working cooperatively with parents, but unfortunately it is not always possible to convince the parents that what they think is right may be harming their child.

What, then, of the situation where a child is born with atypical-looking genitals and surgery holds out the promise of producing genitals that look more typical? Should parents be allowed, and in some cases encouraged, to consent to genital surgery aimed at cosmesis?

As we have already noted, this approach emerged as the standard of care beginning in the 1950s and was theoretically grounded in the assumption that standard-looking genitals were necessary to develop a stable gender identity. Some outcomes have challenged the idea that gender identity arises primarily from nurture; for example, one study of children born XY with cloacal exstrophy who were gender-assigned as girls showed that a substantial number ended up with male identities.[14] *Most* patients with DSD, however, appear to retain into adulthood the gender assigned to them at birth.[15] Does that mean "normalizing" genital surgery is what makes stable gender identity possible? Probably not, because the evidence we have regarding people raised with atypical genitalia also suggests that standard-looking genitals may not be *necessary* for the development of a stable gender identity or for satisfying sexual relations.[9,16–20] Evidence from those who have been surgically "normalized" and those who have not, in the aggregate, thus suggests that most people retain the gender assignment they were given at birth.

So what does pediatric genital normalization accomplish? We're not certain. We do not have systematic evidence that withholding surgery to modify the appearance of atypical-looking genitals represents a risk to psychological development. However, we have substantial historical (albeit incomplete) evidence that people have psychologically survived genital atypicality.[16–20] Might pediatric genital normalization help children by helping their parents cope? About this, the DSD consensus statement says, "It is generally felt [by clinicians] that surgery that is carried out for cosmetic reasons in the first year of life relieves parental distress and improves attachment between the child and the parents. [But] the systematic evidence for this belief is lacking."[1] The DSD consensus statement does not raise the question we would, namely whether it is ethical to deal with parental distress through an intervention on a child.[6] It seems to us, at least, that that should not be the first line of treatment of parental distress, unless there is very good evidence that doing so benefits the child in the long term.

Given the choice, why would any parent *not* opt for genital normalization? The reasons include the following: not wanting to expose the child to the physical costs (i.e., irretrievably lost tissue) and risks of such surgery; recognizing that "surgical reconstruction in infancy will [often] need to be refined at the time of puberty";[1] leaving tissue in place in case the child decides later to opt for no surgical intervention or a surgical intervention different from what the parents would have chosen (e.g., if the child's gender identity changes); choosing to signal to the child acceptance of the physical variation as an acceptable aspect of the child's self; recognizing that, as the AAP policy on children's assent to medical care suggests, allowing children to grow to make optional medical choices signals trust and respect and promotes positive child and familial development.[21]

Meanwhile, parents may opt *for* genital normalization in infancy or early childhood because of a belief (again, not evidence-based) that the child will be spared stigmatization. In a related vein, early surgery is believed to spare the parents discomfort associated with the need to explain the condition to others. It is also assumed (with evidence from studies of wound healing in infants versus adults) that early surgery will leave the child physically better off.[1] Some parents may also think that a child cannot be assigned a gender as boy or girl without surgical "correction" of the genitalia; for this reason, clinicians need to help parents understand the difference between gender assignment, which is a social and legal process, and genital surgery. (Clinicians have achieved a consensus that gender assignment should follow the available data on gender identity outcomes for the type of DSD a particular child has.)[1,8]

The DSD consensus statement supports the consideration of surgeries performed before children can meaningfully participate in the decision but also notes concerns such as the importance of employing a specialist surgeon and the likely outcomes of various options (e.g., it notes "the beneficial effects of oestrogen on tissue in early infancy" and that "vaginal dilatation should not be undertaken before puberty").[1] It does not explore the ethical question of whether parents should be allowed and indeed encouraged to pursue genital normalization. We would note that, as a matter of informed consent, parents typically need help in distinguishing between "medically necessary" interventions (including surgeries) that aim to treat an immediate health problem (e.g., malignancy), those that aim to prevent a known risk (e.g., pain from chordee with erections), and "elective" procedures that aim to prevent what is assumed but not evidenced to engender a risk (e.g., clitoromegaly). Some surgery may be necessary to correct anatomical anomalies incompatible with physical health (e.g., the absence of or an obstructed outlet for urine), but that does not logically imply accompanying cosmetic genitoplasty. A practice among some surgeons has been to convince parents that it is preferable to "do it [i.e., genitoplasty] while we have them on the table [for a necessary surgery]." Although it makes sense, all other things being equal, to reduce the number of exposures to anesthesia, infection, and so on, that consideration should be secondary to the question of whether genitoplasty need be done at that point (or at all). It is critical for the patient's best interests to sort out with families that which is known to be necessary for health and that which is not. A detailed discussion of these issues, on repeated occasions when the parents' emotional state does not constrain decision making, will predictably reduce the likelihood of decisional regret. Here is another example where a behavioral health member of the team could potentially facilitate quality-of-life outcomes: discussions regarding surgical decisions could be introduced in the context of the comprehensive education of the parents about the DSD, including its etiology, management, and contextual factors for the family that may lead them to prematurely rule out options regarding gender assignment or surgery.

On the question of cosmetic genital surgeries, for our part, we would point out that parents must daily make choices about whether and how to make their children conform to societal expectations – for example, having straight teeth for the sake of a nice-looking smile (although an improper bite is a risk factor for tooth and jaw problems).[22] That said, genital surgery is obviously much more serious business than routine orthodontics, and we wish that we had better comparative evidence to guide parents in what to do in cases of atypical genitalia. What we do know is that many former patients are angry about what happened to them, though it is also clear that their anger is often as much about the way in which surgery signaled that they were shameful, abnormal, and unlovable as about the physical effects of surgery.[9] This suggests that, were infant genital normalization followed up in an atmosphere of open, honest, loving acceptance, patients might well find their parents' decision to opt for genital normalization unproblematic, just as patients who have had their cleft lips repaired in infancy seem to.[22] Again, this reflects the importance of attention to the family context and to the importance of actively integrating behavioral health professionals into ongoing care.

Some surgeries associated with DSD are not optional from a medical standpoint and therefore, to our minds, do not present ethical dilemmas. Two examples are surgery preformed to create a urinary opening when a child is born without one and surgery to remove malignant gonadal tissue. The status of some other surgeries, in terms of medical necessity and ethics, is less clear. For example, girls and women with CAIS are at risk for testicular cancer, but the risk appears only at puberty. (The earliest known age of a child with CAIS who developed testicular cancer was 14.)[1] The DSD consensus statement notes that parents can decide to have the testes removed in early childhood and indicates that this "takes care of the associated hernia [if there is one], psychological problems with the presence of testes, and the malignancy risk."[1] Yet the idea that removing the testes removes "psychological problems with the presence of testes" seems problematic, because even women who have had their testes removed may well experience psychological distress from knowing they *had* testes; removal again seems to wrongly assume a surgical remedy for a lifelong psychological issue and might even seem to accidentally promote nondisclosure. (Parents may think that orchiectomy performed before a girl is aware of her condition means she never has to be told.) Moreover, members of the Androgen Insensitivity Syndrome Support Groups have pointed out that leaving testes in place through puberty allows a girl with CAIS to naturally undergo a feminizing puberty – for reasons not germane to this discussion, the bodies of girls with testes and CAIS develop in a fairly typical feminine style during puberty – and allows her the option of avoiding lifelong HRT, should she wish to accept keeping her testes and observing a policy of cancer surveillance. (HRT is not without its own challenges, costs, and risks.)[23]

Whether or not gonadectomy is performed, hormonal treatments may be used, like surgical treatments, to attempt to make some children with DSD more closely approximate social expectations. HRT is used to induce gender-specific puberty when children have had gonadectomy or lack adequate endogenous hormones for puberty. Endocrinologists sometimes also offer parents the option of using hormones to try to make a baby boy's small penis grow larger. Again, the evidence that this improves psychosocial or psychosexual outcomes is lacking, and so we are faced with a question of ethics about whether parents should be allowed or encouraged to opt for such treatments. At the very least, these treatments ought to be specifically described to parents as experimental with regard to the psychological outcomes and ought to be carefully followed up. For consent to be informed, parents would also have to be presented the evidence (or lack thereof) that these children are at increased risk for psychological harm if they remain endocrinologically untreated.

Hormone treatments necessary for the induction of puberty typically occur at a time when the child's maturity level allows her or him to participate in decision making, as facilitated by a behavioral health professional. In the event that a child with DSD is entering puberty without a clear sense of gender identity, endocrinologists may offer puberty-delaying medications to allow the child to determine whether she or he wishes to undergo a feminizing or a masculinizing puberty. Although some of the effects of feminizing and masculinizing puberties can be surgically or hormonally undone later (e.g., breasts can be removed), not all can.

Some endocrinologists promote the administration of dexamethasone (DEX) to pregnant women who might be carrying a genetically female fetus at risk of genital virilization. Congenital adrenal hyperplasia (CAH) exhibits an autosomal-recessive mode of inheritance and may lead to 46,XX children being born with various degrees of "masculinized" genitals (including a large clitoris). Prenatal DEX treatments, administered to the mother and transferred to the fetus across the placenta, are meant to prevent genital atypicality. (Note that DEX does nothing to treat the CAH itself, and so an affected child will still have to undergo lifelong endocrinological care to maintain physical health.) Is the use of prenatal DEX ethically problematic?

We see no evidence that atypical genitalia represent an inherent good (e.g., we see no evidence that they promote tolerance of diversity), and in fact we see evidence that they represent an inherent problem. In other words, we do not see why, all other things being equal, a parent should not elect to promote the growth of typical genitalia and prevent the growth of atypical genitalia. Indeed, the fact that DEX treatments might mean a girl is born with a small clitoris and can thus avoid the risks of clitoroplasty would seem to speak in favor of DEX from an ethical standpoint.

The devil of prenatal DEX treatment is in the details. As already noted, CAH is autosomal-recessive. Thus, if both parents are carriers for CAH, there is a 25% (one in four) chance that any fetus conceived will be affected by CAH. But only XX fetuses risk atypical genital development from CAH; therefore, only one in eight fetuses is at risk for the condition meant to be prevented or minimized by DEX. To be effective, DEX treatment must be initiated before clinicians can know whether a woman is carrying a 46,XX child with CAH, which means that 87.5% of fetuses (and their mothers) who receive DEX treatment (and are thus exposed to the risks) cannot benefit from the treatment. Indeed, the number of those not needing treatment is presumably even higher considering that not all girls with CAH experience significant genital virilization in utero.

Were DEX benign, this would cause little concern. However, as the AAP policy on CAH notes, "Maternal adverse effects ... may be serious and long-lasting. Reported adverse effects include edema, excessive weight gain, irritability, nervousness, mood swings, hypertension, glucose intolerance, chronic epigastric pain, gastroenteritis, cushingoid facial features, increased facial hair growth, and severe striae with permanent scarring." Meanwhile, "mothers with previous medical or mental conditions," including psychosis, hypertension, diabetes, and toxemia, may find those conditions aggravated by DEX.[24] Notably, in one study, "one third of the mothers who received dexamethasone treatment during pregnancy would not elect treatment" again.[24] Animal research has also raised concerns about negative somatic and cognitive effects on children who are treated in utero with DEX. Preliminary research on such children shows "that DEX-treated CAH-unaffected children performed poorer than controls on measures of verbal working memory, which was supported by patient-reported difficulties on the Scholastic Competence questionnaire."[25] DEX-Treated CAH-unaffected children also showed increased social anxiety.[26]

Given the risks, unknowns (including unknown risks of DEX, of genital atypicality, and of genital surgery), and significant number of those who are needlessly treated, we would agree with those who have argued that DEX should be used only as part of multicentered clinical studies in which outcome data are meticulously recorded and disseminated, and in which mothers are appropriately advised of the experimental nature and dangers of the procedure.[24,27] Mothers should also be advised as to what is and is not known about the supposed risks of having atypical genitals.

In summary, ethical considerations in cases of DSD are numerous, and thus it is obvious why the DSD consensus statement suggests that medical ethicists be included in teams that manage DSD. Nevertheless, the basic ethical themes that run through DSD care – disclosure of conditions, the need for clinical and scientific attention to the ultimate goals, management of resources, timing of and decision making for elective procedures – are common to much of pediatric care. For this reason, we hope that, rather than causing the reader to consider how DSD represents a special case in pediatrics, we have illustrated how consideration of DSD may sensitize clinicians to ethical issues that are seen more commonly in pediatric care and that may not receive adequate attention.

References

1. Lee PA, Houk CP, Ahmed SF, Hughes IA. Consensus statement on management of intersex disorders: International Consensus Conference on Intersex. *Pediatrics.* 2006;118:488–500.
2. Dreger AD, Chase C, Sousa A, Gruppuso PA, Frader J. Changing the nomenclature/taxonomy for intersex: a scientific and clinical rationale. *J Pediatr Endocrinol Metab.* 2005;18(8):729–733.
3. Dreger AD, Herndon A. Progress and politics in the intersex rights movement: feminist theory in action. *GLQ.* 2009;5:199–224.
4. Meyer-Bahlburg HF. Hormones and psychosexual differentiation: implications for the management of intersexuality, homosexuality, and transsexuality. *Clin Endocrinol Metab.* 1982;11:681–701.
5. Karkazis K. *Fixing Sex: Intersex, Medical Authority, and Lived Experience.* Durham, NC: Duke University Press; 2008.
6. Dreger, AD. "Ambiguous sex" – or ambivalent medicine? Ethical issues in the treatment of intersexuality. *Hastings Cent Rep.* 1998;28:24–35.
7. Wisniewski AB, Migeon CJ, Meyer-Bahlburg HF, et al. Complete androgen insensitivity syndrome: long-term medical, surgical, and psychosexual outcome. *J Clin Endocrinol Metab.* 2000;85:2664–2669.
8. Consortium on the Management of Disorders of Sex Development. *Clinical Guidelines for the Management of Disorders of Sex Development in Childhood.* Rohnert Park, Calif: Intersex Society of North America; 2006. Available at: www.dsdguidelines.org.
9. Dreger, AD, ed. *Intersex in the Age of Ethics.* Hagerstown, Md: University Publishing Group; 1999.
10. Council on Children with Disabilities, American Academy of Pediatrics. Care coordination in the medical home: integrating health and related systems of care for children with special health care needs [policy statement]. *Pediatrics.* 2005;116:1238–1244.
11. Groveman SA. The Hanukkah bush: ethical implications in the clinical management of intersex. *J Clin Ethics.* 1998;9:356–359.
12. Committee on Pediatric AIDS. Disclosure of illness status to children and adolescents with HIV infection. *Pediatrics.* 1999;103:164–166.
13. Lavin LA, O'Malley JE, Koocher GP, Foster DJ. Communication of the cancer diagnosis to pediatric patients: impact on long-term adjustment. *Am J Psychiatry.* 1982;139:179–183.
14. Reiner WG, Gearhart JP. Discordant sexual identity in some genetic males with cloacal exstrophy assigned to female sex at birth. *N Engl J Med.* 2004;350:333–341.
15. Mazur T. Gender dysphoria and gender change in androgen insensitivity or micropenis. *Arch Sex Behav.* 2005;34:411–421.
16. Dreger AD. *Hermaphrodites and the Medical Invention of Sex.* Cambridge, Mass: Harvard University Press; 1998.
17. Money, J. *Hermaphroditism: An inquiry into the Nature of a Human Paradox.* Doctoral dissertation. Harvard University; 1952.
18. Matta C. Ambiguous bodies and deviant sexualities: hermaphrodites, homosexuality, and surgery in the United States, 1850–1904. *Perspect Biol Med.* 2005;48:74–83.

19. Reis, E. *Bodies in Doubt: An American History of Intersex.* Baltimore: Johns Hopkins University Press; 2009.
20. Reilly JM, Woodhouse CR. *Small penis and the male sexual role. J Urol.* 1989; 142:569–571.
21. American Academy of Pediatrics policy statement: informed consent, parental permission, and assent in pediatric practice (RE9510). *Pediatrics.* 2001;95:314–317.
22. Parens E, ed. *Surgically Shaping Children: Technology, Ethics, and the Pursuit of Normality.* Baltimore: Johns Hopkins University Press; 2006.
23. Sousa, A. Talking with your doctor about HRT. Intersex Society of North America; 2005. Available at: http://www.isna.org/faq/hrt_sousa.
24. Section on Endocrinology, and Committee on Genetics, American Academy of Pediatrics. Technical report: congenital adrenal hyperplasia. *Pediatrics.* 2000;106:1511–1518.
25. Sandberg DE, Cognitive functions in children at risk of CAH treated prenatally with dexamethasone. *Growth, Genetics, and Hormones.* 2007; 23. Available at: http://www.gghjournal.com/volume23/2/ab18.cfm.
26. Hirvikoski T, Nordenstrom A, Lindholm T, et al. Cognitive functions in children at risk for congenital adrenal hyperplasia treated prenatally with dexamethasone. *J Clin Endocrinol Metab.* 2007;92:542–548.
27. Sytsma SE. The ethics of using dexamethasone to prevent virilization of female fetuses. In: Sytsma SE, ed. *Ethics and Intersex.* Dordrecht: Springer, 2006:241–258.

C

THERAPIES

12

Rationality, Personhood, and Peter Singer on the Fate of Severely Impaired Infants

Eva Feder Kittay

"The one thing having a child does is make a philosopher out of a parent." So opens an op-ed piece in the aftermath of the infamous Baby Doe case, an infant with Down syndrome whose parents reluctantly made a decision to let their infant die. If having a child makes every parent a philosopher, having a child with cognitive disabilities makes a philosopher who becomes a parent a far humbler philosopher.

I was a philosophy graduate student when my daughter Sesha was born. She was picture-perfect at birth. It wasn't until Sesha was 4 months old that we suspected a problem. At 6 months, our pediatric neurologist suggested that we visit another doctor for an assessment. This neurologist gave us the news straight – straight up, no soda, no ice, and no palliatives. A two-minute exam and the words "Your daughter is severely to profoundly retarded." When we returned home, I was violently ill. My poor husband had to care for both Sesha and me that terrible night.

Now, I am not suggesting that I took the news worse because philosophy was my chosen trade. But loving Sesha and loving the life of the mind forced me to think – to feel – differently about that latter love. My own child could not share its treasures, could not even remotely approach that which had, I had thought, given my life its meaning. I had to reassess the meaning and value of cognitive capacities as the defining feature of humanity. I discovered that a love for one's child transcended any denumerable set of defining characteristics. What it meant to be human, to have value as a person, would never be the same for me again.

The yardstick I bring to the truth and value of a philosophical position is its ability to embrace a person such as my daughter. Professor Singer's views, I think, fall short. But first let me say that my views are not always at odds with Singer's. Like Singer, I reject the sanctity of a human life ethic

First published in the *APA Newsletter on Philosophy and Medicine*, Winter 2000. Reproduced with the permission of Eva Kittay and the American Philosophical Association.

when it insists on the moral impermissibility of abortion. This ethic also insists that hastening the death of infants and adults who persist in a vegetative state or whose condition is terminal and who face a lingering and painful death is always morally impermissible. I think these positions are wrong and cruel, and that Singer is perfectly correct to challenge them and is courageous to force the argument. Singer takes a quality-of-life ethic in place of a sanctity-of-life ethic. I agree that this approach is preferable. But as Singer deploys it, I find it problematic.

I contrast my views with Singer's, by:

1. disputing that the concept of personhood is given by a denumerable set of attributes, especially ones that privilege cognitive capacities;
2. questioning Singer's coupling speciesism with questions concerning severe human impairments; and
3. challenging the primacy of the impartialist ethics that guides Singer's project.

Instead I argue for a view of personhood in which our relationships to others figure centrally, which affirms species membership as having moral significance, and which affirms partiality as appropriate for certain ethical considerations. I take from a feminist ethics of care a number of key concepts that contrast with the ethics, old and new, that Singer both attacks and adopts. An ethic of care stresses the actual relations we have to particular others and the need to maintain connection and to avoid harm. To privilege an abstract sanctity of human life over the particular concerns of the individuals who live these lives is to fail to attend to the needs of, to fail to be responsive to, those whose lives are affected. The embryo may be human, but it is not a human life. To exclude embryos from moral considerability doesn't commit one, on pain of contradiction, to give up a commitment to the moral specialness of membership in the human species. One can privilege species membership without having to include all forms of human life, only all those humans who live these lives.

An ethic based on the quality of life is less abstract because it is always someone's quality of life that is under consideration. But what is a good quality of life? Whose notion of quality is under consideration? The philosopher's? The physician's? The as-yet-unhumbled philosopher answers as Locke did to the question of what constitutes personhood. With Locke, Singer offers to define a person as one who is "a thinking intelligent being that has reason and reflection and can consider itself, the same thinking thing in different times and places." The physician is hardly less invested in cognitive capacities.

Few would think to say that a good quality of life is getting wonderful hugs and kisses, clapping to your favorite song, giving endless joy to your parents and caretakers, teaching love without uttering a word. Not that the philosopher and the physician couldn't accept this as a life with quality when seeing the joy, but joy – giving it and experiencing it – somehow has rarely made the list of attributes that confer personhood.

Whence does that joy derive? Largely from loving, caring relations with others and with what is beautiful in life, what we can find of beauty in life: a smile, a penetrating look, a mournful strain of music, the cool fluidity of water. Well, the philosopher responds, animals can appreciate some of this as well – isn't Singer right after all then? Isn't it simply speciesism that favors your daughter over the gorilla Koko?

Singer (in *Rethinking Life and Death*) attempts to convince us by conjuring up an institution for the retarded, which it turns out is not for mentally disabled humans, but for full-functioning chimpanzees. However, the preferred setting for a person with retardation is in the community, in the home of her family, or living near where her relationship to her family can be maintained, where she can develop relations with others in the community. If there is no call to integrate chimps into the (human) community, it is because chimps do not have a human community into which to integrate – instead they have a community among "their kind." In contrast, the segregation of retarded persons, it has been argued, is no more morally benign than racial segregation.* So there seems to be a moral difference, after all, between humans who are retarded and chimpanzees. What has gone wrong? Is it that the discrimination against the disabled is not akin to racism, or is it that preference for members of the human community is not akin to racism?

What is left out of the talk of morally relevant attributes is that they, like the ethic they are called upon to overturn (i.e., the ethic of the sanctity of life), are abstracted from the actual lived lives of those who bear them. It is a flawed view that derives, at least in part, from a philosophical hubris, a hubris that vanishes with the birth of a child with severe impairments – impairments that cut directly to the set of attributes put forth in abstraction of the individuals to whom we relate and whose lives and well-being are constitutive of our own identity and happiness.

Living for nearly 30 years with a daughter who arguably does not fit the list of attributions that Singer adopts from Locke, I would have to reject the notion that my child is a person or reject the criteria. It's a simple choice. Sesha, and the many children and adults I have met in these many years who have similarly severe impairments, are persons. Their personhood gives lie to the definitional claims of the list Locke and Singer provide. Perhaps it's just the wrong list. The burden of proof is on the proponent of an attribute criterion of personhood to come up with a better list. But to borrow from Tolstoy, "all unimpaired humans are alike; all humans with severe impairments are impaired in their own special way." We can retain

---

* This idea was recently affirmed in a Supreme Court decision; see *Olmstead v. L.C. and E.W.*

some characteristically human capacities and lose others. What is lost and what is retained determines how much of the scope of human existence we can partake in. It does not and should not determine our personhood.

Who we understand to be persons, I suggest, begins (but does not end) with those to whom we stand in relation, not as generalized others, but as concrete others. Feminist theorists have argued that an "unencumbered" self, a self for whom relations to others is not constitutive of identity, is an abstraction masking multiple dependent and interdependent relations to others. They have argued that the very formation of a self depends on the interrelation with the earliest caregivers, that both our desires and our second-order desires are ineluctably shaped by the communities in which we live and the relationships in which we find ourselves. There is no coherent sense of self, or of oneself as a person, that does not rely for its very constitution on relations with others, beginning with those with whom we are closest. What it is to be a self, what it is to be a person is to be enmeshed in a network of relations that are constitutive of that self.

Just as we come to understand ourselves as persons in and through relations with others, so we come to understand others as persons in and through relationships. But here relationship need no longer be confined to those with whom we are in actual relationship. I propose that this extension is properly made to all those whose possibilities are also our own possibility. Imaginatively extending my relations to those others in whom I see their situation as a possibility for myself is a (if not the) crucial move to seeing our connection to all human beings. Here species membership returns as having moral relevance and distinguishes itself from racism. Any human being – of whatever race, sex, religion, age, ability, limitation, and so on – presents a field of possibilities, which the moral imagination grasps as my own possibilities. This is truer still as I understand myself in relational terms. While I am white, I could have a child or grandchild who is black or of a religion or ethnicity that is not my own. But even the nearest ape does not stand in this relation to me (unless it turns out, as Singer speculates in *Rethinking Life and Death*, that chimpanzees and humans are sufficiently close genetically that they can interbreed). This species partiality in no way suggests that I have any right to wantonly kill, imprison, injure, or mistreat chimps, or any other beings – no more than a partiality to my own child gives me a warrant to mistreat another's child.

The utilitarian principle of the equal consideration of interests seems to suggest that such partiality to our own children is not warranted. Yet even on consequentialist grounds, one could argue that partiality is required in certain sorts of distributions, that an equal consideration of interests in certain contexts would serve everyone rather badly. Imagine having each of us give of ourselves equally to each and every child, whether or not they be our own (biological or adopted). It isn't clear that any child would receive the sort of intense concentration of attention and care that she requires to survive and thrive. So, at the very least, this form of distribution would not be very efficient or effective. Much better to have these vulnerable persons assigned to the care of a relatively few persons who behave not in impartial ways to them, but with partiality.

I understand the above arguments to mean that we cannot claim humans are not properly persons if they do not have the appropriate attributes. Therefore, we cannot claim that infants, whether or not impaired, and severely retarded human are not persons by pointing to their lack of the stipulated attributes. Then, defending the appropriateness of letting infants die or killing them, whatever their condition or ability, by claiming that they are not persons will not do. This of course means that the justification of killing or letting severely impaired infants die because they are not persons also fails.

Singer recognizes that while the attributes necessary for personhood are not fully acquired until well after infancy, there are social considerations that demand that the baby be considered a person prior to their attainment. Yet birth, he claims, is an arbitrary place to mark the beginning of personhood, for the full-term fetus is indistinguishable from the newly born babe, and other cultures often choose a time after birth to confer personhood.

If we take personhood to consist of satisfying a list of attributes, then birth is arbitrary. The full-term fetus differs from the newborn only in its physical separation from its mother – and to the extent that it depends on mother's milk for nutrition, it isn't even all that separate. If personhood is conferred, at least in part, by relationship, then it is less arbitrary. While this being is still within, we don't know it yet. The moment of birth establishes a point where relationship can begin in earnest, so to speak; it is the moment after which the care of a mothering person is necessary to sustain it and bring it into the human community.

Yet birth is arbitrary even for forming a relationship with the baby. Relationship may be established prior to birth. Before birth, prospective mothers will speak of the fetus as "the baby." Alternatively, relationship may be postponed until the infant is welcomed not only by the mother and father, but by the community. Membership into the community solidifies personhood.

The question of whether our own society should move from accepting birth as the socially agreed-upon dividing line should perhaps be split, as it is in Hebraic law, into the case of the full-term baby and the very premature neonate.

I think a close look will reveal that the reasons for which other societies have postponed and still postpone personhood either fail to apply to our own situation (for instance, when the justification has to do with scarcity, harsh living conditions, or the need to space children) or are morally unacceptable on other grounds, such as sex discrimination (as when infanticide is selectively practiced on girls). An affluent society, with access to birth control, with resources to care for disabled persons, and a commitment to gender equality, such as our own, does not share the bases on which traditional societies have justified infanticide. The only remaining justification is based on the emergence of new medical technologies for premature neonatal care. As one mother Singer quotes puts it, "[Sometimes] it is hard to distinguish a premature birth from a late spontaneous abortion." Even here, I am not so sure. Many parents look at the tiny being in its sterile bubble with tubes and wires – looking so unlike a baby – and still see their son or their daughter. Once a parent sees the infant as her child, she sees the infant as a person.

If there are not very strong justifications for moving the line, decisions about the fate of the infant have to be made in light of the infant's personhood. Then, who decides why a very ill and disabled infant should continue to fight for life? I agree with Singer that it must be the parents, together with the physician (although the role of the physician is very problematic). I think that a relational conception of personhood would demand that those who have the responsibility for the care of the child, usually the parents or the mother, must have the first, if not also the last, word about the fate of the infant. If they (and especially the mother) do not or will not take on this responsibility, they can, in generosity, relinquish it to another. Even then, it remains the prerogative of the mother, in particular, to relinquish her responsibility to another. The mother who has made the connection to the child, whose own personhood and interests are now (and so forever) entwined with the child, may judge – perhaps incorrectly, but it must be her judgment – that the child cannot have a worthwhile existence with her or another.

Parents faced with a child with severe impairments at the start of life have to make terrible decisions in a very short period of time. And they have almost no time to educate themselves. The society at large aggravates the situation by providing so little in the form of understanding what a life with disabilities is like, what a family with a disability is like, and, worse still, by providing so few resources to persons with disabilities and to their families. This makes the prospect of having to handle this situation so much more frightening than it need be. Furthermore, society does the family and the child a major disservice in so poorly preparing physicians to understand what it means to raise a child with severe disabilities, what sort of life a person with cognitive disabilities can lead. Such a person, in the best of all worlds, can have a very wonderful life and can be the source of enormous joy for others as well. My daughter has a wonderful life and she, along with my son, is the light of my life, and my partner's and her grandmothers', and a person of central importance to the many who have helped care for her.

What would I say if I were in the nursery with the mother who, learning that her otherwise healthy infant has Down syndrome, says to her husband,

"I don't want it, duck." Do I think it was appropriate for the physician, hearing this, to sign the orders "nursing care only" and allow the child to quietly starve while under heavy sedation? Or to do as Singer suggests would be still better, to actively kill the infant with a lethal injection?

Although I could not say to a mother faced with a very premature infant with severe medical complications, whose survival was uncertain and whose outcome would surely involve significant cognitive damage and medical problems, "Without a doubt, do everything to save this child," I find it very hard to accept the actions of this family and this physician. They seem based on ignorance and prejudice and not on a realistic assessment of the hardships of the family or the life prospects of the child. Furthermore, there are increasing numbers of persons who could relate to a child with Down syndrome, who could find joy here. In this case it would be more decent and generous to allow this particular infant the opportunity to form its connections to another – for the parents to relinquish him to others who could love him.

Birth matters here because birth allows the infant to form relations to persons other than the mother, and when there are others there to fill the void left by the biological parents, there is some very important violation. Perhaps it is that all the consideration here is for the family and none for the infant. If the alternative were to consign the infant to an impersonal and inadequate institution, perhaps such a decision might be justifiable – because the concern was for the happiness or misery of the child that would grow up.

To insist on a relational concept of the person is not to say that when the relationship is not made there is nothing there – one can create a relationship that makes personhood possible only to the sorts of beings who can become persons. Those sorts of beings, I argued earlier, are those whose possibilities are always our own possibilities. I may not become a person with Down syndrome, but I could become a person with diminished cognitive faculties. Once we understand that such a life can still be a fully human life, one well worth living, it is harder to accept the fate of the child of the mother who whispered to her husband, "I don't want it, duck." But hers is a failure of moral imagination that indicts our society and its failure to acknowledge the full personhood and humanity of the many disabled persons. Although I do not mean to accuse Singer of excluding disabled adults from personhood, the marking of severely impaired infants as so easily excluded from personhood works to reinforce a prejudice that, like all prejudice, is vicious and harmful. When we conclude that sometimes an infant's life is best ended, it is a person whose life we are thinking of, just as we sometimes come to this conclusion at other moments in persons' lives. And as in the latter case, it is never only one individual's life that is involved – the decisions are decisions for those individuals whose own personhood is intertwined with the life that hangs in the balance. When we make that choice, when we determine whether that life is a quality life, we must think beyond narrow prejudices.

The life of the mind surely has its charms – and is even an indispensable part of the human project. But thinking, rational reflection, the high cognitive skills required even for rudimentary speech remain a part only, and most surprising to the philosopher, not even the most important part, of what it is to be human and what it means to participate in the highest value. I gleaned this in my early days with Sesha, while still a graduate student. In time, I became a philosopher. Graduate school, colleagues, books, writing, a lot of disciplined thinking turned me into one. However, Sesha, my profoundly cognitively disabled child, has taught me my most important philosophical lessons – if she has not made me a better philosopher, she has surely made me a humbler one.

13

The Ethics of Controlling Reproduction in a Population with Mental Disabilities

Paul A. Lombardo

Human sexuality is a battleground of both law and ethics, and it becomes an even more contentious topic when the sex lives of people with disabilities are at stake. Attitudes toward sexual behavior among the disabled appear to have changed remarkably little recently. As one commentator has put it, the "taboos and stigmas ordinarily associated with sexual behavior are inevitably enhanced when juxtaposed with stereotypes about mental disability."[1]

The potential for discomfort that all parents can face when confronted with the advent of sexual activity on the part of their children is no less present when those children are disabled. In fact, the dependence of some of those children on their parents for support and protection for an entire lifetime can heighten the likelihood of that discomfort and exacerbate parent–child conflicts.

The simultaneous need to respect the autonomy interests of people with disabilities – including their potential for sexual activity and possible parenthood – while not ignoring the very real and often entirely proper paternalism parents and guardians wish to exercise to protect those for whom they care, makes a discussion of contraception or other reproductive issues among this population very complicated. There are very few clear legal and ethical directives that apply to every case. I would like at the outset to assert one principle I do think is clear: people with disabilities have no fewer legal rights and no fewer ethical prerogatives in expressing their sexuality than people without disabilities. Though it takes little effort to imagine a factual context that would make the parent or guardian of a person with a severe physical disability conclude that his or her child or ward was an unlikely or inappropriate candidate for sexual activity, so long as the child or ward is a mentally capable decision maker, the default position remains that such a decision is not one for a caretaker to make. My focus in this chapter is not on people with disabilities generally, but instead on reproduction and contraception among people with a compromised capacity for decision making. I will explore topics that lie at the intersection of sexuality, disability rights, and parental prerogatives, then conclude with a checklist of issues that should be reviewed by doctors and caregivers when decisions about reproduction and contraception are faced by a person with mental disabilities.

SEXUAL EXPRESSION AND MENTAL DISABILITY: AN ETHICAL AND LEGAL QUANDARY

A threshold question when we consider how to approach sexuality among the mentally disabled concerns whether they have the capacity to consent to sexual activity. State laws prescribe minimum ages of consent ranging from 14 to 18. Adults (over 18) having sexual relations with children below those ages may be subject to statutory rape laws, which presume that children do not have the capacity to give meaningful consent to sexual activity. Those laws embody the legal principle of state paternalism (*parens patriae*), which is invoked to protect the young and other vulnerable people from ill treatment by those older and more powerful. Children with disabilities, like other children, are protected by statutory rape laws.

Adults, with or without disabilities, are not necessarily protected by such laws. While almost anyone who is coerced into sexual activity against his or her will may invoke sexual assault or rape laws, prohibitions against such coercion contained in those laws usually do not rely on age as a key factor. For people over the state age of consent, a more important question is the individual's capacity to consent. Sex between two people when only one of them is mentally capable of giving consent can create legal liability for the capable person. Yet whether from the vantage point of psychology or the law, the ability to give consent to sexual activity is not a clearly defined capacity. Thus, while it is widely believed that the right to sexual expression is an important human right available no less to the disabled than to others, defining the contours of that right, and specifically categorizing who may or who may not be capable of exercising it, remain elusive tasks. The role of parents of the mentally disabled must be considered against this uncertain backdrop where paternalism and autonomy are in tension.

PARENTAL PREROGATIVES VERSUS RIGHTS TO REPRODUCTIVE PRIVACY

Parents have long enjoyed extensive powers under U.S. law to decide how their children are raised, including the prerogative to seek and consent to medical treatment on their behalf. Guardians standing in the place of parents may exercise the same powers. The United States Supreme Court has endorsed those rights repeatedly, declaring that parents – not the state – are well equipped to decide what is in their children's best interests.[2] But as early Court decisions made clear,[3] parental powers have never been considered absolute, and parental authority may be restricted in the name of a child's welfare. When a child's well-being is at stake, the protective powers of the state are embodied in laws prohibiting neglect and abuse. Those laws stand in the way of parental decisions that might harm a child's health.

The potential for sexual activity by children, as they develop and go through puberty, highlights another area in which parental authority to control children is not always absolute. The sexual behavior of minors, and related decisions about contraception, pregnancy, and childbirth, are features of the ongoing and vigorous debate about reproductive privacy that began in the United States more than 40 years ago.

In 1965 the Supreme Court ruled that states could not prohibit the distribution of contraceptive information and/or devices or criminalize their use by married couples.[4] Less than a decade later, that decision was extended to give access to contraception to all unmarried adults.[5] The landmark decision of *Roe v. Wade* clarified that the right to reproductive privacy announced in those earlier decisions also prevented states from legislating blanket prohibitions on women's termination of their pregnancies. The authority to end pregnancy granted to adult women was then recognized, at some stages of pregnancy, for unmarried minors.[6] Finally, in 1977, the Court said that the right to reproductive privacy also ruled out many legal prohibitions on distributing contraceptives to minors.[7] In none of these cases did the Court intrude on parental rules and family decisions forbidding sexual activity, contraception, or pregnancy termination. What the Court did prohibit were some laws that required doctors, pharmacists, or other health care workers to solicit parental consent before they could provide products and services directly to minors.

Consequently, in many cases health care providers may legally give birth control information and related medical supplies to minors, and directly receive their consent to terminate a pregnancy without first seeking permission from the parents.* This is, of course, an exception to the usual rule requiring adult status to give consent for medical treatment. And at least in principle, there is no distinction between children with disabilities who might seek access to reproductive health services and any other children with similar needs. Several other key life decisions that affect who will or will not have children are also legally regulated.

---

* This statement is not meant to capture every legal detail of how reproductive rights apply to adults and minors, but merely to summarize the general trend in the law away from complete parental control and toward some independent decision making for minors. Every state has different laws that regulate more specifically how that balance is struck.

LEGAL BOUNDARIES TO REPRODUCTIVE DECISIONS

Marriage

The marriage laws in all states require a minimum age and the ability to enter a civil contract as a condition of receiving a marriage license. Even though they may be adults of sufficient age, people without mental disabilities who do not possess the capacity to understand the significance of marriage may be prohibited from marrying by state laws. Though the existence of a court-ordered guardianship could raise a question about the capacity of an adult contemplating marriage to make a contract, absent guardianship status, parental consent is legally irrelevant in this situation.

Contraception

The law would not prevent a parent from consenting to a child's receiving contraceptives or assisting that child in obtaining them. Barrier methods of birth control and most medications, such as birth control pills and other pharmaceutical agents, are routinely dispensed to adolescents who are sexually active. By the same token, adults with mental disabilities who are capable of interacting with their physicians could receive contraceptive agents without parental consent.

Abortion as Contraception

Though it the most ethically contentious reproductive choice, abortion must be grouped among contraceptive options. Approximately 30 states require the consent of one or both parents as a condition of performing an abortion on a minor, and in a few of those states adult relatives other than parents can also give consent. Many states, while not giving parents the prerogative of consenting, specifically require parental notification before an abortion for a minor may occur. Some five states allow abortion to be performed on minors after the parents have been notified, even in the absence of parental consent. More than a dozen states allow minors to consent to abortion without parental permission.

Despite what appears to be a mandate for parental consent in many states, there are many exceptions, including cases where abuse, neglect, rape, or incest has occurred, as well as medical emergencies. Many states also provide a judicial bypass option, in which a court, exercising traditional juvenile or probate court jurisdiction over family matters, can waive the requirement of parental consent.

Assuming the consent of the parent and the disabled patient, abortion is legally available as a contraceptive method in many states. However, in some states abortion, like sterilization, may not be available to people with mental disabilities without a court order.[8]

Sterilization

Any discussion of the sexual sterilization of people with disabilities must include a reference to the history of the eugenics movement in the United States. That history, which is both complex and troubling, has an inescapable impact on how involuntary sterilization is viewed today.

In the first third of the 20th century, advocates invoked the "eugenic" argument that disabled people were the result of defective heredity and would always have disabled children themselves. They also claimed that prohibiting reproduction among the disabled would eliminate the growing costs of public institutions and support for the agencies that cared for them, and hence lessen the general tax burden on other citizens. Between 1907 and 1937, eugenicists were successful in passing laws that authorized surgical sterilization operations on people with physical and mental disabilities, as well as criminals and the poor, in more than 30 states. By 1980, more than 60,000 documented operations had occurred under the aegis of those laws. Eugenic sterilization laws in the United States provided models for sterilization laws in a dozen other countries as varied as Canada, Sweden, Switzerland, and Japan. Most notably, Nazi Germany passed a law in 1934 that led to involuntary surgery on approximately 400,000. Reflections on this history and the abuse of the disabled it often detailed has led seven U.S. states and several other countries in recent years to issue formal repudiations of past eugenic sterilization laws.

Historical research has also revealed that while many states claimed that their laws were administered only as "voluntary" measures, coercion and deception were regularly at work in the sterilization process. Some patients gave consent when they were told that they would undergo other operations, such as appendectomies. Others agreed to surgery as a condition for release from institutional confinement.

The scope of sterilizing surgery was also controversial. Despite common legal prohibitions on "castrating" operations, many women were subjected to ovarian removal or complete hysterectomies rather than the less radical tubal ligation to prevent conception. And men facing vasectomy were sometimes subjected to testicular removal, ostensibly for therapeutic purposes.

Often those "volunteering" for sterilization were not the patients at all. Family members, in many cases the same people who had initiated institutional commitment for patients, agreed to operations for the convenience of the family or because they believed that, by reducing the number of dependent children, such operations served the interests of society at large. In some cases sterilization was used to hide the results of sexual abuse or to punish adolescents for early sexual activity.

Since the mid-1970s, many states have completely repealed their older sterilization laws; others have dramatically rewritten laws to ensure that disabled patients are shielded from future sterilization abuses. Though a few states continue to allow sterilization of people under antique language targeting the "insane, idiotic, imbecile or feebleminded,"* most states that still allow surgical sterilization of a person with mental disabilities surround the process with common procedural protections. Chief among these is the requirement that operations on people who are unable to give informed consent be approved by a judge.

Sixteen states provide specific legislation describing the standards that must be met before sterilization can take place. Fifteen of those states do not allow an operation to go forward without court involvement. Supreme courts in several other states have declared the need for court control over sterilization decisions involving people who are unable to give informed consent. In almost half the states, no clear legislative or judicial guidance on sterilization exists.

The standards established by courts and legislatures have, in most cases, shared two major points of focus. First, does the potential patient have the ability to give informed consent, and second, is the operation truly necessary to prevent conception? Many states also list subsidiary points related to these two.

Pennsylvania is among the states that are at the most protective end of the spectrum. That state's law is outlined in two decisions from the 1980s and 1990s, providing a lengthy checklist that must be followed and suggesting how those standards can be applied in a specific case. The Pennsylvania standards serve as a model for an ethically scrupulous and legally conservative process, and are a starting point for any practitioner looking for guidance when considering involvement in a sterilization case. It should be noted that the rules laid out in the Pennsylvania cases, though they were applied specifically to females, were meant to apply to males as well.

The first case was *In re Terwilliger*, decided in 1982.[9] In *Terwilliger* a man requested an appointment as guardian of his disabled adult daughter so that he could give legal consent to her sterilization by tubal ligation. The case raised the question of whether a court had the power to decide such issues in a state whose legislature had not specifically regulated sterilization procedures. The Pennsylvania court ruled that the ancient principle of *parens patriae* – the inherent governmental authority to protect the mentally infirm or other vulnerable citizens – also applied to making important and irrevocable decisions for people with mental disabilities. Many other states have announced a similar rationale for taking jurisdiction over sterilization decisions.

---

* Mississippi's law, first passed in 1928, continues to reflect the assumption that cognitive disorders of all types are predictably inherited; Arkansas law includes similar language. The West Virginia Code rests on a similar presumption, that one becomes "mentally impaired" as a result of inheriting such a "defect" because it is of "a genetic nature."

The *Terwilliger* court went on to list procedural safeguards for judges to follow when deciding whether they should order involuntary sterilization:

- after a petition for sterilization has been filed, an independent guardian *ad litem* must be appointed for the individual;
- the patient must undergo a thorough medical, physiological, and social examination; and
- the judge must meet with the patient to assess her ability to make decisions.

If the judge finds that:

- the patient is unable to give informed consent, but able to reproduce; and
- sterilization is the only sensible means of contraception,

the judge will analyze the individual case to determine the best interests of the patient, including:

- the likelihood that she will voluntarily or involuntarily engage in sexual activity;
- her ability to understand pregnancy or contraception, both now and in the future;
- the possibility that she will become pregnant;
- the possibility that the individual will experience trauma or psychological damage as a result of pregnancy;
- the feasibility and medical advisability of less drastic means of contraception, now and in the future;
- the advisability of sterilization now rather than in the future;
- the ability of the patient to care for a child, either on her own or with a spouse;
- evidence that medical advances will occur that will make possible either the improvement of the patient's condition or alternative and less drastic sterilization procedures; and
- a demonstration that the people seeking the sterilization are acting in good faith, for the best interests of the patient, and not merely to further their own interests.

The *Terwilliger* court paid particular attention to the rights of disabled patients, who, like others, have a fundamental right to procreate as well as the right to be free of intrusive bodily interventions such as surgery. It concluded that decisions to authorize the sterilization of people unable to make their own medical decisions should rest only on the best interests of the patient, rather than on the interests or convenience of the patient's parents, guardian, or society, and sterilization must be the only practicable means of contraception.

A second Pennsylvania case, *In re Estate of C.W.*, provided an opportunity for a court to apply these standards in the case of a young woman who had significant mental and physical disabilities that complicated the question of whether sterilization could be in her best interests.[10] C.W. was an adolescent whose mother was caught between two conflicting wishes and also wanted to protect her from a devastating medical outcome. She wanted to give her daughter more freedom but was afraid that freedom would make the girl vulnerable to becoming pregnant. C.W. was unable to speak and had been evaluated as having a mental age of 3–5 years and an I.Q. in the range of 30–50. She suffered from moderately severe retardation, organic brain damage grand mal epilepsy, cerebral palsy, and scoliosis. She communicated in a limited way through minimal signing and making certain noises that those around her learned to interpret.

C.W.'s mother asked to be appointed as her guardian, with specific authority to consent to a laparoscopic tubal ligation. Her reasons reflected her desire to increase the range of experience available to C.W., specifically the wish to allow her to live in a sheltered living facility rather than the socially more restricted environment of her mother's home.

C.W.'s mother realized that there were risks to a fuller life and increased liberty for her daughter. Her seizure disorder was extremely severe. In some years, C.W. endured more than 50 seizures, some of which lasted for over an hour. Her medication regimen included daily doses of Phenobarbital, Dilantin, and Tegretol, some in toxic amounts, to control epilepsy. Over time her doctors learned that even this level of medication did not always control the seizures and that infections or other events that caused a fluctuation in her temperature might also lead to a seizure. Without medication, C.W. could face *status epilepticus* and repeated seizures, and such attacks could be fatal.

With increased freedom, the likelihood of a sexual encounter with either a peer or some other man increased, as did the potential for pregnancy. While C.W. was supervised extensively most of the time, there was evidence that she was not directly monitored during the night while living in the group home and that she could come into contact with men at the homes of relatives, where she frequently visited, at her sheltered workshop, and at social gatherings. There was also some evidence of kissing and a developing relationship with a "boyfriend."

C.W.'s mother realized that her daughter, though very affectionate with any man with whom she came into contact, had no understanding of sexual or reproductive functions. While C.W. was physically sexually mature, she was unequipped emotionally for pregnancy and certainly unprepared for parenthood. There was no way to know what impact pregnancy would have on the fluctuations of her endocrine system and how or whether her ongoing medication would be effective in controlling seizures in such a condition; it was also clear that the medication C.W. took was likely to be teratogenic to any fetus she carried. Added to the risk of pregnancy was the likely inability of C.W. to manage the delivery of a child and the consequent need for a cesarean delivery, with accompanying trauma. The uncertain impact of adding contraceptive hormonal medications – from birth control pills to Depo Provera – to the drugs C.W. already took ruled out other birth control options.

To C.W.'s mother, in the absence of highly restrictive social monitoring, which was probably not feasible in a group living setting, sexual activity for C.W. remained a real possibility; contraception was problematic, and pregnancy was out of the question.

The Pennsylvania court that eventually decided C.W.'s case used the *Terwilliger* standards to analyze her interests. A wide array of professionals testified, assessing C.W.'s situation from the medical, psychological, and social perspectives. The court rejected the suggestion that more training coupled with additional supervision would protect C.W. from pregnancy, saying that such an approach was extremely restrictive and contrary to principles requiring the integration of a person with disabilities into the wider society. It concluded that a mini-laparoscopy in which the fallopian tubes are cauterized in one section could be performed on an outpatient basis, was effective as a contraceptive measure, and was potentially reversible. That procedure was also less problematic and more effective than barrier contraceptive methods and would bypass the potential ill effects of birth control medications on a person with C.W.'s medical history. After a lengthy course of litigation, C.W. was sterilized.

Some judges on the C.W. court panel were critical of the decision and issued a dissent. They believed that other birth control methods should at least be tried before physicians resorted to the surgical option. Perhaps most telling was the objection that sterilization should not be considered when there was no evidence of voluntary sexual activity. Sterilization, they said, would not protect C.W. from the potential for rape or sexual abuse and consequences other than pregnancy, such as sexually transmitted diseases, and an operation could encourage complacency on the part of her caregivers.

Despite the outcome in favor of sterilization, the unusual facts of the C.W. case and the process the court followed in reaching that conclusion make it a good model to review when considering sterilization more generally. The case emphasizes the ethical expectation that surgical sterilization is a dramatic option because it represents a serious invasion of bodily integrity for people with disabilities, no less than for others. We are forced to consider whether sterilization is being proposed "therapeutically" for the benefit of the patient or primarily as a convenience for others. The case reminds us of the lessons of history – that people with mental disabilities have been repeated victims of sterilization policies. They have been subject to deception, coercion, and punishment for expressing their sexuality, often without regard for their level of comprehension or potential for functioning in society.

TWO RECENT CASES

There are a wide range of state laws on sterilization, some lengthy and involving close court oversight, others giving doctors a good deal of discretion in performing sterilization operations on any patient, including one with mental disabilities. Many state court cases have emphasized the need for protecting people with disabilities and other vulnerable patients from sterilization abuse, while others have insisted that making sterilization too difficult is itself an abridgment of rights.[11] Those cases conclude that the right to be sterilized is consistent with the right to choose to marry or have a family, rights that are protected under the general rubric of reproductive freedom. Sterilizing operations have been a focal point of two cases that have appeared in the press and have been the subject of much commentary. One involved extensive surgery, the other a tubal ligation.

Ashley X: The Pillow Angel

In early 2007, news reports detailed a controversy that had developed around what came to be called "the Ashley treatment." The treatment was proposed for a 6-year-old girl in Seattle, Washington, whose parents wished to initiate extensive and radical "medical treatment" that they felt was in their daughter's interests. The girl had been diagnosed at age 3 with static encephalopathy, and her prognosis did not include further mental development. At age 6, she could not sit up, speak, walk, feed herself, or perform any of the behaviors of most children her age. The proposed interventions included surgically removing the girl's breast buds so that her breasts would not develop, giving her a hysterectomy to eliminate the onset of menarche and prevent her from conceiving, and giving her high doses of estrogen that would ensure she would not grow. These steps would ensure that Ashley would not grow larger or develop sexually, making it easier for her family to care for her at home and eliminating many sources of potential discomfort for her.

After consultation with and approval from a hospital ethics committee, doctors performed the interventions the family had requested. When the case became public, the reactions from pediatricians, bioethicists, and others ranged from approval to outrage. Only after the surgery had been completed was it revealed that the hospital where the operations took place was unaware that Washington State law required a court order before the sterilization of a mentally disabled person could take place. The hospital was investigated by Washington State's Protection and Advocacy System, which produced a lengthy report condemning the "Ashley treatment" as a violation of Ashley's legal rights and a process that should not have been initiated without a court order. The hospital admitted to having violated the law and agreed not to sterilize any developmentally disabled person in the future without court authorization and to submit to ongoing monitoring of its policies and procedures.[12] The case ultimately highlighted the difference between surgery that removed organs, like a hysterectomy, and other sterilizing operations, as well as the importance of following state law when proceeding in such cases involving a patient with disabilities.

In re Estate of K.E.J.

A 2008 Illinois appellate court case raised other issues.[13] When she was a child of 8 years, K.E.J. survived a car accident that left her with serious brain damage. At age 24, she was sexually active, but receiving birth control medication. Her mother filed a petition asking the court to order a tubal ligation for K so that she could not become pregnant. K's mother believed that the surgery would not be as great a medical burden for her daughter as was birth control medication (K had endured significant weight gain as a result of the birth control methods she was using) and would obviate the need for the mother to monitor multiple medications for K. After a trial, a judge decided that K was incapable of making the decision on her own but refused to order sterilizing surgery. He said that surgery should be only a last resort after other methods of birth control had been tried and proved unworkable. Before her mother's court petition, K had not used birth control pills or an IUD and had not tried several other types of birth control.

The Illinois appellate court confirmed this result, declaring that K's best interests could be served with a less drastic form of birth control. It quoted from Pennsylvania's *Terwilliger* case in support of the need to measure the best interests of a person unable to give informed consent from that person's perspective, without regard for the needs of his or her family or society at large. The court noted that Illinois had no law specifically regulating sterilization, but its general law regulating the treatment of people with disabilities demanded that guardians attempt to make decisions for people they care for by adhering as closely as possible to what the ward, if competent, would have wished for themselves. The court accepted as good evidence K's repeated protestations against surgery.

CONCLUSION

K.E.J. is the most recent case concerning sterilization to have been decided at the state level. It reiterated several principles that are important for any caregiver to remember when considering a sterilizing operation for a person with mental disabilities.

First, consider the wishes of the potential patient. People with mental disabilities, though not always legally competent or able to give fully informed consent, nevertheless are often able to voice their own desires and fears. Respect for the autonomy of such people requires that we not dismiss their concerns out of hand or give short shrift to their stated wishes for or against surgery.

Second, consider all the alternatives. Permanent birth control in the form of surgical intervention must be justified by something more than a vague concern about future pregnancies. An existing opportunity for sexual activity should be demonstrated and a permanent inability to parent should also be assessed. Many less drastic means of birth control should be considered before surgery is chosen.

Third, enlist the services of other professionals before deciding to perform surgery. The perspectives of other clinicians, social workers, bioethicists, and lawyers will generate a more complete picture of a patient's wishes, rights, and needs than most guardians can provide, and the patient's welfare is paramount in these cases.

Finally, become familiar with state law. For the reasons I have already outlined, in many states sterilization is governed by a specific statute that intentionally makes it more difficult to perform any operation to which the patient does not personally give consent. In other states where no such law exists, there are still serious obstacles to operating without court approval. For important ethical and legal reasons, involuntary sterilizing surgery is not considered a process that should be contemplated without serious deliberation and extensive professional consultation.

References

1. Perlin ML. Hospitalized patients and the right to sexual interaction: beyond the last frontier. *NYU Rev Law Social Change.* 1993–1994;20:517–548.
2. *Parham v. J.R.*, 442, U.S. 584 (1979). The *Parham* case confirmed the rights of parents to commit their children to mental facilities without the full "due process" hearing required for adults.
3. *Prince v. Massachusetts*, 321 U.S. 158 (1944). *Prince* upheld a child labor law that prohibited a woman from using a 9-year-old girl to sell religious literature.
4. *Griswold v. Connecticut*, 381 U.S. 479 (1965). *Griswold* struck down laws prohibiting the distribution of birth control information and devices.
5. *Eisenstadt v. Baird*, 405 U.S 438 (1972).
6. *Planned Parenthood of Missouri v. Danforth*, 428 U.S. 52 (1976).
7. *Carey v. Population Services International*, 431 U.S. 678 (1977).
8. See, e.g, Virginia Code § 54.1–2969 and § 16.1–241.
9. *In re Terwilliger*, 450 A.2d 1376 (Pa. Super Ct. 1982). *Terwilliger* was guided by earlier cases in other states such as *In re Grady*, 426 A 2d 467 (NJ 1981), decided by the Supreme Court of New Jersey.
10. *Estate of C.W.*, 433 Pa.Super. 167, 640 A.2d 427 (1994).

11. Valerie N., 707 P. 2d 760 (Cal. *1985*).
12. Carlson D, Dorfman, DA. Investigative report regarding the "Ashley treatment." Washington Protection & Advocacy System, May 8, 2007. Available at: www. wpas-rights.org. Accessed June 20, 2008.
13. *In re Estate of K.E.J.*, 887 N.E.2d 704, 320 Ill.Dec. 560 (2008).

14

Pediatric Innovative Surgery

Angelique M. Reitsma

INTRODUCTION

Pediatric innovative surgery signifies something of an ethical "double jeopardy," as it incorporates two distinct yet intertwined ethical challenges. First, there is the significant challenge to achieve a proper balance between advancing surgery and offering the appropriate level of protection to children who participate in research.[1,2] Equally challenging is identifying which innovations in essence constitute human subject research, requiring all of the existing mechanisms put in place to protect children as research participants.[1,2] These unresolved ethical issues in pediatric surgery – what constitutes research or innovation generate – persuasive arguments, making innovation in pediatric surgery an especially fascinating and perplexing area of bioethics, attracting public attention and concern.[2] As I will argue in this chapter, current federal regulations and governmental bodies currently do not have a firm grasp on surgical innovation in general, and therefore adult and pediatric patients alike are sometimes at risk of becoming involuntary participants of (informal) research studies, regardless of the otherwise stringent regulations that are in place to protect children as especially vulnerable participants of research. I will also discuss extensively the recent endeavors of both multidisciplinary committees and the surgical community proper to resolve this impasse.

EXISTING PROTECTIONS

During the past decades, there have been major improvements in the area of human subject research protection. Nowadays, it would be unthinkable to enroll a patient or a healthy volunteer, adult or child alike, in a clinical trial without his or her parental consent or pediatric assent, a requirement that was not obvious to early investigators.[1-4] Let us consider the existing regulations that guide research with human subjects, including children.

The Department of Health and Human Services (DHHS) has set forth regulations pertaining to all human subject research in the federal rule 45 CFR 46, which has also been dubbed "the Common Rule"[5] (latest revision, 2005) because it has been adopted by almost all federal agencies. The Common Rule sets out definitions for research (systematic investigations designed to develop or contribute to generalizable knowledge) and for a human subject (a living person from whom data are obtained either through direct interaction or via the use of personal identifiable information or bodily samples). Every person participating in a research study should do so willingly and voluntarily, with prior informed consent, assent where appropriate, and protected by the safeguards that the Common Rule provides (such as prior review of studies by an institutional review board [IRB] to assess the risk–benefit ratio of the proposed trial and the provision that a participant can voluntarily withdraw from the study at any time). For children, the Common Rule has additional provisions as set out in Subpart D (concerning research involving children) and, to a certain extent, also in Subpart B, "Additional Protections for Pregnant Women, Human Fetuses and Neonates Involved in Research." As mentioned before[4,6] this subpart, in a convoluted way, really considers only nonviable newborns and neonates of uncertain viability. This makes it even more difficult for the pediatric researcher and IRB to navigate the review and approval process for studies involving neonates, adding to rather than alleviating the confusion surrounding pediatric surgical research. An excellent exposé on the application of these federal regulations can be found in the *Journal of Pediatrics*[1] as well as in this volume, which provides the pediatric surgical or medical investigator with practical guidance.

All research involving human participants, including children, that is performed with federal support (such as National Institutes of Health grants) or within facilities that receive federal money (e.g., through Medicare and Medicaid) falls under this regulation. This implies that surgical research conducted *without* direct or indirect federal funding is beyond the jurisdiction of the DHHS's Office of Human Research Protections.[7] The development of new drugs and medical devices is closely monitored by the federal government. The Food and Drug Administration (FDA)[8] regulates biological agents, devices, and drugs by reviewing their safety and efficacy for a given indication before granting approval for marketing and distribution. The labeling (package insert) summarizes what the FDA has deemed the safe and effective use of the product, and so-called off-label use of a product, although allowed, may be subject to regulatory scrutiny. When an innovative surgical procedure does *not* include a device, biological agent, or drug, the FDA has no guidance for or jurisdiction over its development and introduction into clinical practice.

IDENTIFYING INNOVATIONS AS RESEARCH

Regardless of these significant advances, informed consent for all surgical research is still not taken for granted. Innovative surgery remains an elusive entity within clinical research. Very often, it somehow evades the currently accepted standards for human subject research, such as obtaining informed consent and assent for research participation and prior IRB approval.[9,10] Every day, surgeons everywhere modify existing operations, attempting to improve their technique and outcomes. Surgeons have historically been idea generators and creative practitioners within their craft.[3] Sometimes this occurs on an individual patient basis; sometimes a group of patients undergoes an innovative procedure. Sometimes a group of patients serves as a prospective or historical control. Innovative surgeries find their way into professional journals and conferences as case reports, case series, or case-control studies, and a very small percentage as prospective clinical trials. But many, perhaps most, of them have one thing in common: they were performed under the heading of innovative therapy, not of research. Whether they started out as spontaneous technique modifications, necessary for a particular patient situation, or as informal studies with or without protocols, most innovations were performed without prior IRB approval and without specific research consent from parents and assent from pediatric patients. In some instances, such review and consent would have been appropriate and necessary; at other times it would not. For some innovations, the need for IRB submission and parental consent and patient assent would have been obvious – for example, in the case of a major surgical procedure carrying high risks – for others, not quite so much – for example, for small or incremental modifications to surgical technique.[11] This uncertainty makes it particularly difficult for surgeons to decide if and when they should seek IRB review and consent in their efforts to improve surgery, unless the study involves an investigational drug or device.[11,12]

Margo[13] confirmed the previously mentioned limitations of current federal regulations when he explained how surgical innovators circumvent outside scrutiny by viewing human research in narrow terms as an activity outlined in a formal protocol. It is only the existence of a protocol that makes the occurrence of research rather than innovative clinical care obvious to the surgeon. It seems that so long as there is no prior intention to learn anything that could be applied to other patients from the process, one cannot be held to be doing research as per the formal DHHS definition that includes "generalizable knowledge" as a prerequisite. The majority of surgical publications involve interventional case reports that concern a series of patients; outcome measures are usually clinical parameters that are obtained during routine clinical follow-up, without any type of formal written protocol. The implicit assumption here is that the clinical hypothesis was not formalized until after the therapeutic intervention. These types of "informal research" are viewed as clinical care and are therefore invisible to IRBs.

The slippery concept of innovation could be applied to all areas of medicine, but surgery has most frequently made use of the term. The somewhat exceptional position of innovative surgery within the realm of research and the apparent lack of ethical regulations specifically governing surgical innovation have been long recognized. Internist Henry Beecher wrote as early as 1961:

Ideally, all surgical interventions should be controlled. When real hazard is involved in a new and unproven procedure, it may be urgent to determine the value of such intervention. This is only possible with a proper plan. One may question the moral or ethical right to continue with casual or unplanned new surgical procedures – procedures which may encompass no more than a placebo effect – when these procedures are costly of time and money, and dangerous to health or life.[14]

A group of surgeons wrote 25 years later:

When large numbers of innovative treatments are being continuously introduced into clinical practice, rigorous testing is mandatory for the protection of individual patients and the just use of limited resources. This holds true with even greater force in light of the evidence that many innovations show no advantage over existing treatments when they are subjected to properly controlled study. They may even be less effective, or harmful.[15]

The pediatricians Frader and Caniano[16] suggested:

The era of limitations on health care expenditures and renewed concern about the human burden of unproven medical interventions may herald a sea change in attitudes toward surgery.

Frader and Flanagan-Klygis[17] repeated the call for formal assessment of surgical interventions. Increasingly, from the surgical community proper, there is a call for vigilance toward cavalier innovators and reckless acceptance of procedures and techniques that have not been scientifically tested, some authors even offering solutions.[11,18–31] In her 2007 presidential address to the American Pediatric Surgical Association (APSA), Dr. Donahue discussed the mandate for innovation in pediatric surgery, calling for the maintenance of excellence while effecting change.[32] The APSA already complies with the evolving National Surgical Quality Improvement Project to help accomplish that.[32] Concurrently, the call for evidence-based surgery is growing stronger.[2,33,34] The American College of Surgeons, the most authoritative professional fellowship representing U.S. surgeons, has made it one of its important goals. In 2004, the director of the Association of American Medical Colleges' (AAMC) Council of Academic Societies Affairs contacted the presidents of five major surgical societies, suggesting that leaders of the surgical community provide guidance on this issue.

The objectives of this project were to (1) clarify the distinction between variations (minor modifications not requiring specific disclosure), innovations (modifications of potential significance to the patient, requiring disclosure), and research (systematic investigations designed to develop or contribute to generalizable knowledge); and (2) suggest guidelines to surgeons and hospitals for appropriate implementation and oversight of surgical innovations. The Society of University Surgeons (SUS) chose to pursue this initiative, and a statement, composed by a working group that included surgeons and a bioethicist, recently appeared in a surgical journal.[35]

A few years before this initiative was taken, bioethicists from the University of Virginia conducted a two-year study of the ethics of surgical innovation. The results and conclusions of this project were published in the surgical literature,[11,12] and recommendations for policy change appeared in a book published in the summer of 2006.[36] The rising demand for more ethically sound innovation in surgery from the surgical, the bioethical, and the lay arena appears to be an open invitation for increased and better applicable regulation of clinical surgical research.

THE MORAL PROBLEM

The ethical issues that pediatric surgical innovation may bring about are indeed multifaceted. Surgical innovation is not an unequivocally negative entity but rather an intrinsic part of surgery that is necessary for progress and future improvement of the practice of surgery. As such, it has decidedly positive moral elements. However, other elements and some forms of surgical innovation *do* give rise to moral concern.

The first and perhaps most obvious concern is the threatened respect for a patient's *autonomy*. Respect for autonomy is not a mere ideal in health care; it is a professional obligation.[37] Autonomy, or self-determination, is expressed in the doctrine of informed consent. In the pediatric situation this means that the parent(s) or guardian(s) gives informed consent to participate in research, and the child has an opportunity to voice his or her assent. Essentially, a patient's and the parents' right to self-determination is in jeopardy when he or she is not presented with complete information about the nature of the procedure (experimental vs. accepted) and given the opportunity to elect or reject an offered treatment or participation in an experiment. Good clinical practice in surgery and the standard of professional practice dictate that every surgeon present a patient and his or her parents with all the pertinent information about and alternatives to a suggested procedure, including the nonoperative treatment modalities. This becomes particularly stringent if the suggested procedure is experimental. Information that is necessary for coming to an informed decision includes knowledge about the expected outcome and the risks and benefits of a certain procedure. If such information is unavailable because the procedure has not yet been adequately evaluated, true informed consent and subsequent autonomous decision making are hampered. However flawed and incomplete the informed-consent process may be, it still is an important way to add to the layers of protection surrounding children as study subjects.

A *paternalistic* act occurs when decisions that are necessarily within the scope of patient and parent preferences and a duty to disclose are overridden by the physician. It seems apparent that the consideration of risks and benefits involved in a surgical procedure is necessarily a part of a patient's preference and should be readily disclosed by the treating surgeon. This is unfortunately not always a given in the case of surgical innovation.[2] When risks and benefits are partly or largely unknown, as in the case of innovative procedures, they cannot be fully disclosed or adequately considered. The authorization process would still be ethically acceptable so long as all factors were laid out and a patient's parents were willing to voluntarily have their child undergo a procedure with a (partly) unknown risk–benefit ratio. A possible scenario would be a desperate situation, where no other therapies were available and the surgeon, parents, and patient agreed on using an experimental procedure in a last effort to treat the patient, who would otherwise be facing certain worsening of symptoms or perhaps even demise. In a less dramatic situation, however, a surgeon may not feel as compelled to share every bit of information about an innovative procedure. In general, risk assessment should involve the child and parents as decision makers and, when the procedure is highly experimental, the insight of an IRB as well.

The principle of *nonmaleficence* dictates that a physician refrain from causing harm to the patient and also includes obligations not to impose *risks* of harm. In cases of risk imposition, law and morality recognize a standard of due care that determines whether the agent that is causally responsible for the harm is legally or morally responsible as well. What constitutes harm in the case of surgical innovation can vary. When performing an experimental procedure of unproven utility, a surgeon exposes a patient to unknown risks. These risks can be of great magnitude (the ultimate being death) or of relatively small impact. Jones termed this practice "reckless experimentation," adding that it should always be condemned, regardless of estimated risks.[38]

The principle of *beneficence* consists of three moral norms: (1) one ought to prevent evil or harm, (2) one ought to remove evil or harm, and (3) one ought to promote or do good. Applying these norms to surgical innovation leads to a multifold analysis. When no other therapy is available for a particular patient or diagnosis, performing an experimental procedure, as opposed to doing nothing, can be an act of beneficence. Also, striving to improve surgical care is an act of beneficence and is a trait of the virtuous surgeon. The good surgeon, as determined by most U.S. professional surgical societies, should always aim to better his or her practice and the profession as a whole. Promoting the well-being of future patients is a beneficent act. If it fails to make improvements, surgery eventually becomes outdated, leading to a situation where a surgeon can offer only obsolete and old-fashioned operations to patients. In essence, innovation is an intrinsic and vital part of surgery. Without it, there would be no progress. But progress is never linear; sometimes a few sidesteps are taken. Such sidesteps might be clinical trials in which a surgical technique is put to the test to establish its efficacy and safety. Or they might include monitoring the outcomes of a newly developed procedure clinically, perhaps not in a formal study but nonetheless via a model that is experimental in nature. Patients involved in these very sidesteps deserve adequate protection because the procedures are not of proven utility. In the case of children as a vulnerable population, these protections are appropriately more stringent, although some argue that they are perhaps too stringent, limiting or preventing trials that may involve risk to the child. It is thought that important studies, in which parent and child would participate with fully informed consent, may never be approved.[2]

The principle of *justice* mandates that health care and (scarce) resources be distributed evenly and fairly. In the context of research, it demands that research subjects be selected fairly and without undue pressure being placed on one particular gender or social or racial group. If a medical experiment is formulated into a research protocol, which is subsequently submitted to an IRB for review, attention will be given to fair subject selection. IRBs have guidelines and formulas for even distribution among the various population denominators, to ensure a just selection system. When experimental surgeries are not submitted to IRBs and are performed without protocol and without prior patient population determination, it is highly unlikely that patients will be selected randomly, fairly, or evenly across the general population. This not only may confound the scientific results of the informal study, but also represents an unjust method of patient selection. Certain patient groups may be more heavily burdened, depending on the expected outcomes of the procedure.

When a surgeon presents an innovative procedure as an accepted therapy, the information she is giving is arguably *deceptive*. Unintentionally, the patient and his parents are given a false sense of security that the procedure he is undergoing is of proven utility, when in fact it is not. The surgeon in turn may subconsciously mislead herself into thinking she is doing the right thing for the patient by submitting him to an experimental procedure. The underlying assumption leading to this is, again, that new equals better, when in fact this has not yet been scientifically proven. This is usually done as a framing error, where a procedure is termed a *new treatment*. This situation is not unique to surgery; it occurs often in medicine as well. For example, the off-label use of FDA-approved drugs by physicians is in fact a clinical experiment presented as a validated treatment.

Another way of thinking about the self-deception a surgeon experiences is the existence of bias toward the innovative therapy. This is illustrated by a lack of equipoise.

Equipoise is the existence of true uncertainty about the effectiveness of therapeutic modalities, and it is the basis and prerequisite of any (randomized) clinical trial. If equipoise exists, it is considered ethical to randomize patients or healthy volunteers to test the hypothesis that the new therapy is better than the old one. If in the heart and mind of a surgeon bias exists toward an innovative procedure, true equipoise is absent. This is an added impediment to innovative procedures finding their way into a formal research protocol and through IRB review. Even if the effectiveness, safety, and long-term outcomes of the innovation are unknown, when the performing surgeon is biased toward its (supposed) merits, it will not be put to the test.

SAFETY AND EFFICACY

If history generates concern over experimentation in pediatrics, concern for the field of pediatric surgery should be even more stringent. Surgery, in contrast to other areas in medicine, has been free to develop new operations and treatments without strict requirements of animal testing and prospective human clinical trials. ... Many operations in children were developed without prior study; current outcomes are all too often unknown because of a lack of prospective data.[2]

Many of the operations that are currently in use have never been formally tested in a rigorous scientific trial. They were originally introduced into clinical care as were so many other procedures before and after them: as innovative therapies. As such, they were simply implemented in surgical practice without additional safeguards to protect the patients who underwent these experimental procedures. This has been and largely still is accepted and constitutes everyday surgical practice. Only when the implications of the procedure are enormous, and the risks and stakes are high (life and death issues, e.g., in the case of fetal surgery, heart surgery, and live liver graft transplantations), are the surgical profession and the public alike alerted about their introduction and only then do they rightfully demand that first studies be done to establish efficacy and safety.[39-41] Live donor liver graft transplantations, for example, have received a lot of attention from professionals and have sometimes caused outrage.[42,43] This was especially the case when two healthy donors died after donating a portion of their livers. Transplant surgeons such as Cronin complain that the true morbidity and mortality, let alone the overall efficacy of this innovation, are still largely unknown, while the procedure gains widespread use and popularity regardless.

The less high profile innovative surgeries, however, escape this added scrutiny and eventually find their way into standard clinical care. After a while, the novelty wears off these innovations and they become established techniques, with or without scientific testing. While the *safety* of these procedures will eventually be established through the regular surgical mechanisms (e.g., morbidity and mortality conferences and case reports) and by way of malpractice suits if necessary, their true *effectiveness* may never be known if a randomized controlled clinical trial is never done. When put to the test, some of these much-hyped procedures may prove partially or completely ineffective, at times no better than a placebo. This was shown in the case of internal mammary artery ligation for angina pectoris in the 1950s and, more recently, in adult arthroscopic knee surgery trials.[44,45] The latter trials are perfect examples of how a new procedure gains wide acceptance and is reimbursed by third-party payers even in the absence of strong scientific evidence. When the evidence was finally sought, it turned out that the procedure was no better than the sham surgery: the placebo (Moseley) or the nonoperative treatment modality (Kirkley). The problem in the pediatric situation is that surgical placebo-controlled trials cannot easily be conducted. IRBs would most likely not approve exposing a child to sham surgery, such as in the earlier knee arthroscopic study, as it would constitute a greater than minimal risk, in the absence of justification by anticipated benefit. A randomized trial that compares an existing technique – for example, the currently accepted standard of care – with an innovative procedure may have a better chance of being approved, so long as the risks are justified by the prospect of direct benefit to the participant/ patient. Achieving evidence-based surgery in the pediatric situation is even more complicated than in the adult arena, due to the increased research protections for children.

ULTERIOR MOTIVES

There are several reasons that surgical innovations are continually introduced into practice outside the research realm and without prior formal scrutiny, and reimbursement is one of them. The cost of an experimental technique may not be covered by insurance companies, while the standard of care is. Modifying a procedure to the point of making it highly experimental but still booking it as standard technique will (hopefully) ensure needed reimbursement. The financial incentives to study new drugs (heavily sponsored by pharmaceutical companies) are absent in surgery; this significantly reduces the external entrepreneurial push to innovate within the clinical trial model. Unless a drug or medical device is involved, there is no financial gain for companies to be made; hence, the surgical community has a hard time finding the money to conduct clinical trials involving an experimental procedure alone. These financial disincentives to innovate within the scientific model are considerable and a formidable obstacle to change. Especially for the pediatric situation this appears to be a valid concern, as pediatric surgery has less funding and fewer resources for innovation than do fields with a higher clinical volume.[2] Another motivation is the "cutting edge" factor. As Chisholm et al. found, children's hospitals are more likely than other facilities to adopt innovative surgical procedures, such as laparoscopic appendectomies, even when clear benefit over standard treatment has not been established.[45] In their 2006 study, Chisholm and colleagues reviewed 50,825 pediatric appendectomies and postulated:

Children's hospitals, nearly all of which were teaching facilities, may take a certain pride in offering services that are *perceived* to be better than existing procedures *before* the evidence to prove such superiority exists. In fact, many may want to be part of implementing the procedure early with the goal of helping develop the evidence supporting its value." (emphasis added)

While it is certainly laudable to want to gather data to generate knowledge about a new procedure, the value of such results may be questioned in the absence of true equipoise and a protocol, including a statistical design with adequate power. In effect, the early patients of such innovations serve as human research subjects – guinea pigs – without the necessary protections and perhaps partly in vain, as the true efficacy of the innovation may not be fully established via this informal research route.

As laid out in this chapter, it has been possible for surgical innovations, including those in pediatric surgery, to evade the scrutiny of existing safeguards for human subject research. This has been partly because surgeons *themselves* do not always regard their modifications and innovations as clinical research.[11] As outlined in *Ethical Guidelines for Innovative Surgery*,[36] part of the problem most likely stems from a deficit in education. Some surgeons lack a thorough understanding of federal requirements and the role of IRBs in the conduct of human subjects research.[11,46] More fundamentally, there is uncertainty and disagreement among surgeons about what constitutes routine variation on a surgical technique to accommodate a specific patient's unique circumstances, which requires no prior approval, versus a planned new or innovative technique that warrants specific informed consent, versus an experimental research study that requires formal IRB approval.[11,47] Innovations are therefore not assessed within a formal research protocol and are not submitted for IRB review before implementation of the procedure. Invisible to IRBs, innovations go forward without external oversight. Innovations are not readily defined as research, especially if they constitute incremental modifications. Also, standard of care is more difficult to define in the surgical domain because every surgeon may have a preferred style of performing the same procedure.

The first and foremost problem for the effective oversight of surgical innovations is therefore their vague definition. To aid in the identification and definition of research-like innovations, using certain criteria may be helpful. Sometimes the nature of the innovations is such that they become quite experimental and necessarily enter the realm of research activities. Criteria that would make an innovation a research activity have been discussed by several experts on the matter and have been narrowed down to a few common denominators. Important criteria, as formulated by the Reitsma–Moreno working group in 2006,[48] that distinguish incremental improvements from experimental innovations are the following: intent (if the surgeon plans to perform an innovation with the intent of testing a hunch, informal hypothesis, or theory about it), extent of departure from the standard of care (if significantly different from currently accepted procedure), outcomes (risks and benefits are largely unknown or not adequately described in the international professional literature), and risks involved (greater perceived risk indicates greater need for scientific scrutiny).

In 2008, a group from the SUS came out with recommendations for guidelines rooted firmly in the earlier Reitsma–Moreno criteria. The group, in collaboration with Reitsma and Moreno as well as with a number of prominent U.S. surgeons, including pediatric surgeons, recommended that all innovative surgery that falls short of being true research still be reviewed by a committee and submitted to an online registry. Building on previous work,[49] the SUS group offered a working definition for such innovations:

An "innovation" is a new or modified surgical procedure that differs from currently accepted local practice, the outcomes of which have not been described, and which may entail risk to the patient. Many innovations are used on an ad-hoc basis as dictated by the clinical situation. Some innovations, however, may be developed in a more systematic fashion and may ultimately meet the criteria for human subject research, although they do not meet the criteria at the time they are performed. Example: A surgeon decides to perform Natural Orifice Translumenal Endoscopic Surgery, removing an appendix via a patient's vagina.[35]

The following details and provisions were added:

Innovations that are necessitated by the clinical situation are ethically appropriate. In the interest of full disclosure and trust essential to the physician–patient relationship, it is recommended that the surgeon disclose the innovation to the patient or patient's surrogate. This disclosure should take place before surgery – as part of the informed consent process – if it is a planned innovation, or postoperatively if an unanticipated innovation takes place during the operation.

The informed consent process should include specific discussion of the innovative aspect of the procedure. Any omission of such discussion arguably involves deception and violates patient autonomy-based rights to submit to care, and could create potential liability for surgeons and their institutions.

If the surgeon uses an unapproved drug or device in an emergency, it is expected that the surgeon abide by FDA guidelines for emergency use of unapproved medical devices (http://www.fda.gov/cdrh/manual/unappr.html).

If a drug or device is used "off-label" – i.e., with a patient population, dose, route of administration, or preparation that is different from the labeling – it is the responsibility of the physician to determine the relative risk and to disclose it to the patient as part of the informed consent process.

When possible, surgeons are encouraged to first perform the innovative procedure in a simulated or animal model, rather than first attempting a new procedure or skill on a patient.

If a procedure is not described in surgical textbooks published in the United States, its novelty should be described to the patient as an integral part of the informed consent process, even if it is a common practice in other parts of the world.

Some innovations may not meet the definition of research – and thus be exempt from formal IRB approval – but require some form of oversight and more-than-routine informed consent by the patient. Such oversight should occur when: (a) an innovation is not yet part of a formal investigation; (b) the surgeon seeks to assess a hunch, hypothesis or theory (e.g., that the innovation is an improvement of technique); (c) the new approach differs significantly from current practice; (d) the outcomes of the innovation have not been previously described; or (e) the innovation entails risks for complications. If the innovation involves a planned activity with essentially unknown outcomes and risks, the innovation requires additional oversight AND submission to a national registry, publicly available to surgeons (described below). This additional oversight should come from a local Surgical Innovations Committee (SIC), as described below.

If it is the intent of a surgeon to perform a particular innovation repeatedly, the SIC should review early outcomes – with consideration of a potential proficiency-gain curve – to determine if this is appropriate, and whether a formal research protocol should be initiated to assess the value of the innovation. The surgeon has a professional and ethical obligation to review the outcomes related to the innovation. If they are notable, either in a positive or a negative sense, the results should be broadly disseminated. This will allow other patients to benefit from useful innovations, and help other surgeons avoid implementing harmful or fruitless innovations. Dissemination of results should conform to the regulations Standards for Privacy of Individually Identifiable Health Information, also known as the Health Insurance Portability and Accountability Act of 1996 (HIPAA) Privacy Regulations found at 45 CFR Sections 160 and 164. Note that both the Federal regulations governing research and the HIPAA Privacy regulations have rules governing the conduct of research as well as the need for patient/subject confidentiality.[35]

With regard to the surgical innovations committee, or SIC, Biffl et al. recommended the following:

The SIC should be appointed by a responsible leader of the institution, such as the Chief of Staff, and should provide periodic written reports to the institutional leader. The SIC should have no conflicts of interest with the innovator and be comprised of (1) a Department of Surgery representative who is certified by the American Board of Surgery, and a Fellow of the American College of Surgeons;

(2) individual(s) with a vested interest in patient safety, including a designated patient advocate; and (3) other community stakeholders as deemed necessary and appropriate. The SIC should enlist local or national experts with experience relevant to the proposed innovation, as necessary. The SIC would be responsible for reporting the outcomes related to any approved innovation back to the institutional leadership that convened the committee.[35]

In addition, the SUS group adopted a table that was originally developed by Reitsma, Moreno, et al. to aide surgeons in the process of deciding which innovations should be submitted for additional review (Table 14.1).

Finally, in collaboration with the American College of Surgeons, the group established a national registry for innovations.[49] This registry contains a listing of ongoing and completed surgical innovations and provides contact information for the innovator, allowing surgical innovators to consult the registry before embarking on their own innovation, facilitating sharing of information, and minimizing duplicative effort on multiple fronts – particularly for those innovations that are unsuccessful and are unlikely to be described in the literature. The SIC would require the

TABLE 14.1. *Surgical Innovations Requiring Formal Review*

If the innovation is planned[a] *AND:*

The surgeon seeks to test a hunch, theory, or hypothesis about the innovation;
OR:

The innovation differs significantly from currently accepted local practice;
OR:

Outcomes of the innovation have not been previously described;
OR:

The innovation entails risks for complications;
OR:

Specific/additional patient consent *appears* to be appropriate;

Then:

(a) The described review by a local surgical innovations committee is required, plus

(b) submission to the national innovations registry is required, and

(c) additional informed consent is required of the patient specific to the experimental nature of the proposed innovation.

---

[a] If an innovation occurred but was *unplanned*, it should be regarded as having been performed on an individual as-needed basis for the benefit of that particular patient, unless it meets any of the five other criteria listed in this table. In such instances, postoperatively, the patient or patient's surrogate should be informed of the innovative nature of the procedure. If it does not meet any of the criteria, the innovation falls under acceptable modifications of surgical technique.

Source: Biffl et al.;[35] adapted from Reitsma and Moreno.[48]

innovator to review the national registry prior to submission of his or her proposal and to list the innovation with the registry, once approved, as part of the review process.

The fact that two separate groups of professionals could come up with and essentially agree on how to view, deal with, and ensure ethically appropriate innovative surgery is a clear signal that the professional leaders in surgery, bioethics, and other relevant disciplines have taken a strong and yet very pragmatic stance with respect to the responsible regulation of surgical innovation, solving some of the major ethical, surgical, and scientific challenges that had lingered unresolved for so long. This is a promising and encouraging situation that should inspire pediatric surgeons to feel comfortable about continuing to innovate – responsibly.

CONCLUSION

In 1986, pediatrician Harry Shirkey described infants and children as "therapeutic or pharmaceutical orphans" because so few interventions had been developed and studied in the pediatric population. There is a moral imperative to continue innovation in pediatric surgery and prevent children from once again becoming "therapeutic orphans." Appropriate studies and progress must be promoted.[1]

Some 40 years have passed since Shirkey[50] made this astute remark, and since then many thoughtful pediatricians and pediatric surgeons have tried to present solutions to the formidable challenge of pediatric surgical innovation. It is abundantly clear that surgical innovation must proceed, for the benefit of both current and future pediatric patients. Children should no longer be treated as "orphans" but should be offered the best surgical treatments that have been developed especially for children and investigated by using children as patients and research subjects. Yet innovations will need to proceed in a controlled, ethically and methodologically sound manner that allows for solid progress while conscientiously protecting some of the most vulnerable and scientifically neglected patients in the surgery realm: children.

References

1. Diekema DS. Conducting ethical research in pediatrics: a brief historical overview and review of pediatric regulations. *J Pediatr.* 2006;149 (July, Suppl. 1): S3–S11.
2. Riskin DJ, Longaker MT, Krummel TM. The ethics of innovation in pediatric surgery. *Sem Pediatr Surg.* 2006;15(November):319–323.
3. Riskin DJ, Longaker MT, Gertner M, Krummel TM. Innovation in surgery: a historical perspective. *Ann Surg.* 2006;244:686–693.
4. Moreno and Kravitt, Chapter 5, this volume.
5. 45 CFR 46: Code of Federal Regulations, Title 45, Public Welfare, Department of Health and Human Services. Part 46: Protection of Human Subjects. Available at: http://www.hhs.gov/ohrp/humansubjects/guidance/45cfr46.htm.

6. Reitsma AM, Moreno JD. Maternal–fetal research and human research protections policy. *Clin Perinatol.* 2003;30:141–153.
7. Office of Human Research Protections, U.S. Department of Health and Human Services. Available at: http://www.hhs.gov/ohrp.
8. U.S. Food and Drug Administration. Available at: http://www.fda.gov/.
9. Reitsma AM. Evidence based surgery: a growing need for a limited enterprise [open editorial]. *Virtual Mentor, American Medical Association Online Ethics Magazine.* 2004. Available at: http://www.ama-assn.org/ama/pub/category/13072.html.
10. Reitsma AM, Moreno JD: Surgical research, an elusive entity. *Am J Bioethics.* 2003;3:52–53.
11. Reitsma AM, Moreno JD. Ethical regulations for innovative surgery: the last frontier? *J Am Coll Surg.* 2002;194:792–802.
12. Reitsma AM, Moreno JD. Ethics of innovative surgery: US surgeons' definitions, knowledge, and attitudes. *J Am Coll Surg.* 2005;200:103–110.
13. Margo CE. When is surgery research? Towards an operational definition of human research. *J Med Ethics.* 2001;27:40–43.
14. Beecher HK. Surgery as placebo: a quantitative study of bias. *JAMA.* 1961; 176:1102–1107.
15. Roy DJ, Black P, McPeek B. Ethical principles in surgical research. In: Troidl HW, Spitzer O, McPeek B, Mulder DS, eds. *Principles and Practice of Research: Strategies for Surgical Investigators.* New York: Springer-Verlag; 1986:581–604.
16. Frader JE, Caniano DA. Research and innovation in surgery. In: McCullough LB, Jones JW, Brody BA, eds. *Surgical Ethics.* New York: Oxford University Press; 1998:216–241.
17. Frader JE, Flanagan-Klygis E. Innovation and research in pediatric surgery. *Sem Pediatr Surg.* 2001;10:198–203.
18. Bunker JP, Hinkley D, McDermott WV. Surgical innovation and its evaluation. *Science.* 1978;200:937–941.
19. Casler JD. Clinical use of new technologies without scientific studies. *Arch Otolaryngol.* 2003;129:674–677.
20. Cronin DC, Millis JM, Siegler M. Transplantation of liver grafts from living donors into adults: too much, too soon. *New Engl J Med.* 2001;344:1633–1637.
21. Jones JW. Ethics of rapid surgical technological advancement. *Ann Thorac Surg.* 2000;69:676–677.
22. Josefson D. University must tell patients that they were research "guinea pigs." *Brit Med J.* 2000;321:1487A.
23. Love JW. Drugs and operations: some important differences. *JAMA.* 1975; 232:37–38.
24. McKneally MF. Ethical problems in surgery: innovation leading to unforeseen complications. *World J Surg.* 1999;23:786–788.
25. Moore FD. Ethical problems special to surgery: surgical teaching, surgical innovation, and the surgeon in managed care. *Arch Surg.* 2000;135:14–16.
26. Anonymous. Qualms about innovative surgery. *Lancet.* 1985;1(8421):149.
27. Strasberg SM, Ludbrook PA. Who oversees innovative practice? Is there a structure that meets the monitoring needs of new techniques? *J Am Coll Surg.* 2003;196:938–948.

28. Ward CM. Surgical research, experimentation and innovation. *Brit J Plast Surg.* 1994;47:90–94.

29. Waring GO. A cautionary tale of innovation in refractive surgery. *Arch Ophthalmol.* 1999;117:1069–1073.

30. Kornetsky S. *Guidelines, Concepts and Procedures for Differentiating Between Research and Innovative Therapy.* Boston: Children's Hospital Boston; 2001. *Internal memo.* Available at: https://courses.law.washington.edu/mastroianni/H536a_Wi09/private/boston_children_hospital_guidelines.pdf.

31. McKneally MF, Daar AS. Introducing new technologies: protecting subjects of surgical innovation and research. *World J Surg.* 2003;27:930–937.

32. Donahoe PK. The mandate for innovation in pediatric surgery: creating the environment for success, parity, and excellence. *J Pediatr Surg.* 2008;43:1–7.

33. Jarvik JG, Deyo RA. Cementing the evidence: time for a randomized trial of vertebroplasty. *Am J Neuroradiol.* 2000;21:1373–1374.

34. Petrelli NJ. Clinical trials are mandatory for improving surgical cancer care. *JAMA.* 2002;287:377–378.

35. Biffl WL, Spain DA, Reitsma AM, et al. Responsible development and application of surgical innovations: a position statement of the Society of University Surgeons. *J Am Coll Surg.* 2008;206(6):1204–1209.

36. Reitsma AM, Moreno JD, eds. *Ethical Guidelines for Innovative Surgery.* Hagerstown, Md: University Publishing Group; 2006.

37. Beauchamp TL, Childress JF. *Principles of Biomedical Ethics. 5th ed.* New York: Oxford University Press; 2001.

38. Jones JW. The surgeon's autonomy: defining limits in therapeutic decision making. In: Reitsma AM, Moreno JD, eds. *Ethical Guidelines for Innovative Surgery.* Hagerstown, Md: University Publishing Group; 2006:75–92.

39. Lyerly AD, Mahowald MB. Maternal–fetal surgery: the fallacy of abstraction and the problem of equipoise. *Health Care Anal.* 2001;9:151–165.

40. Lyerly AD, Cefalo RC, Socol M, Fogarty L, Sugarman, J. Attitudes of maternal–fetal specialists concerning maternal–fetal surgery. *Am J Obstet Gynecol.* 2001;185:1052–1058.

41. Lyerly AD, Gates EA, Cefalo RC, Sugarman J. Toward the ethical evaluation and use of maternal–fetal surgery. *Obstet Gynecol.* 2001;98:689–697.

42. Moreno JD. Donation disaster: a high price for the gift of life. AbcNews.com. Available at: http://abcnews.go.com/Health/story?id=116999&page=1. Accessed January 25, 2002.

43. Moseley JB, O'Malley K, Petersen NJ, et al. A controlled trial of arthroscopic surgery for osteoarthritis of the knee. *N Engl J Med.* 2002;347:81–88.

44. Kirkley A, Birmingham TB, Litchfield RB, et al. A randomized trial of arthroscopic surgery for osteoarthritis of the knee. *N Engl J Med.* 2008;359:1097–1107.

45. Chisolm DJ, Pritchett CV, Nwomeh BC. Factors affecting innovation in pediatric surgery: hospital type and appendectomies. *J Pediatr Surg.* 2006;41(November):1809–1813.

46. Rutan RL, Deitch EA, Waymack JP. Academic surgeons' knowledge of Food and Drug Administration regulations for clinical trials. *Arch Surg.* 1997;132:94–98.

47. Angelos P, Lafreniere R, Murphy T, Rosen W. Ethical issues in surgical treatment and research. *Curr Prob Surg.* 2003;40:345–448.
48. Reitsma AM, Moreno JD. Ethics guidelines for innovative surgery: recommendations for national policy – a position statement from the Committee on the Development of National Policy Recommendations for Innovative Surgery. In: Reitsma AM, Moreno JD, eds. *Ethical Guidelines for Innovative Surgery.* Hagerstown, Md: University Publishing Group; 2006:150–170.
49. American College of Surgeons Innovations Registry. Available at: http://web.facs.org/innovations/innovationsdefault.htm.
50. Shirkey H. Therapeutic orphans. *J Pediatr.* 1968;72:119–120.

15

Conjoined Twins

Alice D. Dreger and Geoffrey Miller

The major ethical question we shall address in this chapter is, Under what conditions should conjoined twins be separated? Before we address that question directly, some background is in order.

Most types of conjoined twins appear to result from incomplete splitting of a single fertilized ovum, but some conformations termed "conjoined twinning" may involve a fusion of closely approximated embryos. The term "parasitic twin" refers to a conjoined twin lacking a functional brain. For example, "parasitic twins" sometimes appear in the form of extra arms or legs or as an essentially undeveloped embryo contained within the body of its fully grown twin ("fetus in fetu"). Nonparasitic conjoined twins have traditionally been classified according to where they are joined; thus, the nomenclature of conjoinment relies chiefly on the suffix *pagos*, a Greek term meaning "that which is fixed or joined." For example, craniopagus twins are joined at the skull; thoracopagus twins share part of the chest wall and often the heart; pyopagus twins are usually back to back, joined at the rump; ischiopagus twins are joined at the sacrum and coccyx; and omphalopagus twins are joined at the abdomen and sternum.[1] "Dicephalic" refers to twins who appear to have two heads on one body, though the actual number of appendages and internal organs varies from set to set. Indeed, the degree of shared anatomy and associated congenital malformations varies in all types of conjoined twins.[2] The majority of conjoined twins throughout history have been stillborn or have died during the neonatal period because of congenital malformations.[3] Today many are diagnosed prenatally and aborted.

Conjoined twins inevitably engender some degree of fascination and curiosity in others, at least upon first encounter. Surely this is in part because people who are conjoined challenge many generally unspoken assumptions about personhood, individuality, independence, sexuality, and privacy.[4] Their very difference may in itself be perceived by some as a threat. Nevertheless, when nonparasitic in form, they should be considered human beings worthy of the same respect and justice – that is, the same kind and degree of ethical consideration – as other humans.[5] The challenge can be how to apply to conjoined twins ethical considerations that, in theory and in practice, have generally assumed individuals who are physically independent. Clearly, conjoined twins with separate heads and central nervous systems should be viewed as two individual persons, as they invariably see themselves that way.[6] But they are obviously one physical entity, a *set* of conjoined twins – two in one, so to speak – and those who remain conjoined inevitably develop intensely close relationships with their twins, such that it is typical when one is dying for the other to readily accept a shared death.[4] Philosophers of conjoined twinning have thus reasonably asked whether the ethical approach ought to address the one physical being, or whether the ethics that we might apply to a separate individual apply to each of the twins, without primary consideration of the fact that they share one expanse of skin.[7]

Removal of a so-called parasitic twin is generally uncontroversial, particularly if it is likely to leave the sentient person with less physical impairment and disfigurement. Separation of autosomic twins is, however, sometimes controversial, particularly when (1) separation will introduce high risk or will necessarily physically harm those who are functioning well conjoined and (2) separation will necessarily result in the death of one, as when surgeons cut one away from a shared heart. The latter type of separation has been called "sacrifice surgery." Sacrifice surgeries have typically been performed when physicians have believed that, left conjoined, one twin will ultimately cause profound suffering and/or the death of the other. Sacrifice surgery raises a medicolegal question about whether the surgery, because the surgeons knowingly bring about the death of a person, constitutes a crime.[8] Additional legal questions may also arise in cases of conjoinment when there is disagreement between parents and physicians, or if the concept of informed consent in this situation is challenged.[9]

As technology and experience increase, more attempts at separation are made. But most separations remain serious and difficult interventions that very few are experienced at performing. Thus, one ethical question involves whether institutions that lack experience with separations ought to undertake them. Institutions are apt to gain enormous positive publicity from separations; one physician confessed that his institution enjoyed approximately $20 million worth of free publicity from a highly publicized separation.[10] Meanwhile, surgeons who perform separations are often hailed as heroes in the media (even if their patients die or are left profoundly disabled). This kind of self-interest is one reason institutions that are inexperienced may attempt separations. This situation may also result in families being pressured to participate in far more media coverage than may be in their best interests, as they are told the hospital "needs" the media to help defray the costs of these enormously expensive endeavors. In short, the stakes of separation can be so high that, if a separation is to be made public, an independent group of ethics consultants should be engaged in order to avoid conflicts of interest skewing the decision making.

The surgical, medical, and social challenges of separations speak to the need to provide thoughtfully integrated health care for conjoined twins and their families. Physical therapy for the twins and professional mental health support for the twins and their families should be provided as standard practice, whether or not separation is being considered. In other words, these critical services ought not to be offered only in preparation and follow-up to separation, but in all cases. That many separations are motivated by the belief that they will improve psychosocial functioning highlights the relevance of professional psychosocial care provision regardless of whether separation is to happen. Psychologists and social workers who have dealt with issues of disability and chronic illness (e.g., those on craniofacial teams) may be tapped for help with these cases, as many of the concerns in these cases parallel other, less dramatic situations.

The history of those who have lived conjoined and those who have undergone separation challenges the common assumption that separation is always the best choice. We are unaware of any individuals who regret their parents' decision to separate them from a twin; even those who have lost twins and bodily functions have not spoken against their separations, and several have spoken in their favor.[4] On the other hand, among twins who have remained conjoined into adulthood, only one set, Laleh and Laden Bijani, has ever elected separation for themselves; these twins died from separation at the age of 29 in 2004. The Bijanis (discussed in more detail later) were truly extraordinary for conjoined twins. The typical claim of conjoined twins who have grown together into adulthood is that their condition is normal for them. Like most people, conjoined twins accept the bodies into which they were born as the right ones for them, even if the situation is socially disadvantageous. Many have even suggested that their situation left them in a state superior to that of singletons.[11] Meanwhile, neither the medical nor the popular literature bears out what has been termed by Dreger the singleton assumption, that is, that conjoinment necessarily results in psychosocial harm. (Whether it does depends on social and familial context.) Nor does either the medical or popular literature bear out the assumption that separation necessarily improves psychosocial outcome. Separation in many cases *increases* the risk of morbidity and mortality, and often results in harm.[4] Thus, what seems intuitive in these cases – that conjoinment is unlivable and separation is always the right choice – simply is not true.

When separation is considered, surgeons need to determine the extent and nature of the conjoinment, including whether there is a shared vascular circulation or shared organs. They also must determine the chances of success for either of the twins and assess their degree of certainty in the matter. Furthermore, as already suggested, they need to step back from the situation and ask themselves whether the patients' best interests or their own hubris and competitive instincts drive them on. A principled approach to the moral questions would dictate that, for fully informed adults, we respect the autonomy of each twin, provided that health professionals are not asked to act against their conscience, knowledge, or the law. Health professionals would also be required to honor their duty to protect the vulnerable should one or both twins be viewed as not competent to make a decision concerning separation; it would seem they would be required to act in a way that was good for each twin and to avoid irreparable harm. Justice would require that we would want to treat each twin equally, from an ethical standpoint, and in the same manner as we would treat nonconjoined individuals.[8]

Yet, as noted earlier, conjoined twins may present an extraordinary medical ethical situation, namely when separation may ultimately help one while inevitably harming or killing the other. If surgeons have separated twins with the knowledge that they have inevitably caused the death of one of the twins, have they murdered that person and are they legally responsible? Can parents give consent to "sacrifice surgeries"? Who decides? Interpretations of this situation have differed in differing contexts.[4]

The first sacrifice surgery appears to have occurred in 1955 in the United States,[12] and, to date, the procedure has occurred at least 11 times.[4] Well-known examples include the separation of Amy and Angela Lakeberg, born in 1993, and sharing a liver and a six-chambered heart. Separation necessarily entailed the death of one and risk to the other, but physicians believed that long-term survival was unlikely if they remained conjoined. Surgeons at the Children's Hospital of Philadelphia decided that Amy was the weaker twin and performed the sacrifice separation. Angela died, too, a few months later, never having left cardiac intensive care.[13] A significantly more positive outcome resulted in 2000 when, immediately after birth, Sandra Ivellise Soto was separated by sacrifice surgery from her sister, Darielis Milagro, in a procedure planned during their gestation. Prenatal scans had shown that Sandra lacked a heart and aorta and that, because of a twin reversed-arterial perfusion sequence, leaving them together would cause both to die soon after birth unless they were separated.[14] At last report, Darielis was said to be doing very well.[15] The sacrifice surgery involving Rosie and Gracie Attard, in which the parents raised objections, is discussed in more detail later in this chapter.

As we have suggested, even separation surgeries not involving an intentional sacrifice of one can be fraught with ethical challenges. For example, separation of craniopagus twins is inevitably a high-risk endeavor, which raises the question of whether it should be attempted. Similarly, separation of dicephalic twins necessarily results in severe damage to urinary, reproductive, and sexual organs, again raising the question of whether separation really leaves patients better off. In cases of dicephalic boys, the surgical intervention is even more dramatic than in girls, as the practice has been to sex-reassign one twin. In one case of dicephalic boys, parents who checked a pair of sons into the hospital for separation surgery ultimately left only with one daughter.[16] (The boy given the penis died.) Did the risk–benefit ratio really justify the choice made? It is difficult to say, especially because reporting of follow-up has been so inconsistent and seemingly biased toward the cases involving more positive outcomes. A true evidence-based comparison of the risks of separation and conjoinment would require health care professionals to publish honest longitudinal data and would require them to study not only those who are separated, but those who live conjoined. Parents could then seriously consider, in the case of dicephalic girls, whether to opt for separation, as the parents of Katie and Eilish Holton did,[17] or to accept conjoinment as part of their daughters' lives, as the parents of now-teenagers Abagail and Brittany Hensel have. We would not have to rely on the media to tell us what's happened to separated and conjoined twins to contrast life with craniopagus conjoinment, as in the case of Yvonne and Yvette McCarther,[6] with craniopagus separation, as in the case of Carl and Clarence Aguirre.[18]

We shall now present two recent cases that demonstrate in more depth the complex ethical and legal arguments that can attend cases of separation, namely the cases of the Bijanis and the Attards.

The Iranian sisters Ladan and Laleh Bijani, adult craniopagus conjoined twins, actively sought physicians who would agree to separate them. Initially they went to Germany, but the physicians they consulted there declined to perform the separation because they judged that it would very likely result in the sisters' deaths. Their clinical judgment was based on scans showing that the sisters' cranial blood supply was intensely intertwined. The sisters also shared a major cranial vein.[19] Had the German team opted to go ahead, knowing or believing that death would ensue, they would have made a moral judgment that would have required very strong justifications. Such justifications, which are not necessarily sufficient, could have included deciding that the twins' quality of life was so bad that any risk was worth it or that the medical professionals must respect the twins' autonomy, against their own better judgment, by complying with their demands.[20]

Clearly, a moral argument can be made in favor of attempting the separation of conjoined twins, provided that the risks are reasonable and appropriate consent is obtained. All other things being equal, separation would seem to promote lives endowed with more choice and maximal privacy and, especially, lives free from the morbid curiosity of others (presuming surgery does not result in notable disfigurement). But as we have noted, the lives of many conjoined twins are not so intolerable as to justify separation regardless of risk. Indeed, there was no evidence that the life of either of the Bijani twins was in imminent danger, nor was there evidence that their lives were intolerable. They were described as happy and intellectually accomplished. Both had law degrees, though they did prefer that their lives proceed in independent directions.[19]

Nevertheless, eventually a team in Singapore agreed to attempt separation. It took more than 50 hours to complete the separation, but within about 2 hours, both women were dead from uncontrollable blood loss. The team told reporters that they had considered halting the operation when it became clear that the cranial blood supply was so intertwined as to cause serious complications, but they decided to press on, believing it was what the sisters would have wanted.[21] The lead surgeon, Keith Goh, told the press, "At least we helped them achieve their dream of separation."[22] Ladan and Laleh Bijani's father, a physician, expressed profound outrage at the loss of his daughters to what he considered from the start to represent a hopeless operation. It probably did not allay the father's anger that the stock price of the privately traded hospital where the surgery took place went up in response to all the publicity.[4]

As we have noted, the Bijani twins were unique in history in that they were conjoined adults who agreed to physical separation. No other twins in history, including those sets in which one was dying or dead, have ever consented to separation.[4] The questions that arise in the Bijani case, then, are whether the surgeons were morally justified in taking such a tremendous risk in an attempt to satisfy this preference and whether the women's consent was adequately informed.

To take the second question first, it can be argued that a patient's consent is always influenced by faith and trust in the patient's caregivers; this places a greater moral weight on medical professionals to be clear that faith in one's surgeon cannot change risk. King, in writing about the Bijani twins' death, states, "Overestimation of benefit [and underestimation of risk] is common in medical innovation, perhaps especially in surgery."[23] For the Bijani twins, the involvement of the media and the inability of medical professionals to counsel the twins separately raises the possibility of coercion. Could they have been swept along by a wave of inappropriate hopeful expectation or a driving need for one twin not to disappoint the other? The moral balance returns again to the physicians involved and is a dilemma found in other examples of so-called pioneer surgery. Human nature in the form of academic ambition or intellectual curiosity may cloud the issues. Surgeons may argue that, even if they fail, the lessons learned may later lead to acceptable levels of success. (For example, after the Bijanis died, Johns Hopkins University neurosurgeon Benjamin Carson, who went to Singapore to assist, told the press, "No act is a failure if you learn from it.")[24] In such a situation boundaries must be recognized.

The approach to the moral question should include necessity and proportionality. Although law courts might consider proportionality (as we shall see later), it is not easily quantified. It is a moral matter that weighs an act with a likelihood of causing death or severe disability against allowing the opportunity for an individual to live a preferred life. In the case of the Bijani twins, how necessary was it to perform the operation, and if there were degrees of necessity, were the risks of the surgery disproportionate to the preferred need?

It is unclear from the public record what the Bijanis were actually told with regard to risk. What we do know is that, in advance of the surgery, members of the surgical team quoted to the media significantly lower odds of disability and death than the most recent published literature suggested was likely for craniopagus separations.[4] The most comprehensive study at the time concluded that "mortality and morbidity after surgical separation are horrendous; of the 60 infants operated on, 30 died, 17 were impaired, 6 were alive but ultimate status unknown, and only 7 were apparently normal."[1] Yet before separation, members of the surgical team named only a 50% chance that one or both of the Bijanis would be disabled or die from the surgery.[23–25] This is especially curious given that the difficulty of craniopagus separation is generally considered to increase exponentially with age, so that the risk for the Bijanis would presumably have been even higher than the risk in previous cases, all of which were pediatric separations. A group of Iranian neuroscientists who studied the case in hindsight concluded the operation should have been staged, if done at all: "The most complex communication was in the major cerebral superficial sinuses which made separation a distant reality and a utopian dream."[19]

Despite the commodification of medicine, physicians should be more than mere purveyors of technical skills. They have a duty to refuse to provide treatment if they truly believe it is likely to cause death or extreme harm, and a duty to perform treatment in a way they believe to be the most likely to lead to the outcome sought by a patient. The surgeons who conducted the operation on the Bijani sisters apparently believed that the hope of improving quality of life justified proceeding with the surgery.[20] The judgment made by the surgeons in this case raises the question of how we view disability or difference from our own perspectives; what could have convinced them that the Bijanis' lives were so poor as to justify the risks taken?

How anatomical and functional difference is viewed is necessarily tainted by weighted language and misconception. For example, describing someone as "suffering from an affliction" clearly weights an argument in favor of intervention. In the case of the Bijanis, the sisters' pleas to be separated would surely have pressed the surgeons to try to intervene to remedy an affliction. Did this pressure – along with the pressure of public attention at a time of strained international relations between the West and Middle East – diminish medical reasonableness and the important medical virtue of prudence, or *phronesis*? Annas quotes Carson as saying, when the decision was made not to perform the operation in phases, "[A]t that point

I felt like a person heading into a dark jungle to hunt a hungry tiger with no gun."[9] But why should a surgeon agree to these terms when two healthy women's lives are at stake? Whether the twins themselves were willing to accept the risk (presuming they understood the real risk) begs the question of whether physicians should always follow the instructions of their competent adult patients despite the odds of success. Adults are free to choose or refuse a course of treatment even if this is irrational in others' eyes. But the converse also applies. Physicians are free to refuse to attempt a treatment if they reasonably believe it to be unethical or irrational.

Another ethically complex separation involved the Attard twins and their encounter with English law courts. As we shall demonstrate, consideration of the concepts of necessity and proportionality played an important role in deciding their outcome. The case of the Attard twins[26] differs in several ways from that of the Bijanis. They were infants; the parents disagreed with the physicians; surgery meant the inevitable death of one twin, and no surgery was believed to mean the early death of both twins; and the case for surgery was decided in the law courts.

Michelangelo and Rina Attard, from Malta, had been sent to St. Mary's Hospital in Manchester, England, following a prenatal ultrasound showing that Rina was carrying conjoined twins. The family was sent to St. Mary's not because the hospital had experience with conjoined twins, but simply because that was the institutional affiliation of a physician who consulted in Malta. The mother, afraid of giving birth to the children, refused medical advice to give birth early and was finally delivered two weeks after her due date, in August 2002.[27] The twins were known in the public sphere as Jodie and Mary (though their given names were Gracie and Rosie, respectively). Born ischiopagus, the girls were joined at the abdomen and lower pelvis. Jodie's heart and lungs (i.e., those nearest Jodie's head) supplied much of the cardiac and pulmonary function for their conjoined body, as Mary's side lacked an adequately functioning heart or lungs. Mary also had an abnormally formed brain, the specific consequences of which were uncertain. The only midline shared organ was a large urinary bladder.

Medical opinion held that, if the twins were not separated, both would die from Jodie's heart failure within several months. If they were separated, Mary would inevitably die during the operation.[28] Jodie appeared neurologically typical for her age and was described as bright and flourishing, while Mary was less interactive and viewed less favorably.[29] The parents were devout Catholics, and because of their religious convictions, they were unwilling to sacrifice the life of one of their children, even for the sake of the other, and would not consent to an attempted separation. What was missed in many media accounts was that the parents had another reservation about the separation: they were clearly afraid of having to raise the survivor given the profound disabilities she would be left with, especially given that in their culture parents tend to be blamed for their children's disabilities.[30] Thus, the parents appear to have been willing to accept the natural death of both daughters rather than face the prospect of raising one or two daughters. (It is typical of media reports – which like to valorize surgeons, parents, and "heroic" babies – to oversimplify the psychological, social, and surgical complexity of attempts at separations.)[4]

Because the physicians involved wanted to try to save Jodie and give her a more normal body, the Central Manchester Health Care Trust petitioned the High Court (Family Division) as to whether an operation would be legal. Justice Johnson ruled that it would be lawful, being (so he said) in the best interests of both the children. He concluded that Jodie would be better off without Gracie and that Gracie would be better off dead sooner rather than suffering needlessly.

The parents immediately appealed, and the dilemma went to the Court of Appeal (Civil Division). This case, known as *Re A*,[26] was heard by Justices Ward, Brooke, and Walker, who also judged that the separation was lawful, but for different reasons. We will analyze their judgments in depth later. For now we note the outcome of the case. The surgery went forward and, as expected, Mary died during the operation. Jodie underwent the first stages of reconstruction and rehabilitation and then returned to Malta with her parents, who, in a story they sold to the media to help pay for Jodie's care, expressed gratitude toward the surgeons (who had acted against their will) for saving Jodie.[31] Much of British public opinion seemed to support a morally intuitive response that the judgment was correct.[28]

The questions raised by this complex medical drama might be thought of as twofold. The first is the moral question of whether sacrificing one person for another can ever be right. The second is the legal question of whether the court can allow such an operation to proceed knowing that the judgment would seem to condemn an innocent, defenseless person to death. For this not to be prosecuted as a case of murder, the defense must be that either the apparent person to be condemned is in fact not a person or there is an absolute necessity to proceed.[32]

An argument in favor of the separation could have been that Mary was merely a parasite deriving her life from Jodie. Yet we believe that both Mary and Jodie were persons (we do not, in other circumstances, recognize personhood merely by applying some vague I-know-it-when-I-see-it neuropsychological standard) and that this was self-evident – and evident to their parents, as well as to the surgeons who acted in an appropriately grave fashion when they made the cuts that meant Mary's death.[33] Both Mary and Jodie thus had the right to live. That Mary was dependent on the heart on Jodie's side, although detrimental to Jodie's health, does not mean she was not a person.

Given that Mary was as much a person as Jodie, moral theory asks whether the separation represents an unjust action that must not be taken despite the consequences, or whether one should determine what will lead to the greatest good when there is a choice of unsatisfactory outcomes. These are, in Cowley's words, "the lumbering dragons of deontology and consequentialism."[34] The English court in this case assumed that it had a duty to rule on this matter of life and death and based its decision on a strained best-interests test and the doctrine of necessity. Contrasting scripts arose because of the different perspectives of the players and were not necessarily negated by claiming a rational objective approach. To quote Cowley again, Justice Ward saw "a potentially healthy child being drained of life blood by a parasite ... and [could] (then) see what ought to be done. The parents [saw] two children and the children are theirs, whom God in his inscrutable mystery ... condemned to die."[34]

Some might argue that the intention of the physicians and the judges who agreed with them was to save Jodie and not to kill Mary – that is, that we are dealing with what is known as the doctrine of double effect. The moral distinction is that, had Mary survived, the surgeons would have been delighted. But the inevitable outcome argues against this moral distinction. The doctrine of double effect says an action that causes harm may be justified only in certain circumstances:

1. The action in itself must be good or at least morally indifferent.
2. The agent must intend only the good effect and not the evil effect. The evil effect is foreseen but not intended.
3. The evil effect cannot be a means to the good effect.
4. There must be proportionality between the good and evil effects of the action.

But these criteria are not all satisfied when the separation of conjoined twins is certain to lead to the death of one. The aim of the doctrine is to promote a good, but not intend an evil. (Evil in this context does not mean nonpreferable.) Nor is the aim to reach a utilitarian conclusion. Wenkel argues that the doctrine does not allow for killing one twin instead of losing both twins. He states:

1. the action of killing one or both of the twins is not morally indifferent;
2. the essence of care is removed from the child who is killed causing an evil effect;
3. the evil effects of the child's death, caused by the hand of the doctor, are the means to an end;
4. the evil effects are parallel to or out of proportion.[35]

We shall now examine and comment on the *Re A*[26] proceedings. Some of the legal principles in English case law were summarized by Judge Ward. There are similarities to other international jurisdictions. They can be itemized as follows:

- "[T]he fundamental principle ... is that every person's body is inviolate."[36]

- "English law goes to great lengths to protect a person of full age and capacity from interference with his personal liberty."[37]

The common law, as it relates to consent to treatment for children, was stated by Lord Scarman in *Gillick*:

It is abundantly plain that the law recognizes that there is a right and duty of parents to determine whether or not to seek medical advice in respect of their child and having received advice, to give or withhold consent to medical treatment.[38]

Thus, to treat a child without the appropriate consent, or against the wishes of the parents, could constitute trespass to person or assault.[39] But parents also have a legal duty and responsibility to care for their children, and if it is deemed that they are not exercising this, the courts can override their rights.[38,40] Parents and the courts are required to act in the best interests of the child, from the perspective of the child.[41,42] The English courts allow an interpretation of best interests to be based on broad medical and psychosocial grounds, including emotional and all other welfare issues.[42]

Arguably, this type of court judgment may be governed by personal bias as well as the social mores of the day. This is not necessarily an adverse criticism, as law, morality, value judgment, and social need are intertwined and are a reflection of social mores. However, such judgments should be tempered by a constitution or human rights convention. Judge Ward could not justify bringing the life of Mary to an end on the basis of the argument that it would be in her best interests. But he felt compelled, indeed duty-bound, to render a judgment using a rationale reminiscent of the situation portrayed in the novel *Sophie's Choice*, wherein a woman is forced by a Nazi officer to choose which one of her two children will be sent to the gas chamber.[43] Ward argued that it was clearly in Jodie's best interests to survive and that the least detrimental choice was to allow her life rather than take a course of action that would lead to the early death of both children. This may highlight the moral dilemma, but it is questionable whether it bolsters the legal argument.

It was furthered argued that the doctors would be coming to the rescue of Jodie, albeit by killing Mary. But if it can be argued that coming to the defense of Jodie justifies killing Mary, it can also be argued that not performing the surgery is coming to the defense of Mary.[44] Perhaps Jodie might have been morally justified in saving herself from Mary, if she was able, but she was not, and Mary, as an innocent individual, did have a right not to have her life deliberately shortened.[45] The self-defense argument might seem to apply if we view the organs on Jodie's side of the body as hers, rather than there being one organism in which two persons share the organs. But there were two hearts and two sets of vasculature, for the most part. One set was working well; the other, on Mary's side of the body, was not. Even so, as Wasserman writes:

But conceding this does not eliminate the moral ambiguity about Mary's claim to the continued use of these organs. The fact that we are inclined to speak of the organs as Jodie's hardly compels us to treat her as having the same rights in these organs against Mary that a normally embodied child would have in her organs against the rest of the world ... even if the organs in Jodie's body cavity can be said to be hers, the kind of property she has in those organs, and her right to exclude Mary from their use, is by no means clear.[46]

In *Re A* the court had to demonstrate that, by allowing the intended death of Mary by a positive act, they were not authorizing murder. Clearly, with the very act of performing the operation, the death of Mary was a known certainty and satisfied the English criminal law on intention[47] demonstrating *mens rea* for murder, which should be separated from motive.[48] As a defense against this, the court used the legal doctrine of necessity. To quote Uniacke, it "applies to cases in which a person breaks the letter of the law, but where in so doing they act in accordance with a value judgment that the law endorses."[49] It is the courts that make that judgment, and they must identify four requirements in order to justify criminal conduct:

1. there must be no other choice;
2. the act must be done to avoid inevitable and irreparable evil;
3. no more must be done than is reasonably necessary;
4. and the act must not be disproportionate to the evil avoided.[49]

It was Judge Brooke who analyzed this doctrine of necessity in *Re A*. He noted a notorious 1884 incident involving lifeboat murder and cannibalism and the trial of the perpetrators (*R v. Dudley*).[50] In this case, four men escaped a sinking ship on a lifeboat. After 19 days, the three eldest killed and devoured 17-year-old Richard Parker so that they could survive. The three men were charged with murder and their defense against this was one of "necessity." This was rejected on the basis that the young man was not a direct threat, and it was no more necessary for him to be killed than the other three.[51] The Victorian court denied the defense of necessity for murder in *R v. Dudley* on the basis of two objections: (1) Who was to be the judge of necessity? By what measure is the comparative value of lives to be measured? (2) To permit such a defense would mark an absolute divorce of law from morality.

Judge Brooke, in *Re A*, addressed these objections by arguing that this was not a case where both children had a chance of living, as Mary was already "designated for death." As for the second objection, he argued that it would be immoral to save Jodie if this meant the premature end of Mary's life, but it could also be said to be immoral not to save Jodie if there was a good prospect of a fulfilling life ahead. He concluded that the court was not equipped to choose between the competing arguments (but choose it did), and the situation was not one in which there was a clear-cut divorce of law from morality.

The problem with this is that, if this was going to be the approach, there should be consideration, or even acceptance, of other morally tenable arguments, such as those held by the parents. If the law cannot choose between these moral choices, it is arguable that the courts are where the choice should be made. However, Judge Brooke justified his legal decision by applying the doctrine of necessity and concluded, by sanctioning the operation, that the requirements were satisfied. There is moral ambiguity in *Re A*, and perhaps in *R v. Dudley*, but the question is whether this ambiguity is, to quote Wicks, "a legal justification for homicide."[48] By allowing the doctrine of necessity as a defense, the court was stating that it preferred the murder of one to save another to the naturally unpreventable death of both at some time in the future.

Judge Walker also supported the defense of necessity. He stated:

I would extend it, if it needs to be extended, to cover this case. It is a case of doctors owing conflicting legal, and not merely social or moral, duties. It is a case where the test of proportionality is met, since it is a matter of life and death, and on the evidence Mary is bound to die soon in any event. ... It should not be regarded as a step down a slippery slope because the case of conjoined twins presents a unique problem.[26]

So in the case of conjoined twins, the defense of necessity for murder is allowed to save the life of one by intentionally killing the other, provided that the other will die anyway. Can one escape the flaws in this argument by saying that it applies only to conjoined twins when one is bound to die anyway?

Ultimately, in the Attard case (i.e., *Re A*[26] proceedings), the court ruled that case law dictated that a best-interests approach should apply to the consideration of sacrifice surgical separation to which parents object. The surgery was justified on the basis that it was in the best interests of the twin who had the capacity to survive, and one judge even argued, improbably, that it was acknowledged that it was also in the best interests of the twin who would inevitably die. The legal decision was made in the belief that there was a moral obligation to make that decision. Judge Ward did not make it clear whether there was a legal obligation to decide between competing best interests, although Judge Brooke concluded that the court was not equipped to choose between competing moral arguments in the case.

As far as the criminal law was concerned, it was judged that the doctrine of necessity justified Mary's death, despite the fact that this had been rejected in the past as a defense of murder. The court decided that this rejection did not apply, as Mary was going to die anyway. We are uncertain whether this is a legal or moral justification and suspect that even the court was uncertain. We also suspect that the English judges believed their position in society, including their level of education, enabled them to make a difficult moral decision rather than a legal one (despite pronouncements that their arguments were legal). This hubris is fraught with danger for individual freedoms. The law should define and proscribe boundaries of behavior. However, where there are reasonable, although undesirable, choices concerning the medical or surgical treatment of a child, most people would allow for the choice to be made by truly informed, competent parents. One is left wondering, in the case of the Attards, whether supportive education of the parents with regard to disability and a commitment to financially and socially support the family through the intended survivor's rehabilitation and life would have led the parents to agree to the separation without any need to go to court.

In summary, the ethical (and even legal) considerations that arise in cases of conjoinment are often complex, yet often they mirror considerations in other realms of care. Too often we are so focused on the unique aspects of conjoinment that we forget to consider how it is *like* what else we know. Most notably, the history of conjoinment highlights the need for medical professionals to take very seriously what they know about the likely outcomes of an intervention versus those without intervention and to put the best interests of their patient above the interests of their careers and institutions. Health care professionals dealing with children and adults who are conjoined would do well to hold themselves and each other to as high a moral and professional standard as they would when dealing with those not conjoined.

References

1. Spencer R. *Conjoined Twins: Developmental Malformations and Clinical Implications.* Baltimore: Johns Hopkins University Press; 2003:310–311.
2. Pearn J. Bioethical issues in caring for conjoined twins and their parents. *Lancet.* 2001;357:1968–1971.
3. Kaufman MH. The embryology of conjoined twins. *Child Nerv Syst.* 2004; 20:508–525.
4. Dreger AD. *One of Us: Conjoined Twins and the Future of Normal.* Cambridge, Mass: Harvard University Press; 2004.
5. Annas GJ. Siamese twins: killing one to save the other. *Hastings Cent Rep.* 1987;17(2):27–29.
6. Smith JD. *Psychological Profiles of Conjoined Twins.* Westport, Conn: Praeger; 1988.
7. Barilan YM. One or two: an examination of the recent case of the conjoined twins from Malta. *J Med Philos.* 2003;28:27–44.
8. Sheldon S, Wilkinson S. Conjoined twins: the legality and ethics of sacrifice. *Med Law Rev.* 1997;5:149–71.
9. Annas GJ. *American Bioethics: Crossing Human Rights and Health Law Boundaries.* New York: Oxford University Press; 2005:81–94.

10. Personal communication, anonymous to Alice Dreger, 2006.
11. Dreger AD. The limits of individuality: ritual and sacrifice in the lives and medical treatment of conjoined twins. *Stud Hist Philos Biol Biomed Sci.* 1998;29:1–29.
12. Kiesewetter WB. Surgery on conjoined (Siamese) twins. *Surgery.* 1966;59: 860–871.
13. Thomasma DC, Muraskas J, Marshall PA, Myers T, Tomich P, O'Neill JA Jr. The ethics of caring for conjoined twins: the Lakeberg twins. *Hastings Cent Rep.* 1996;26(4):4–12.
14. Norwitz ER, Hoyte LP, Jenkins KJ, et al. Separation of conjoined twins with the twin reversed-arterial-perfusion sequence after prenatal planning with three-dimensional modeling. *N Engl J Med.* 2000;343:399–402.
15. Grady D. A "miracle" saves one of conjoined twins who shared a heart. *New York Times.* August 11, 2000:1.
16. O'Neill JA Jr, Holcomb GW III, Schnaufer L, et al. Surgical experience with thirteen conjoined twins. *Ann Surg.* 1988;208:299–312.
17. Spitz L, Stringer MD, Kiely EM, Ransley PG, Smith P. Separation of brachio-thoraco-omphalo-ischiopagus bipus conjoined twins. *J Pediatr Surg.* 1994;29: 477–481.
18. Abraham L. Separation anxiety. *New York Magazine.* August 22, 2005.
19. Khan ZH, Hamidi S, Miri SM. Craniopagus, Laleh and Ladan twins, sagital sinus. *Turk Neurosurg.* 2007;17(1):27–32.
20. Wilkinson S. Separating conjoined twins: the case of Laden and Laleh Bijani. In: Gunning J, Holm S, eds. *Ethics, Law and Society.* Burlington, Vt: Ashgate; 2005:257–260.
21. Grady D. 2 women, 2 deaths and an ethical quandary. *New York Times.* July 15, 2003.
22. Anonymous. Nation in shock over death of Iranian twins. *Belfast News Letter* (Northern Ireland). 2003(July 9):14.
23. King NMP. The stories we tell. *Hastings Cent Rep.* 2003:33(5):49.
24. Arnold W, Grady D. Twins die trying to live two lives. *New York Times.* July 9, 2003.
25. Interview with Benjamin Carson on *Nightline*, July 11, 2003. Transcripts available from ABC News Transcripts at: http://abcnews.go.com/NIGHTLINE.
26. *Re A (children) (conjoined twins: surgical separation)*[2000] 3 F.C.R. 577 (C.A.).
27. A family's faith. *ABC News Prime Time.* December 14, 2000. Available at: http://abcnews.go.com/primetime.
28. Jenkins R. Siamese twin Jodie is bright and flourishing. *Times* (London). December 16, 2000:5.
29. Hill DJ. The morality of the separation of conjoined Attard twins of Manchester. *Health Care Anal.* 2005;13:163–176.
30. Justice Johnson in the High Court Justice Family Decision, case no. FD00P10893, 2000 (August 25).
31. Anonymous. Siamese twin returns home. *BBC News.* June 17, 2001.
32. McCall Smith A. The separating of conjoined twins: a human life has the greatest value, but its loss may be justified. *BMJ.* 2000;321:782.
33. Anonymous. Siamese twin op details revealed. *BBC News.* December 7, 2000.

34. Cowley C. The conjoined twins and the limits of rationality in applied ethics. *Bioethics.* 2003;17:69–88.

35. Wenkel DH. Separation of conjoined twins and the principle of double effect. *Christian Bioethics.* 2006;12:291–300.

36. *Re F (mental patient: sterilization)* [1990] 2 AC 1, [1989] 2 WLR 1025, 72 per Lord Goff.

37. *SvS; W v. Official Solicitor* [1972] AC 24, [1970] 3 ALL ER 107, 43.

38. *Gillick v. West Norfolk Area Health Authority* [1986] 1AC 112, [1985] 3ALL ER 402, 184G.

39. *Re R (a minor) (wardship: consent to treatment)* [1992] 2 FCR 229, [1992] Fam 11, 22.

40. *Re B (a minor) (wardship: medical treatment)* [1981] 1 WLR 1424.

41. *Re MB (medical treatment)* [1997] 2 FLR 426, 439.

42. *Re A (medical treatment: male sterilization)* [2000] 1 FLR 549, [2000] 1 FCR 193,555.

43. Styron W. *Sophie's Choice.* New York: Random House; 1979.

44. Harris J. Human beings, persons and conjoined twins: an ethical analysis of the judgment in *Re A. Med Law Rev.* 2001;9:221–36.

45. Watt H. Conjoined twins: separation as mutilation. *Med Law Rev.* 2001; 9:237–45.

46. Wasserman D. Killing Mary to save Jodie: conjoined twins and individual rights. *Philos Pub Q.* 2001;21:9–14.

47. *R v. Nedrick* [1986] 1 WLR 1025.

48. Wicks E. The greater good? Issues of proportionality and democracy in the doctrine of necessity as applied in *Re A. Comm Law World Rev.* 2003;32:15–34.

49. Uniacke S. Was Mary's death murder? *Med Law Rev.* 2001;9:208–220.

50. *R v. Dudley & Stephens* (1884) 14 QBD 273.

51. Annas GJ. Conjoined twins: the limits of law at the limits of life. *N Engl J Med.* 2001;344:1104–1108.

16

Ethics and Immunization

Joel E. Frader and Erin Flanagan-Klygis

INTRODUCTION

Without question, immunization against many infectious diseases has dramatically reduced mortality and morbidity, especially among children in both industrialized and developing areas of the world. The impact grew over the last half of the 20th century, with major reductions in disease burden caused by polio, measles, rubella (with respect to congenital defects), and varicella viruses and by invasive bacteria such as *Haemophilus influenza*, various pneumococci, and *Bordetella pertussis*, among others. The long-term effect on serious disorders such as liver cancer, caused by the hepatitis B virus, or cervical cancer, caused by the human papilloma virus (HPV), remains to be seen. Despite this clear medical success, vaccines have become the focus of considerable social and ethical controversy.

MORAL JUSTIFICATION FOR IMMUNIZATION

Immunization has two principal purposes: (1) the prevention of harm to individuals who receive vaccines and therefore develop protective immunity and (2) a reduction in social burdens associated with infection. The latter occurs both because of the economic savings associated with the direct cost of care, as well as such things as lost time and income on the part of caregivers, and because of the phenomenon of herd immunity, which reduces the spread of disease throughout a population, even to those not vaccinated or to those whose immunity has waned or become impaired as a result of unrelated diseases or treatment (e.g., HIV infection, cancer chemotherapy, and the use of steroids for rheumatological disorders). Thus, we justify vaccination primarily on the basis of its direct beneficial effect: the development of immune protection against disease, in individuals and in populations.

Of course, we must balance the beneficent interventions against the nearly inevitable kinds of harm that the actions produce. In the case of vaccines, potential harm arises from possible adverse medical reactions to the agents (allergy or other excessive immune responses, such as postimmunization arthritis, induced by the vaccine's antigens; inadvertent wild-type disease caused by genetic reversion of live virus vaccines, as occurs in roughly 1 in 3 million doses of oral polio vaccine; or viral illness from live virus vaccine in immunocompromised hosts or their contacts). Another potential hazard includes the high economic costs of vaccines. Much of the current controversy about vaccine use also involves scientifically unsubstantiated fears of direct side effects of vaccines, such as weakening of the immune system from "too many" vaccinations, especially in young children; the rising incidence of autistic symptoms in childhood populations, wrongly attributed to both measles vaccine and the use of ethyl mercury containing thimerosal; and behavior changes brought about by the feeling of being "protected" against disease, as some worry might occur following the use of the HPV vaccine, in this case the development of promiscuous sexuality.

Other ethical concerns that arise in the modern vaccine wars include (1) the fact that, at least in the immunization of children, the decision to vaccinate generally rests with a surrogate rather than an autonomous individual and (2) social justice, primarily entailing the problem of unvaccinated populations who become "free riders," receiving the benefits of herd immunity but accepting none of the possible medical or financial risks incurred by immunized children and families. This chapter will consider these issues.

KNOWN AND PERCEIVED HARM CAUSED BY IMMUNIZATION

As noted earlier, vaccines do have risks, some serious. Earlier whole-cell preparations of the pertussis vaccine produced substantially more complications than the current acellular vaccine. Those reactions included high fever with associated seizures, inconsolable crying, or a syndrome of hypotonia and hyporesponsiveness. None of these presaged permanent neurological injury, however. Some believed that pertussis vaccine precipitated severe encephalopathies, including seizure disorders, cognitive impairment, and other chronic central nervous system conditions, though careful epidemiological studies found no such association. Oral polio vaccine, which uses an attenuated live virus, can cause full-blown polio in individuals receiving the vaccine or in immunocompromised contacts, usually those who change diapers, if the live virus reverts to the genetic wild type. This rare occurrence, estimated to be one case of polio per 3 million administered doses, stimulated the change from oral polio vaccine to injected inactivated-virus vaccine in the United States. Other examples of serious vaccine-related adverse events include anaphylaxis (e.g., approximately one case per 600,000 doses of hepatitis B vaccine) and encephalitis/encephalopathy following inoculation with measles vaccine, occurring fewer than one time in 1 million doses, compared with one in a 1,000 cases associated with measles infection.[1] Fever, rashes, and local irritation or sterile abscesses are relatively common minor reactions to modern vaccines.

This information, available in much greater detail in many sources, including standard textbooks of pediatrics and the *Red Book*[2] of the American Academy of Pediatrics (AAP), relies on considerable scientific evidence. In spite of this, the media, the Internet, and anti-vaccination groups stir fear in the hearts of parents with sensationalized and biased information linking vaccinations to everything from autism to diabetes. To a certain degree, this problem flows from the success of widespread immunization: with disease burdens so low, rates of events temporally related to vaccination appear more common than the diseases themselves.[3] Fear of adverse events has eclipsed fear of disease for some parents, bringing them to view vaccination not as protective, but as risky. Beliefs about the hazards of immunization, especially brain damage, may be growing. As a consequence and despite actions like the switch to the less "reactogenic" acellular pertussis vaccine, immunization rates for pertussis have fallen in some places in the United States and in Great Britain, with a rising incidence of disease. More recently, the media and cultural wars over immunization have focused on the measles vaccine and/or the use of thimerosal and their alleged relationships to autistic behavior.

It seems worth mentioning that at least some of the uproar about a purported link between the measles vaccine and autism stems from an infamous, now-retracted[4] publication by Wakefield and colleagues[5] of "[i]leal-lymphoid-nodular hyperplasia, non-specific colitis, and pervasive developmental disorder in children." The study attempted to elucidate intestinal pathology in 12 children with bowel inflammation and recent onset of neurological and behavioral problems. The authors reported that 8 of the children had developed their symptoms after receiving measles–mumps–rubella (MMR) vaccination and that 1 child had recently been infected with measles. The first author has gone on to assert a causal relationship between measles virus nucleic acid and the development of autistic behaviors. Moreover, additional epidemiological and, most recently, blinded case-control pathological and virology studies have refuted the link between measles, colitis, and autism.[6]

While MMR vaccine used to contain thimerosal, the original discussion of a relationship between measles vaccine and autism did not implicate the compound. However, concern about neurological toxicity from mercury, especially to fetuses and young children, from mercury-containing compounds rose in the late 1990s, around the time of the Wakefield[5] paper. In 1997, with the FDA Modernization Act, the U.S. Congress required that the agency study the effects of mercuric compounds on children, among others. Various government and other studies noted toxic effects of mercury on developing nervous systems; the increasing environmental exposure to mercury, from food sources such as fish, as well as from general environmental contamination; the presence of mercury compounds as antiseptics and as preservatives in childhood vaccines; and a rising incidence of autism spectrum disorders (ASDs). In 1999, the AAP and the U.S. Public Health Service published a joint statement[7] (under the auspices of the Centers for Disease Control) calling for manufacturers to phase out the use of mercury-containing compounds in vaccines and for deferral of the use of hepatitis B vaccine containing thimerosal in newborns. In 2001, an Institute of Medicine report[8] on thimerosal in vaccines and neurodevelopmental disorders concluded that, while no information established a causal relationship, the hypothesis of harm from thimerosal was "biologically plausible." That statement fueled the already fired-up fears of many. Subsequent studies have noted that the incidence of ASDs has continued to rise despite the removal of thimerosal from vaccines and have otherwise rejected the causal hypothesis.[9] Of note, hypothesis testing cannot definitely prove that no relationship exists.

Thus, parents, even scientifically sophisticated ones, continue to rely on heart-wrenching anecdotes about children who have experienced either an apparently sudden onset of neurodevelopmental symptoms or, among those with known disorders, a notable decline in cognitive and behavioral function following immunization. The case of Hannah Poling provides a poignant example. The child developed fever and neurological symptoms at the age of 19 months within two days of receiving four vaccines against nine diseases on the same day. She subsequently regressed developmentally and eventually had a muscle biopsy that resulted in the diagnosis of an unspecified mitochondrial disorder.[10] In the spring of 2008, her parents reached a settlement in a vaccine compensation suit claiming damages, including the precipitation of autistic behavior, stemming from her immunizations at 19 months. Hannah's father is a neurologist who believes that "regressive encephalopathy with autistic features follows vaccination in susceptible children."[11] By this Dr. Poling appears to suggest that the immunizations *cause* encephalopathy in some children with metabolic disorders. Dr. Poling does not stand alone, apparently. A 2005 publication showed that 10% of Swiss pediatricians and a higher percentage of non-pediatricians would not follow recommended vaccination schedules, and non-pediatricians "were more likely not to have immunized their children against measles, mumps, hepatitis B, or *Haemophilus influezae* type b" because of safety concerns.[12] One can perhaps better understand non-physician fears and beliefs, especially when encountering stories of children who develop autistic symptoms after immunization, given the worries of scientifically trained doctors.

While fears associated with thimerosal may be declining, given the compound's removal from most vaccines used in the United States, new targets of anti-immunization activists arise all the time. Aluminum has risen to the top of some lists of toxins in vaccines. A 2004 article in *Medical Veritas: The Journal of Medical Truth* [*sic*] claims that aluminum in vaccines plays a role in the development of autism.[13] Despite such anti-vaccine campaigning by some physicians and scientists and the media's unsophisticated reporting of "all sides" of the controversy, Americans still generally rely on their physicians for advice about immunization, with sufficient participation to keep vaccination rates at levels that maintain herd immunity in most communities.[3]

Another prevalent parental phobia concerns the potential for the growing list of immunizations to "overwhelm" or damage the immune systems of their young children.[14,15] However, modern vaccines actually contain fewer antigens than those used as recently as 1980, with the total number of immunogenic proteins and polysaccharides in the vaccines given to children as of 2000 numbering approximately 125, compared with more than 3,000 in 1980, despite the addition of the *H. influenzae*, varicella, pneumococcal, and hepatitis B vaccines over that interval.[16,17] Encounters with viruses, bacteria, food, and other elements of the natural world expose infants and young children to many more antigens that stimulate immune responses than those acquired through vaccination. Of course, the expressed fears about too many vaccines may have more to do with parental concerns about the number of injections children receive and the pain, fear, and minor reactions brought on by the shots. Additional attention to pain control and continued efforts to combine vaccines into single injections may help demonstrate to parents that professionals share families' desires to protect their children from medical assault.

Finally, some of the objection to the HPV vaccine arises from worry that administering protection against a sexually transmitted virus will somehow alter the status or behavior of the immunized girls.[18] Whether this effect will occur because health care professionals or parents will have to discuss sex with those receiving the injection, thus raising the patient's awareness and interest in intercourse, or whether protection against cancer 30 or 40 years later will free some girls from their disease-avoiding tendency to abstain from sexual relations, or whether this effect will take place through some other sexually liberating mechanism, remains somewhat mysterious.[19] The concerns over disinhibition[18,19] apparently struck enough people as problematic to induce some anti-HPV vaccine crusaders to shift their opposition to efforts to include HPV in school-based or other vaccine mandates, citing the importance of parental choice. This strategy has the important effect of excluding at least some potential recipients, regardless of their or their parents' sexual politics, as many children receive mandated vaccines without charge. The HPV vaccine, which requires a course of three injections, is quite expensive: up to $160 an injection. Without availability through state-mandated programs, some adolescent girls will not have access to the vaccine, limiting its effectiveness and raising important justice considerations.[19,20]

LAW, POLICY, AND PARENTAL PREFERENCE: THE ETHICS OF VACCINE REFUSAL AND PUBLIC HEALTH

Pediatric immunization programs undoubtedly stand as one of the most important U.S. public health initiatives of the 20th century. Most authorities attribute this success largely to state mandates to complete many childhood vaccinations before children enter child care and/or school. In the year 2000, the United States achieved its highest rates of immunization coverage and the lowest rates of vaccine-preventable disease ever documented.[21] As noted earlier, with low community disease burdens, the society can easily tolerate a proportion of nonimmunized children, whether or not nonvaccination depends on medical, religious, philosophical, or "personal" (fear, false scientific beliefs, etc.) reasons cited by parents. So do we have good justification for current immunization mandates? Should we, as some anti-vaccine crusaders desire, rescind the laws and policies requiring immunization and expand parental liberty to exempt their children from vaccination?

Opel, Diekema, and Marcuse[22] examined the Washington State Board of Health school immunization policy and noted several important points. When some new vaccines, like HPV, become available, one should not readily add them to school vaccine programs because we may not yet have adequate data on longevity of antibody status, long-term safety, and cost effectiveness. The last-named especially applies, as in the case of the HPV vaccine, when a primary aim of immunization pertains to very long term goals, such as the development of cancers in adults. Opel and colleagues[22] also observe that some vaccines, with HPV again serving as a good example, contribute little, if anything, to the health or safety of the school-age population or the state's duty to provide an education to children. In addition, school vaccine mandates do not fully protect many of the most vulnerable, that is, young children at risk from pertussis, *H. influenzae*, and pneumococcal disease. Whether states should have laws mandating vaccination for entry into child care, which could or should provide better protection for infants and toddlers than we now have, is partly an empirical question and partly one of ethics and politics. Empirical concerns have to do with such matters as the proportion of young children in child care rather than at home and the available mechanisms and support for enforcing such laws and regulation, especially since most child care takes place in private, rather than tax-payer-supported, settings. Thus, Opel et al.[22] help us distinguish between mandates for immunization for school entry, and by implication entry into child care, and other kinds of mandates that might seek to achieve widespread child immunization. The latter, then, involve core political and ethical questions regarding state power and parental liberty.

Some see the laws almost entirely through the lens of public health. Others regard vaccination laws as an unnecessary affront to parental autonomy. Legally mandated vaccination in the United States emerged in the late 19th century in Massachusetts, during the epidemic of smallpox. In *Jacobson v. Massachusetts*,[23] the Supreme Court upheld the Massachusetts law in 1905, ruling that state police powers include the right to protect the public against infectious disease by enacting universal vaccination requirements, which paved the way for all states to adapt their own immunization legislation.[24] Laws requiring vaccination for school entry were upheld in 1922 by the Supreme Court in *Zucht v. King*.[25] Modern school-related childhood immunization initiatives began in the 1970s with efforts to eliminate the transmission of measles at the major sites of disease transmission among the predominant age group – school-age children – affected by the disease.[26] Evidence showed that states with school immunization laws had measles incidence rates 40–51% lower than states without such laws.[27] As a result, the late 1970s saw school vaccination statutes broadened and more strictly enforced. The provision of free vaccine and the threat of exclusion from school without proof of vaccination proved highly successful in eradicating repeated, sustained measles outbreaks.[27] By the second year after the implementation of strong measures, the incidence of measles in states strictly enforcing vaccination laws fell to one-tenth of the incidence in other states.[27] From a public policy perspective, states have clear legal authority to mandate vaccination, and such measures have succeeded in dramatically reducing the incidence of disease and complications from many important infectious agents.

However, parents may avoid vaccinating their children by invoking personal exemptions. Three types of legally recognized exemptions exist – medical, religious, and philosophical – and each has recognition under state laws. All 50 states have adopted medical exemptions for children who would be placed at significant risk by vaccination, such as those with compromised immune systems who could become ill from live virus vaccines. Religious exemptions exist in 48 states and permit individuals, or parents for their children, to refuse vaccination on religious grounds, regardless of their affiliation with a specific religious community. In addition, 19 states permit philosophical exemptions from school-entry vaccine requirements. These allow for deep-seated alternative beliefs, not clearly qualifying for religious exemption, to justify the refusal of vaccinations. (Ross and Aspinwall[28] suggest that the courts may regard many, if not most, philosophical exemptions as qualifying under religious exemption laws.) Despite the apparent ease of parental invocation of exemption in most states, such actions account for a small fraction of unvaccinated children. In 1998, the average percentage of children unvaccinated as a result of personal (nonmedical) exemption was less than 1%.[29]

Laws in the United States generally assume that parents make decisions with the best interests of their children in mind. Indeed, parents have great latitude to raise their children in accord with family beliefs and personal values. With regard to health care, laws generally require government agencies and courts to override parental authority only when parental decisions amount to abuse or neglect of children, and the neglect provisions typically entail only situations involving a substantial threat to the life and safety of a child.[30] The situation can become especially difficult for state officials and judges when parents find the support of state licensed health care professionals, even when the long-term health or life of the child may be at stake.[31]

Few argue that, under current conditions of generally high immunization rates for the relevant contagious diseases, parental refusal to vaccinate one or more children in a family places the unimmunized children at high risk of life-threatening illnesses. When coverage rates for certain vaccines stay at or above 85–95% depending on the vaccine, herd immunity allows nonvaccinated individuals to enjoy protection from infection. Concern arises from the fact that most states make use of religious and personal exemptions quite easy, raising the risk that vaccination rates will fall. In addition, parental exemptions raise the problem of free riders.[32–35]

Those in a defined population who depend on others to provide community protection (herd immunity) assume no risks or costs of the vaccines yet are recipients of the collective benefit, creating an injustice. Moreover, their action, if enough parents refuse vaccines and erode herd immunity, makes the larger community more susceptible to morbidity and mortality from contagious diseases. Feiken and colleagues[29] studied records in Colorado for an 11-year period to determine what, if any, increased risk of measles and pertussis disease correlated with religious and philosophical exemptions to vaccine use. They found that children aged 3–18 years who were unvaccinated due to religious or philosophical exemptions had a 22-fold increased risk of acquiring measles and a 6-fold greater risk of acquiring pertussis than immunized children. The annual incidence of measles and pertussis among *vaccinated* children aged 3–18 years positively correlated with the frequency of children whose parents had invoked an exemption to vaccination, with relative risks of 1.6 and 1.9, respectively. The study confirmed what physicians and epidemiologists fear: vaccine refusal poses risks of disease to unvaccinated individuals and adds risks for the entire population.

As Field and Caplan[20] note, "Mandating a vaccine can alleviate disparities in access. It would be difficult to implement or to justify a public policy that conditioned school attendance on vaccination, if availability of the vaccines involved were restricted." Vaccine mandates often prompt private insurers to cover the cost of the vaccine and its administration, or they bring about inclusion of the vaccine in publicly funded programs. While mandates limit parental liberty, they serve the interest of fairness by making the benefits of vaccines widely available. As with many matters of law, policy, and ethics, public and personal actions involve balancing competing interests and rights with their correlative duties.

CONCLUSION

As many others have noted, vaccines are neither 100% effective nor 100% safe. In the mumps outbreak in Iowa in 2006, more than half of the cases occurred in individuals who had received the recommended two doses of vaccine.[36] As we indicated earlier, both minor and, rarely, major adverse reactions do occur, and physicians who put their heads in the sand to avoid acknowledging the unintended negative aspects of immunization will only undermine public trust in the vaccination project. Physicians' dismissal of children from their practices when their parents refuse vaccines raises the risk of denying access to ongoing care when disease strikes and may not foster the best interests of children.[35,37] The question remains, how do we balance the scientifically established personal and public health benefits of immunization against the protection of individual and family liberties so cherished in the United States?

Feudtner and Marcuse[38] examined this question, concluding, and we concur, "Public health programs involve more than just issues of health. In recent decades the medical literature has reflected a societal emphasis on economic considerations, but public health is also a morally-laden medical venture. Concerns for individual liberty and social equity permeate public health policy, and should be incorporated into mainstream analysis of health care programs." Public perception (or misperception) of vaccine safety, influenced by media-flamed worry, seems to increasingly resist the conclusions of the medical and scientific community. A fear of adverse events has eclipsed the fear of disease for some parents, who view vaccination not as protective, but as risky. If parents misperceive the risks of vaccination as exceeding the risks of vaccine-preventable disease, then many of these parents will view vaccine laws as forcing them to put their children in harm's way. Attempting to change public policy to make laws and regulations governing vaccine refusal more stringent may precipitate a backlash, with adverse effects on disease prevention, as well as on the universal education of children, and the withdrawal of more children from needed medical interventions.

A successful childhood vaccination program must balance constitutionally protected parental liberties with social responsibility. Right now we find little justification for policy changes such as the repeal of religious exemption laws, though we acknowledge that a decline in immunization rates to the point of undermining herd immunity could tip the balance the other way.

References

1. Ada G. Vaccines and vaccination. *N Engl J Med.* 2001;345:1042–1053.
2. American Academy of Pediatrics. *Red Book: 2006 Report of the Committee on Infectious Diseases.* 27th ed. Elk Grove Village, Ill: American Academy of Pediatrics; 2006.
3. Smith MJ, Ellenberg SS, Bell LM, Rubin DM. Media coverage of the measles–mumps–rubella vaccine and autism controversy and its relationship to MMR immunization rates in the United States. *Pediatrics.* 2008;121:e836–e843.
4. Murch SH, Anthony A, Casson DH, et al. Retraction of an interpretation. *Lancet.* 2004;363:750.
5. Wakefield AJ, Murch SH, Anthony A, et al. Ileal-lymphoid-nodular hyperplasia, non-specific colitis, and pervasive developmental disorder in children. *Lancet.* 1998;351:637–641.
6. Hornig M, Briese T, Bauman ML, et al. Lack of association between measles virus vaccine and autism with enteropathy: a case-control study. *PLoS ONE.* 2008;3(9):e3140. Available at: http://www.plosone.org/article/info:doi/10.1371/journal.pone.0003140.
7. Centers for Disease Control, and Prevention. Notice to readers: thimerosal in vaccines – a joint statement of the American Academy of Pediatrics and the Public Health Service. *MMWR.* 1999;48:563–565.
8. Stratton KR, Gable A, McCormick MC. *Immunization Safety Review: Thimerosal-Containing Vaccines and Neurodevelopmental Disorders.* Washington, DC: National Academy Press; 2001.
9. Madsen KM, Lauritsen MB, Pedersen CB, et al. Thimerosal and the occurrence of autism: negative ecological evidence from Danish population-based data. *Pediatrics.* 2003;112:604–606.
10. Poling J, Frye RE, Shoffner J, Zimmerman AW. Developmental regression and mitochondrial dysfunction in a child with autism. *J Child Neurol.* 2006;21:170–172.
11. Poling J. Vaccines and autism revisited. *N Engl J Med.* 2008;359:655.
12. Posfay-Barbe KM, Heininger U, Aebi C, et al. How do physicians immunize their own children? Differences among pediatricians and nonpediatricians. *Pediatrics.* 2005;116:e623–e633.
13. Buttram HE. Vaccine scene, 2004 update: still MMR vaccination, mercury, and aluminum. *Medical Veritas: The Journal of Medical Truth.* 2004. Available at: http://www.medicalveritas.com/images/00018.pdf.
14. Gellin BG, Maibach EW, Marcuse EK. Do parents understand immunizations? A national telephone survey. *Pediatrics.* 2000;106:1097–1102.
15. Wolfe R, Sharp L, Lipsky M. Content and design attributes of antivaccination web sites. *JAMA.* 2002;287(24):3245–3248.
16. Offit PA, Quarles J, Gerber MA, et al. Addressing parents' concerns: do multiple vaccines overwhelm or weaken the infant's immune system? *Pediatrics.* 2002;109:124–129.

17. Gregson AL, Edelman R. Does antigenic overload exist? The role of multiple immunizations. *Immunol Allergy Clin North Am.* 2003;23:649–664.

18. Gibbs N. Defusing the war over the "promiscuity" vaccine. *Time.* June 21, 2006. Available at: http://www.time.com/time/nation/article/0,8599,1206813,00.html.

19. Casper MJ, Carpenter LM. Sex, drugs, and politics: the HPV vaccine for cervical cancer. *Sociology of Health and Illness.* 2008;30:886–899.

20. Field RI, Caplan AL. A proposed ethical framework for vaccine mandates: competing values and the case of HPV. *Kennedy Inst Ethics J.* 2008;18:111–124.

21. Anonymous. National, state and urban area vaccination coverage levels among children aged 19–35 months – United States, 1999. *MMWR.* 2000:49:585–589.

22. Opel DJ, Diekema DS, Marcuse EK. A critique for evaluating vaccines for inclusion in mandatory school immunization programs. *Pediatrics.* 2008;122:e504–e510.

23. *Jacobson v. Massachusetts*, 197 U.S. 11 (1905).

24. Jackson CL. State laws on compulsory immunizations in the United States. *Pub Health Rep.* 1969;84:787–795.

25. *Zucht v. King*, 260 US 174 (1922).

26. Centers for Disease Control, and Prevention. Measles and school immunization requirements – United States. *MMWR.* 1978;27:303–304.

27. Orenstein WA, Hinman RA. The immunization system in the United States: the role of school immunization laws. *Vaccine.* 1999;17:S19–S24.

28. Ross LF, Aspinwall TJ. Religious exemptions to the immunizations statutes: balancing public health and religious freedom. *J Law Med Ethics.* 1997; 25:202–209.

29. Feiken DR, Lezotte DC, Hamman RF, et al. Individual and community risks of measles and pertussis associated with personal exemptions to immunization. *JAMA.* 2000;284:3145–3150.

30. Diekema DS. Parental refusals of medical treatment: the harm principle as threshold for state intervention. *Theoret Med.* 2004;25:243–265.

31. Frader JE, Michelson K. Ethics in pediatric intensive care. In: Fuhrman BP, Zimmerman JJ, eds. *Pediatric Critical Care.* 3rd ed. Philadelphia: Mosby Elsevier; 2006:7–16.

32. Hershey JC, Asch DA, Thumasathit T, et al. The roles of altruism, free riding, and bandwagoning in vaccination decisions. *Org Behav Hum Decision Process.* 1994;59:177–187.

33. Meszaros JR, Asch DA, Baron J, et al. Cognitive processes and the decisions of some parents to forego pertussis vaccination for their children. *J Clin Epidemiol.* 1996;49:697–703.

34. Veatch RM. The ethics of promoting herd immunity. *Fam Commun Health.* 1997;10:44–53.

35. Diekema DS, Committee on Bioethics of the American Academy of Pediatrics. Responding to parental refusals of immunization of children. *Pediatrics.* 2005;115:1428–1431.

36. Marin M, Quinlisk P, Shimabukuro T, et al. Mumps vaccine coverage and vaccine effectiveness in a large outbreak among college students – Iowa, 2006. *Vaccine.* 2008;26:3601–3607.

37. Flanagan-Klygis EA, Sharp L, Frader JE. Dismissing the family who refuses vaccines: a study of pediatrician attitudes. *Arch Pediatr Adolesc Med.* 2005;159:929–934.
38. Feudtner C, Marcuse EK. Ethics and immunization policy: promoting dialogue to sustain consensus. *Pediatrics.* 2001;107:1158–1164.

17

Psychotropic Drug Use in Children

The Case of Stimulants

Ilina Singh

INTRODUCTION

Rising rates of stimulant drug use among children have been accompanied by a vigorous social and ethical debate over the relative harm and benefits of psychotropic drugs for children.[1] Of these drugs, the stimulants methyl phenidate (e.g., Ritalin) and amphetamine (e.g., Adderall) are the most frequently used. In a medical context, stimulants are almost always prescribed to treat attention deficit/hyperactivity disorder (ADHD); therefore, debates about stimulants have included concerns about the validity and overdiagnosis of ADHD. ADHD is the most common child psychiatric diagnosis in the world and is characterized by core symptoms of inattention, hyperactivity, and impulsiveness.[2] Most children are first diagnosed when they reach school age; approximately 75% of those diagnosed are male.[3]

The debate over ADHD and stimulant drugs is characterized by polemical positions that can misrepresent scientific understanding of ADHD, on the one hand, and dismiss valid social and ethical critiques of the disorder and drug treatment, on the other. This chapter encourages a balanced perspective. After a background section in which some of the controversies over ADHD and stimulant drug treatment are reviewed, the discussion will focus on the identification and analysis of key ethical issues that pediatricians and mental health care providers need to be aware of in order to provide the best care for young people and their families.

BACKGROUND CONTROVERSIES

Validity of ADHD Diagnosis

Two definitions are currently used in the diagnosis of ADHD. American psychiatry follows the ADHD diagnosis described in the *Diagnostic and*

Statistical Manual of Mental Disorders, 4th ed. (DSM-IV).[2] DSM describes two primary categories of behavioral symptoms: inattention and impulsivity-hyperactivity. These are used to diagnose one of three subtypes of ADHD: inattentive type, hyperactive-impulsive type, or combined type. The World Health Organization's manual, the *International Classification of Diseases,* 10th ed. (ICD-10), calls the condition hyperkinetic disorder (HKD or HD).[4] Studies have shown that a diagnosis of ADHD is significantly more likely if DSM-IV criteria are used rather than ICD-10 criteria.[5]

Because of its prevalence in the United States, ADHD is sometimes thought of as a North American disorder. However, a meta-analysis by geographic region suggests that South American countries have the highest prevalence (11.8% of school-age children), and European countries have the lowest prevalence (4.6%).[3] The United States does have a larger proportion of school-age children who are actually diagnosed with ADHD than other countries (approximately 5–6%), but this national figure conceals the significant regional variation in diagnosis rates.[6] Geographic region, as well as a child's ethnicity, socioeconomic status, and gender, are factors associated with lower or higher rates of ADHD diagnoses. In certain areas of the United States, such as in the Great Smoky Mountains, ADHD is underdiagnosed.[7]

Where Americans take a clear lead is in their spending on ADHD drugs: in 2006 the United States had 83% of the global market share.[8] But the rest of the world is catching up. Economists have found that, in the past decade, the consumption of ADHD medications in countries of the Organization for Economic Cooperation and Development increased ninefold, exceeding rates of increase in consumption in the United States. In developing world nations, increases in annual use and spending on ADHD medications are greater than 20%.[8]

Treatment of ADHD

Despite the diagnostic and definitional complexities that surround the ADHD diagnosis, there are effective treatments for children diagnosed with ADHD. In the United States and increasingly in Europe, psycho-stimulants are the first line of treatment for the disorder. These drugs have been shown to be more effective than behavioral therapy alone in treating ADHD symptoms, and more effective than behavioral therapy combined with drug treatment.[9] Stimulants such as Ritalin have been used to treat behavior problems in children since the 1950s.[10] In the 1970s, researchers showed that a positive response to stimulants is not limited to children with ADHD; "normal" children show improvements in attention and focus as well.[11] The largest study of drug efficacy to date showed that methyl phenidate use is associated with short-term improvements in cognitive tasks. However, it is not clear whether sustained use of methyl phenidate is associated with long-term improvements in academic achievement.[12]

Stimulant drug treatment for children was long considered relatively safe. Common side effects are usually mild and include appetite suppression and insomnia. Recently, however, more serious side effects have been the subject of new warnings by the U.S. Food and Drug Administration (FDA). Since February 2007 all drugs used to treat ADHD (e.g., Ritalin, Concerta, Adderall, and Strattera) have carried an FDA warning of risks of serious cardiovascular side effects (including death), growth suppression, and the development of psychosis or other psychiatric conditions.[13]

The Debate over ADHD and Stimulant Drugs

The complexities that practitioners face in defining and coming to a scientific understanding of ADHD are not unique; they exist for most mental disorders due to the absence of biological markers of disease. ADHD is a special case because the incidence of global diagnoses is rising rapidly and sharply, alongside increasing rates of consumption of stimulant drugs by children. The following section outlines some of the key social and ethical considerations that grow out of the ADHD phenomenon.

Is ADHD Real?

The validity of the ADHD diagnosis is at the core of the debate over ADHD and stimulant drugs. The anti-ADHD position finds its most extreme expression in the Scientology movement; scientologists believe that ADHD is a myth and that psychiatric diagnosis and drugs are forms of oppression forced on children by neglectful parents, greedy pharmaceutical companies, or inept teachers.[14] Scientology and other anti-psychiatry forces have a significant national and international influence, and their public propaganda can perpetuate incorrect, harmful, and stigmatizing notions about ADHD and other mental disorders. On the other hand, these arguments remind us that classifying and labeling young children's behavior as abnormal has a subjective, and a moral, dimension and that at present the scientific evidence for the validity of the ADHD diagnosis is too weak to justify, or to curtail, the growth in rates of diagnosis and stimulant drug use among children.

The science side of the debate over the validity of ADHD has tended to respond to the anti-ADHD argument by asserting the biological and genetic evidence for the "realness" of the disorder. This strategy relies on the persuasiveness of expert scientific language and argumentation and tends to avoid the problems of cultural and social bias in ADHD diagnoses.[5] Moreover, such arguments have a tendency to reify diagnoses, which is to say that they represent psychiatric classifications as though they have an absolute correspondence to concrete, biological dysfunctions. Though useful, psychiatric classifications are abstract approximations of complex and heterogeneous biological conditions that interact with environmental factors to produce behavioral outcomes.

Given the complexity of ADHD at the genetic and neurobiological levels, and the phenotypic heterogeneity, it is important not to elevate biological accounts of ADHD, or indeed the diagnosis itself, to inflexible truths or facts. It is just as important not to relegate scientific evidence and the ADHD diagnosis to myth or fictions.

Are ADHD Diagnosis and Stimulant Drugs Used to Treat Socially Based Dysfunctions and Deficiencies?

It is possible to believe that ADHD may be a real disorder, yet simultaneously to have significant concerns about the causes of ADHD behaviors, as well as about the overdiagnosis and overuse of stimulant drugs. The rapid growth of ADHD diagnoses has been attributed to various factors, including parents, psychiatrists, teachers, schools, cultural trends, and environmental toxins. As a thoughtful sociological critique has shown, some of these claims deserve consideration and further research. Social or cultural factors can serve as primary instigators of behavior problems in young children. For example, academic performance pressures on young children, developmental expectations of young boys, and expectations of "good" mothers to produce successful sons are hypothesized to increase problem behaviors, especially in young boys.[1,15] Such factors may also increase the need for medical resources that boost children's and families' capacities to meet social expectations. In order words, these social and cultural factors can influence children's behavior directly, or they can influence rates of diagnosis. Demographic factors certainly influence rates of diagnosis: race and socioeconomic status are predictors of both ADHD diagnosis and underdiagnosis of ADHD, depending on the community.[16]

An active area of research involves pre- and perinatal influences on children's behavioral outcomes. In some cases, ADHD may have primary environmental causes: lead exposure (whether lead paint, lead dust, or lead in the soil) and cigarette smoking by the mother during pregnancy are significant predictors of ADHD.[17–19] The impact of these environmental factors tends to be mediated by genetic and biological mechanisms that are not yet well understood.

ETHICAL IMPLICATIONS FOR CHILDREN

Contemporary ADHD is part of an era of neurobiogeneticization of behavior in which stimulants must be seen as potential options and opportunities for children, parents, teachers, and clinicians. There is considerable pressure to use them. Indeed, drugs may be a relatively primitive harbinger of neuroenhancers to come. Realistic and pragmatic – not ideological and speculative – assessment of the social and ethical consequences for children is critical.

The primary ethical concern for children taking stimulant drugs – or any other psychotropic medications – is safety. More and more children are not taking just a single psychotropic drug, but a combination of these drugs.[20] There is no base of evidence on the safety of common drug cocktails, and prescribing relies largely on physician experience. The international evidence base may be corrupted, as the pharmaceutical industry has been found to selectively publish psychotropic drug trial results and has concealed unfavorable safety data on psychotropic drug effects in children.[21] Even as psychotropic drug treatment in childhood is becoming increasingly common, it is imperative to continue to monitor children's physical responses to the drug(s) over time. Recent studies also suggest that children taking stimulant drugs for ADHD may be at greater risk for substance abuse and delinquent behaviors, although it is not possible to know whether diagnosis and/or drug treatment are causal factors in these outcomes.[22]

The protection of children from unsafe substances is paramount. However, if the risks of stimulant drug use in children do not outweigh the benefits (decades' worth of clinical and anecdotal evidence suggests that this is the case when stimulants are used in appropriate doses and not in combination with other drugs), then a secondary set of ethical concerns must be evaluated. This set of concerns includes the potential types of social and moral harm to children of stimulant drug use. This potential harm has been the subject of much public and ethical debate: There is a concern about the stigma associated with ADHD diagnosis and/or stimulant drug treatment[23] and the degree to which diagnosis is a label that a child carries all of his or her life. There are concerns about whether stimulant drug treatment presents a threat to a child's ability to exercise autonomy and to make decisions (agency). It has been suggested that stimulants may threaten what is natural or authentic in children.[24] Some observers question whether stimulant drug treatment complicates a child's ability to develop an appropriate conception of personal responsibility for behavior.[25]

Few positions in the passionate debate over the potential ethical harm of ADHD diagnosis and drug treatment are supported by empirical evidence. This is because the debate itself has been largely philosophical – that is, abstracted from the world of experience. As a consequence, stimulant drugs and childhood have become the focus of a particular style of ethical argumentation – that of "nurture-neuroethics."[26] Nurture-neuroethics is an ethics that bases notions of responsibility for care (nurture) of the child on a set of largely unexamined ideas about the nature of childhood and the nature of children. Childhood is frequently depicted as a state of idealized innocence, and children are viewed as disempowered and passive subjects in need of protection. These arguments leave little room for the assertion of children's ability to make choices and to have an impact on the world with their choices (agency). Yet evidence from in-depth empirical studies of the ethical implications of psychotropic drug treatment suggests that children are able to successfully negotiate agency and responsibility around ADHD diagnosis and stimulant drug treatment. Children even express a desire for psychotropic drugs, and they successfully negotiate the stigma around psychiatric diagnosis and/or drug treatment. Moreover, the majority of young children interviewed in these studies do not tend to associate taking stimulants with threats to their personal identity or authenticity. However, this may change as children enter adolescence.[23,24]

Until we know more about the balance of ethical harm and treatment benefits, caution regarding the ethical use of stimulant drug treatments in children is important. At present, the evidence base from which to create ethical practice guidelines for stimulant drug treatment in children is relatively weak. However, it is possible to point out some key areas where pediatricians can be especially observant of factors that may compromise the ethical use of stimulant drugs and the treatment of children with them.

Pediatricians' Ethical Practice with Respect to Stimulant Drug Use in Children

Social Influences in Stimulant Drug Treatment for Children. Due to time considerations, an evaluation for ADHD does not typically involve a discussion with parents and the referred child about the social factors that could be driving the desire for an ADHD diagnosis and/or a course of stimulant drug treatment. An initial consultation with a pediatrician is, however, an ideal time to gauge the influence of such factors as part of a clinical assessment of the child's needs. Is the school or a teacher pressuring the family? Does one parent or both parents feel the need to "normalize" the child's behavior because it has become socially embarrassing; or does the family simply not have the personal resources to deal with the child's behavior? Are the parents driven by performance pressures to produce a very successful child? A general discussion with the family that includes the child him- or herself can help a pediatrician assess the relative influence of such concerns. If they are present, they will need to be weighed against the extent of the child's behavioral impairments.

The pediatrician should also understand that a child living in a high-pressure family or school environment may be exhibiting behavioral problems as a response to the environment, rather than because of the presence of organic disorder. However, it is most often more difficult to change the environment than it is to provide a course of treatment that will help the child function better. Often there is an ameliorating impact on the environment as the child's behavior is improved and the environmental pressures lift somewhat. The pediatrician who decides to medicate a child in circumstances where the environment is clearly contributing to the child's behavior makes a justifiable ethical decision to act in the immediate best interests of the child. It is also imperative in such cases, however, to note and discuss the sources of environmental stress or pressure and to highlight these in the case notes as points to follow up in subsequent meetings with the child and family. High-pressure contexts can over time create psychological problems in children. It is important that pediatric care engage parents and caregivers in efforts to change these contexts, rather than simply prescribe additional psychotropic medications for these children as problems accumulate.

Coercive Factors Influencing the Request for ADHD Diagnosis and Drug Treatment. As already noted, it is not unusual for a child's school to exert a certain amount of pressure on a family to pursue an ADHD diagnosis and stimulant drug treatment, although in several U.S. states teachers are now forbidden from discussing stimulant treatment with families.[29] There may also be more subtle coercive factors operating, such as the promise of additional educational resources if the child receives a diagnosis that provides disability benefits or the promise of a place in a child care center if the child is taking stimulant drugs. Competition within the school or on the playing field may contribute to the desire to medicate a child, because stimulants can improve cognitive function and concentration. The pediatrician's evaluation should include an attempt to identify potential coercive factors that may be exerting pressure on the parents and/or the child to pursue medical treatment.

This raises the question of the child's right to refuse treatment in situations where the parents are being coercive. Until the child is the age of majority, parents or a legal guardian are empowered to make medical decisions on behalf of the child. Technically, therefore, a child under the age of 18 in most countries does not have the right to refuse drug treatment. However, it is becoming increasingly clear that children from a very young age have the capacity to understand their medical conditions and are competent to judge treatment decisions.[30] Children are too often left out of such decisions because it is assumed that they do not have capacity to understand when in fact they do. Therefore, good medical decisions will take a child's view into account. If the treatment decision goes against the child's desire, it is necessary to take the time to help the child understand why the decision has been made. This will also ensure better treatment compliance over time.

MARKETING INFLUENCES

The influence of the pharmaceutical industry on drug consumption and physician prescribing is both insidious and enormous. Most pediatricians have had the experience of drug representatives coming into the clinic to discuss new treatments on almost a daily basis. In addition, the drug industry funds all the major clinical trials for drugs; it pays academic researchers handsomely to perform these trials; it ghost-writes scientific articles that educate physicians and the public about new drugs; it provides funds for major research centers and positions at the world's most prominent universities; it organizes and pays for cutting-edge research conferences; and it spends billions of dollars on public advertising campaigns.[31,32] Studies suggest that busy clinicians receive a good deal of their information from industry promotional materials and that this affects their prescribing practices.[33] During these visits, drug reps also leave behind samples of drugs, notepads, pens, and a variety of other goodies that serve as advertisements for their drug.

It is certainly the case that, without pharmaceutical industry funds, our understanding of diseases and the rate of innovation and progress in treatments would be severely curtailed. However, drug industry influence is one of the major ethical problems facing physician and patient autonomy today. In the case of treatments for ADHD, this arguably has an influence on children's consumption of psychotropic drugs. Children in the United States are the world's largest consumers of ADHD drugs and of psychotropic drug cocktails. They are prescribed these at ever younger ages, with rising rates of psychotropic drug treatment among preschoolers.[34] Pediatricians have an ethical responsibility to protect their patients from drug company influences and to refuse drug company involvement in their practice when this involvement could threaten their ability to provide treatment that is in the best interests of the child. Some argue that this ethical responsibility means that drug companies should no longer be allowed access to physicians' offices for any reason, and certain offices either severely limit or refuse access to drug representatives. This is a decision that each pediatrician must reach. It is also necessary to be aware of the insidious drug advertising that pediatricians could pass on to their patients. Vehicles for such advertising include the pens, tissue boxes, and trinkets that are made to look like toys but actually carry drug advertising. They also include educational information leaflets about childhood disorders and drug treatments that provide useful information to families but that may also skew information in such a way as to make drug treatment seem necessary.

Finally, pediatricians can help to educate parents to be critical consumers of drug advertising, whether they encounter it on television, in magazines, or on the Internet. Print advertisements for ADHD drugs tend to promise women a highly idealized relationship with their little boys, a relationship that sustains an oppressive mothering ideology linking successful sons to good mothers.[35] Pediatricians can help parents become aware that these advertisements manipulate consumer longing for a highly desirable lifestyle by linking that lifestyle directly to drug treatment. With their awareness and discussion of such coercive social factors, pediatricians can help to reduce physician compliance with socially generated, industry-sanctioned norms of behavior for parents and for young children.[36] This will help to create a more thoughtful, and more critical, public understanding of drug advertising and more careful take-up of ADHD drug treatments for children.

EXPANDING THE NOTION OF SIDE EFFECTS AND
INVOLVING CHILDREN IN FOLLOW-UP CARE

Contemporary practice in pediatrics and in child psychiatry is increasingly burdened by costs and burgeoning caseloads. Children with ADHD in both the United States and the United Kingdom feel the impact of these clinical practice pressures; they tell researchers that they have difficulty getting in to see their doctors and that, when they do see a doctor, he or she talks only to the parent(s), performs some quick medical checks on the child, and then writes out the next prescription for stimulants. Children would like to see more of their doctors, they would like to see the same doctor more often than they do, and in many cases, they would like to talk to their doctors about what is going on for them around their diagnosis and treatment.[27]

One way to increase pediatricians' interactions with children themselves during follow-up appointments is to include the social and ethical impacts of ADHD drug treatments in the scope of the assessment of side effects of treatment. Pediatricians could ask a child a short series of age-appropriate questions that invite him or her to discuss stigma, coercion, personal responsibility, and identity issues. Children as young as 8 or 9 years old are likely to be able to respond to such questions, if the language is kept simple. Children are likely to be less inhibited in responding to such questions if the parent or caregiver is not present. If such questions are asked in all follow-up meetings – which are mandated for continued prescription of stimulant drugs – even reticent children should become more responsive, and the quality of the relationship between the pediatrician and the child will be much improved. This can serve as an important base for the pediatrician's ability to discern later social and ethical problems around drug treatment, including noncompliance, which increases in adolescence, as well as more serious violations, such as black market sales of stimulants.

STIMULANT DRUG TREATMENT FOR THE PURPOSES
OF ENHANCEMENT

The problem of valid ADHD diagnosis and stimulant drug use in children must be seen against a sociocultural landscape of increasingly fluid ideas about normalcy, identity, and individual improvement. In this context, the broad benefits of stimulant drugs mean that a valid diagnosis is no longer the only justification for stimulant consumption. Among U.S. university students, stimulants are increasingly used as performance enhancers in exam and other academic situations.[37] Academics in the United Kingdom admit to using stimulants and admit to desiring more performance-enhancing drugs.[38] Another extraclinical form of justification for stimulant drug use is associated with a style of thought called "transhumanism."[39] Transhumanism may represent an extreme – the desire to enhance the function of the human body and mind by any and all means – but it exists within an emerging spectrum of desire for human cognitive enhancement. Indeed, venture capitalists are already projecting billion-dollar futures for neurotechnology companies that successfully enhance worker productivity through "neuro-enablement" technologies.[40]

Stimulant drug use among children for purposes of enhancement is very different than such use among consenting adults. Key physical and moral risks would have to be addressed if enhancement became a legitimate justification for prescribed treatment with stimulants. At present, there is no regulatory framework for overseeing the use of stimulants in children for enhancement.[41] However, it is clear that the use of stimulants for cognitive enhancement is increasingly common among adolescents, and it is likely that such use will become more common among younger children as well. Without management and oversight of stimulant drug use, children are at increased risk of harm; therefore, it is appropriate to consider the benefits of clinical oversight of cognitive enhancement practices. At present this can be said only of stimulant drugs and no other psychotropic drugs that could be used for enhancement purposes, such as memory-enhancing drugs. There are sufficient safety data on stimulants to warrant clinical management of enhancement use, whereas there are not sufficient data on other psychotropic drugs for use in children. Any pediatrician who is aware that cognitive enhancement may be a reason for a family seeking treatment must be particularly careful to investigate the ethical areas outlined in this chapter.

CONCLUSION

Pediatricians play a major role in shaping the future of ADHD diagnosis and stimulant drug treatment in children. They are a key resource in the effort to increase our understanding of the potential moral and ethical harm of ADHD diagnosis and stimulant drug treatments, and they can take the lead in implementing ethically responsible stimulant-drug-prescribing practices. Children will benefit enormously from a socially conscious and ethically aware doctor who takes the time to talk to them and listens to their reports about the ways in which their behavior, their diagnosis, and their treatment affect their lives. As more and more children come to take stimulants and other psychotropic drugs, it is ever more necessary to change a system that does not provide physicians the time to build trust and a relationship with their young patients. In time, scientists will have a much better understanding of what ADHD is at the biogenetic level. This will no doubt have an important impact on clinical practice, but genes and biomarkers ought never to become a substitute for the physician–patient relationship, especially not when a child's development and future are at stake.

References

1. Conrad, P. *The Medicalization of Society.* Baltimore: Johns Hopkins University Press; 2007.
2. American Psychiatric Association. *Diagnostic and Statistical Manual of Mental Disorders.* 4th ed. Text revision. Washington, DC: American Psychiatric Association; 2004.
3. Polanczyk G, de Lima, MS, Horta BL, Biederman J, Rohde LA. The worldwide prevalence of ADHD: a systematic review and metaregression analysis. *Am J Psychiatry.* 2007;164:942–948.
4. WHO. *The ICD-10 Classification of Mental and Behavioral Disorders.* Geneva: World Health Organization; 1992.
5. Moffitt TE, Melchior M. Why does the worldwide prevalence of childhood attention deficit hyperactivity disorder matter? *Am J Psychiatry.* 2007;164:856–858.
6. Olfson M, Gameroff MJ, Marcus SC, Jensen PS. National trends in the treatment of attention deficit hyperactivity disorder. *Am J Psychiatry.* 2003;160:1071–1077.
7. Costello EJ, Mustillo S, Erkanli A, Keeler G, Angold, A. Prevalence and development of psychiatric disorders in childhood and adolescence. *Arch Gen Psychiatry.* 2003;60:837–844.
8. Scheffler RM, Hinshaw SP, Modrek S, Levine P. The global market for ADHD medications. *Health Affairs.* 2007;26:450–457.
9. Jensen P, Hinshaw S, Swanson J., et al. Findings from the NIMH Multi-modal Treatment Study (MTA): implications and applications for primary care providers. *Develop Behav Pediatr.* 2001;22:60–73.
10. Singh I. Bad boys, good mothers and the "miracle" of Ritalin. *Science in Context.* 2002;15(4):577–603.
11. Rapoport JL, Buchsbaum MS, Weingartner H, Zahn TP, Ludlow C, Mikkelsen EJ. Dextroamphetamine: its cognitive and behavioral effects in normal and hyperactive boys and normal men. *Arch Gen Psychiatry.* 1980;37:933–943.
12. http://clinicalevidence.bmj.com/ceweb/conditions/chd/0312/0312_I5_HARMS.jsp. Accessed November 20, 2008.

13. http://www.fda.gov/cder/drug/infopage/ADHD/default.htm. Accessed November 15, 2008.

14. Mieszkowski K. Scientology's war on psychiatry. Available at: http://dir.salon.com/story/news/feature/2005/07/01/sci_psy. Accessed November 13, 2008.

15. Singh, I. Doing their jobs: mothering with Ritalin in a culture of mother-blame. *Social Sci Med.* 2004;59(6):1193–1205.

16. Stevens J, Harman JS, Kelleher KJ. Ethnic and regional differences in primary care visits for attention-deficit hyperactivity disorder. *J Develop Behav Pediatr.* 2004;25(5):318–325.

17. Mill J, Petronis A. Pre- and peri-natal environmental risks for attention deficit-hyperactivity disorder (ADHD): the potential role of epigenetic processes in mediating susceptibility. *J Child Psychol Psychiatry.* 2008;49(10):1020–1030.

18. Altink ME, Arias-Vasquez A, Franke B, et al. The dopamine receptor D4 7-repeat allele and prenatal smoking in ADHD-affected children and their unaffected siblings: no gene–environment interaction. *J Child Psychol Psychiatry.* 2008;49(10):1053–1060.

19. Millichap JG. Etiologic classification of attention-deficit/hyperactivity disorder. *Pediatrics.* 2007;121:e358–e365.

20. Safer DJ, Magno Zito J, dosReis S. Concomitant psychotropic medication for youths. *Am J Psychiatry.* 2003;160:438–449.

21. Kendall T, McGoey L. Truth, disclosure and the influence of industry on the development of NICE guidelines: an interview with Tim Kendall. *BioSocieties.* 2007;2:129–140.

22. Molina B, Flory K, Hinshaw S, et al. Delinquent behavior and emerging substance use in the MTA at 36 months: prevalence, course, and treatment effects. *J Am Acad Child Adolesc Psychiatry.* 2007;46(8):1028–1040.

23. President's Council on Bioethics. *Beyond Therapy: Biotechnology and the Pursuit of Happiness.* New York: Dana Press; 2003.

24. Sandel M. *The Case Against Perfection: Ethics in the Age of Genetic Engineering.* New York: Belknap; 2007.

25. Fukuyama F. *Our Posthuman Future: Consequences of the Biotechnology Revolution.* New York: Picador; 2003.

26. Singh I. Beyond polemics: science and ethics of ADHD. *Nat Rev Neurosci.* 2008;9:957–964.

27. Singh I, Keenan S, Mears A. The experience of treatment and care for ADHD: the NICE ADHD Diagnosis Draft Guideline. Available at: http://www.nice.org.uk/nicemedia/pdf/ADHDConsFullGuideline.pdf. 2008.

28. Singh I. Clinical implications of ethical concepts: the case of children taking stimulants for ADHD. *Clin Child Psychol Psychiatry.* 2007;12:167–182.

29. http://www.agbell.org/docs/pipefile.pdf. Accessed November 22, 2008.

30. Miller VA, Drothar D, Kodish E. Children's competence for assent and consent: a review of empirical findings. *Ethics Behav.* 2004;14(3):255–295.

31. Angell M. *The Truth About the Drug Companies: How They Deceive Us and What to Do About It.* New York: Random House; 2004.

32. Moynihan R, Cassells A. Selling sickness: how the drug companies are turning us all into patients. Sydney: Allen & Unwin; 2004.

33. Caudhill TS, Johnson M., Rich EC, et al. Physicians, pharmaceutical sales representatives, and the cost of prescribing. *Arch Fam Med.* 1996;5(4):201–206.

34. Zito JM, Safer DJ, dosReis S, Gardner JF, Boles M, Lynch F. Trends in the prescribing of psychotropic medications to preschoolers. *JAMA.* 2000; 283:1025–1030.
35. Singh. I. Not just naughty: 50 years of stimulant drug advertising. In: Watkins E, Toon A, eds. *Medicating Modern America.* New York: New York University Press; 2007:131–155.
36. Little MO. Cosmetic surgery, suspect norms and the ethics of complicity. In: Parens E, ed. *Enhancing Human Traits: Ethical and Social Implications.* Washington, DC: Georgetown University Press; 2000:162–176.
37. Bronwen CC, McLaughlin TJ, Blake DR. Patterns and knowledge of non-medical use of stimulants among college students. *Arch Pediatr Adolesc Med.* 2006;160:481–485.
38. Tysome T. Pills provide brain boost for academics. *Times Higher Education Supplement.* June 29, 2007. Available at: http://www.timeshighereducation.co.uk/story.asp?sectioncode=26&storycode=209480
39. http://www.transhumanism.org/resources/FAQv21.pdf. Accessed November 22, 2008.
40. http://brainwaves.corante.com. Accessed November 19, 2008.
41. Singh I, Kelleher KJ. Brain enhancement in children. In: Farah M, Chatterjee A, eds. *Neuroethics in Practice.* Oxford: Oxford University Press; forthcoming.

D

END OF LIFE

18

Brain Death, Minimal Consciousness, and Vegetative States in Children

Geoffrey Miller and Stephen Ashwal

Various groups treat death in different ways. Medically, death is the diagnosis of a biological event. To the philosopher, people's interests and the obligations owed them are usually thought to depend on certain qualities possessed only by the living. In religious traditions, death may simply be a transition. To the anthropologist, it is a social event and the beginning of a ceremonial process.[1] Legally the presence and determination of death are necessary when the decision is made as to whether the cause was natural, accidental, homicide, or suicide; when vital organs can be harvested for transplantation; when burial, cremation, or autopsy can occur; when inheritances must be determined; when a spouse can remarry; and when an individual can bring an action in his or her own right. Every culture has customs, norms, rituals, and ethical requirements and prohibitions surrounding death. In modern society, these requirements and prohibitions have been complicated by the ability to keep alive individuals who, in previous circumstances, would have died without intervention. In times past, the traditional approach to the recognition of death relied on the irreversible cessation of heart and lung function. A person would be seen to be unconscious and in a state resembling death, and another person, who was not necessarily a physician, would feel for a pulse, listen with his or her ear to the chest, and look for condensation on a mirror placed close to the nose and mouth. If no evidence of heartbeat or respiration was heard, felt, or seen, death was presumed present, and the passage of time would usually confirm this. There was not absolute public trust in this method, and some feared premature burial.[2] This was alleviated, to a great extent, by the introduction of the stethoscope and later the electrocardiogram. Thus, increased medical expertise cemented faith in the cardiopulmonary criteria for death. However, as medical technology improved, it became possible to maintain respiratory and cardiac function in circumstances where previously this would not have been possible. The question that then arose concerned whether death was present, or could be declared, when medical intervention was responsible for respiration and circulation, and whether there another way of diagnosing death. To some extent, this question was driven by a need for organ donation and transplantation.[3] But in the 1950s, there was acknowledgment of the role of brain function in determining death and in defining the pathological states of the brain that were such that life could be maintained only with assistive technologies.[4] About 10 years later, an ad hoc committee of the Harvard Medical School described this pathological state of irreversible coma and proposed a definition of brain death.[5] There were to be two means of determining biological death; one was cardiopulmonary, and the other neurological. As will be seen later, the coherence of this concept is problematic. We will outline these two means and provide support for the continued use of the brain death concept based on operational usefulness and its moral rightness in that it can provide good in the absence of harm and, for most, in the absence of offense to intuition or moral sense.

The recommendations of the committee were that cardiopulmonary death was the irreversible cessation of cardiac and respiratory function, which would be followed by brain death. Brain death was the irreversible cessation of whole-brain function, which would be followed by the cessation of cardiopulmonary function without the institution of artificial measures. As brain function cannot be sustained in the complete absence of brain stem function, in the United Kingdom brain death is taken to be equivalent to brain stem death. But proposing these two means of recognizing death does not imply that there are two forms of biological death, only that there are two forms of recognition.[6] The concept of irreversible neocortical death does not equate with biological cardiopulmonary death, although it has been considered an alternative,[7,8] However, it is considered by many to be equivalent to philosophical or social death. To appreciate our understanding of the determination of death requires that we eschew metaphysical nuances. To diagnose death requires that it be understood to be a biological phenomenon that can be reliably and repeatedly determined. As Bernat argues,[6] other concepts, spiritual, legal, and philosophical, are important in their own contexts but are not relevant to the biological concept, which should be unambiguous and rest on the determination of irreversibility. Bernat's argument is that the presence of death does not occur when the heart and lungs stop functioning or when there is no evidence of brain activity, but when the absence of these functions is irreversible. When irreversible brain death occurs, the organism has died, even though parts of that previously alive organism can be artificially maintained.[6] The concept of brain death is now almost universally accepted,[9] both because of the increasing technological ability to maintain circulation and ventilation following irreversible loss of brain function and because of the dead-donor requirement for organ transplantation. Clinical determination of brain death can be reliable and repeatable, and is an acceptable means of determining death, although there is variability in its performance.[10–13] In the United States, the present criteria for brain death are as follows: (1) a proximate cause for the coma must be known and has to be sufficient to account for the irreversible loss of all brain function; (2) any abnormal metabolic parameters should be insufficient to account for the comatose state; (3) the effects of any central nervous system–depressant drugs and neuromuscular blocking agents must be excluded, and the patient must have a core temperature of greater than 32°C and a mean arterial blood pressure of greater than 55 mm of mercury; (4) any movement must be attributable to spinal cord function, that is, there are no other spontaneous movements or motor responses; and (5) brain stem reflexes must be absent, and these include absent cough and pharyngeal reflexes, corneal and papillary light responses, caloric responses to iced water, and a positive apnea test. This last test is the one that most validates and determines the clinical diagnosis of brain death. It is conducted after all other evaluations are completed and is performed in such a way as to minimize the risk of hypoxia or hypotension by delivering a high concentration of oxygen to the airway before and during the test. The apnea test is positive if, after a minimum duration of five minutes, there are no respiratory movements with a documented concentration of carbon dioxide in the blood of greater than 60 mm of mercury; results are confirmed by two examinations separated by at least six hours in a patient older than 1 year. Confirmatory tests allow confirmation of whole-brain death. The most reliable are those that demonstrate an absence of cerebral blood flow. If, for technical reasons such as cardiopulmonary instability or physical constraints, the formal brain death examination cannot be completed (usually the apnea test), the diagnosis can be confirmed by demonstrating an absence of intracranial blood flow by angiography or radionuclide scanning. The demonstration of electrocerebral silence on electroencephalography (EEG) is a common confirmatory test but is subject to false positive findings.[14] In children the diagnosis of brain death may require confirmatory tests and longer observation periods.[15] In the United States, for those infants 34 weeks gestation to 2 months, the EEG and clinical examination should be repeated after 48 hours. For children 2 months to 1 year of age, the observation period is 24 hours, and for those older than 1 year the observation period is 12 hours,[16,17] The EEG is not necessary in the older child.

In many international jurisdictions, statutory and common law set the general legal standard for determining death, but not the medical criteria for doing so. For example, the United States Uniform Determination of Death Act states that "an individual who has satisfied either (1) irreversible cessation of circulatory and respiratory function, or (2) irreversible cessation of all functions of the entire brain, including the brain stem, is dead. A determination of death must be made in accordance with acceptable medical standards." This leaves the area free for medical science to improve the maintenance of life and the determination of death. In the United States, two states (New York and New Jersey) also take religious considerations into account, stating that death must not be declared in violation of an individual's religious beliefs. If a neurological determination of death violates those beliefs, death is based on cardiopulmonary criteria. Not everyone agrees with the present medical recognition that brain death is equivalent to death, and in a free society consideration should be given to religious and cultural traditions. For example, in 1990, the Danish Council of Ethics declared that death should be defined by how a community identifies it. The council believes that irreversible loss of cardiac function is death and that brain death, when it occurs while a patient is on a ventilator, is a condition that precedes death when the ventilator is removed.[18] Thus, cardiac transplantation is not permissible. The views of the Japanese community are also reflected in the behavior and beliefs of the Japanese medical profession, where transplant operations involving brain-dead patients are rare.[19] In Japan it is reported that about 30% of the population does not accept brain death as death.[20] Vital organ transplants from brain-dead children younger than 15 years are not allowed. This is because Japanese law allows organ donation from brain-dead individuals only if they have previously declared that they would give permission. Children are viewed as not legally competent to complete a donor card. Furthermore, health professionals will continue caring for brain-dead children until cardiac arrest occurs. Some of these children have "survived" for months and years.[20] If these views are held by some in non-Japanese countries, they should be respected. However, our opinion is that through sensitive counseling health care professionals should attempt to gain permission for the withdrawal of life-sustaining treatment, without coercion, recourse to the courts, or even quasi-legal rulings from ethics committees.[21]

Although the core features of the clinical determination of brain death are very similar worldwide, there is variation with respect to the need for and type of ancillary testing, as well as variability in the performance recommendations for tests such as the apnea test. This variability is also seen in the required type and number of physicians involved and in hospital policies. This is poorly explained and does not have a firm empirical explanation or scientific basis.[22,23] The variability is seen within countries and between institutions[9,24,25] and in brain death determination practices with children.[26–28] Furthermore, the concept of brain death is understood differently within professional groups. For example, in Canada pediatric intensivists were surveyed on their understanding of the concept and how it was equivalent to death.[27] In this group, 48% chose as the major reason that it was equivalent to death was the death of the person, that is, they chose a higher brain concept; 31% chose a prognosis concept, that is, brain death inevitably leads to death; and 35% believed brain death was equivalent to death because there was a loss of integration of the organism. Because of this variability in practice and understanding, Greer et al.[24] have suggested that guidelines be rewritten with emphasis on practical details and that individual institutions be held more accountable for closely following national guidelines.

Even though the concept of brain death and its inevitable correspondence to biological death is widely accepted, there continue to be detractors who argue against its equivalence to a biological or theological death.[8,29,30] By reporting the continued existence of cardiopulmonary function, artificially maintained, for prolonged periods in individuals who were brain dead, as well as the maintenance of pregnancy in and delivery of an infant from a woman who was brain dead, Shewmon has suggested that, given the right circumstances, brain death is not the same as the complete cessation of function of the organism.[31-34] This is supported by Taylor, who states that brain death is really only "near death" and is a legal fiction that allows for organ procurement and transplant.[35] Shewmon's argument that loss of somatic integrative unity is not a physiologically tenable rationale for equating brain death with the death of the organism as a whole is persuasive. But that does not disqualify the continuing use of the concept of brain death. Rather, it may demonstrate that the concept and its determination were created by academic medical bodies that would want to justify their reasoning purely on a scientific basis and avoid notions of personhood. That the scientific rationale has flaws should not take away from its broad acceptance, and this acceptance comes from a utility that does not offend the moral sense of most people. Of course, a different noncoercive approach is necessary when surrogate decision makers do not accept the concept. But does this matter? Are we doing something wrong by using the concept of brain death as equivalent to biological death? We would argue strongly that we are not, because biological death will inevitably follow in the absence of artificial support. The ethical questions relate to the use of artificial support and when and for what this may be justified. Considerations of the metaphysical questions concerning philosophical death, and death in a social sense, may take different paths. But as McMahan writes, "Most people seem to agree, however, that when we die we cease to be here, though normally our dead bodies remain, for a while anyway."[36]

There are some who argue that, because there is widespread ethical and legal acceptance of the withdrawal of life-sustaining treatment from individuals for whom death is both imminent and inevitable but who are not brain dead, these individuals should be available for organ donation prior to the determination of death.[37] But even if this could be conducted in a rigorously correct ethical and clinical manner, the danger of undermining public trust would not allow it. How we determine and define death may have as much to do with subjective standards as with some degree of scientific certitude, and these subjective standards are required to satisfy social and moral legitimacy.[38] The use of the concept of brain death is not an attempt to redefine death. Rather it is a way of determining death that is acceptable as equivalent to death by cardiopulmonary criteria and has as its basis that this is an irreversible cessation of life. There are those who question this concept and state that artificial ventilation delays death, which then occurs when the ventilator is removed or cardiac arrest occurs. Whatever one believes, there is a broad consensus that it is morally reasonable to equate irreversible whole-brain death with death for very practical purposes, but that this moral reasonableness does not extend to the irreversible absence of neocortical activity, for the same practical purposes. We call this neocortical death the vegetative state and will discuss it next.

THE PERMANENT VEGETATIVE STATE

Recognition of the vegetative state (VS) entails a clinical diagnosis. The Multi-Society Task Force on the Persistent Vegetative State has defined the criteria for its recognition.[39] These include:

1. No evidence of awareness of self or environment and an inability to interact with others.
2. No evidence of sustained, reproducible, purposeful, or voluntary behavioral responses to visual, auditory, tactile, or noxious stimuli.
3. No evidence of language comprehension or expression.
4. Intermittent wakefulness manifested by the presence of the sleep–wake cycle.
5. Sufficiently preserved hypothalamic and brainstem autonomic function to permit survival with medical and nursing care.
6. Variably preserved cranial nerve and spinal reflexes.

Irreversibility is believed to be very likely when the condition has been present for more than 3 months following a nontraumatic brain injury and 12 months after a traumatic brain injury. This is acknowledged by the use of the term "permanent vegetative state."[8] Individuals in a permanent VS are neither medically nor legally considered dead. However, they are, by present definitions, considered to be irretrievably close to death without artificial hydration and nutrition. Patients in this chronic state of wakefulness without awareness[39] have no cerebral cortical function and are unconscious. They do exhibit sleep–wake cycles with either full or partial hypothalamic and brain stem function. The VS is considered permanent when the chances that the patient will regain consciousness are exceedingly small. The distinguishing feature is an irregular but cyclic state of sleep and wake cycles, unaccompanied by any detectable expression of self-awareness.[39] Autonomic function is maintained, and the patients may be aroused by certain stimuli, opening their eyes if they are closed, changing their facial expressions, or moving their limbs. They can smile and vocalize (grunt, moan, scream). Their heads and eyes can briefly follow a moving object or move toward a loud sound.[40] The most difficult area, for many, with which to come to terms is the prediction of irreversibility. As opposed to brain death, this is based on probabilities and not absolutes.[41]

With regard to a permanent VS in children, a report from the American Child Neurology Society stated that it could be diagnosed based on the appropriate proximate cause and an appropriate period of observation.[42] The core findings are wakefulness without awareness, unconsciousness with eyes open, and an absence of voluntary behavior and language and any cognitive response. The estimated average prevalence of a VS in children is estimated worldwide to be 49 per million.[43-46] Causes include trauma, hypoxia-ischemia, neurometabolic and neurodegenerative disorders, and developmental malformations. As in adults, recovery from a VS after traumatic brain injury is unlikely after one year, and the degree of recovery appears to be very limited.[43] Outcomes of a VS after a nontraumatic injury are, as in adults, worse than those after traumatic brain injury. After 3 months only 3% are reported to regain awareness.[43] Good or moderate functional recovery is extremely unlikely, but may occur. The conclusions of the Multi-Society Task Force[39] are that after 3 months children in a post-traumatic VS have a 56% chance of recovering consciousness, in contrast to only 3% of children in a nontraumatic VS. The VS is likely to be permanent 12 months after traumatic brain injury and 3 months after nontraumatic injury in children. The chance of recovery after these time periods is rare, and the outcome is almost always a severe disability.[43]

Some may argue that the permanent VS, where there is neocortical death, is equivalent to not being alive. The argument is that "consciousness is the most critical moral, legal, and constitutional standard, not for human life itself, but for human personhood,"[47] and thus permanent unconsciousness is a state in which a human no longer exists as a person, although he or she is biologically alive. But it is unlikely that an individual in a permanent VS could be considered medically or legally dead. However, when this state is certified, actions might be taken that allow the individual to die. Such reasoning for allowing an individual to die is probably more acceptable to the general public and the constraints of law than is declaring a VS to be death. But it is a compromise between keeping an individual in a permanent VS alive as long as possible and acknowledging that the permanent VS represents a loss of human existence, as we know it. Even so, there are some who would argue that there are some forms of life, including those in a permanent VS, who exert no moral claim on us to be preserved.[3] This thorny end-of-life issue remains controversial and contentious, as there is not really a moral distinction, in cases of a permanent VS, between allowing an individual in such a state to die and ending the life of that individual. But to accept the permanent VS as medicolegally equivalent to death would mean that a neocortical death was the same as the present agreed-upon medical and legal definitions of death. For this to occur, it would be necessary to equate a biological death with the philosophical concept of a social death.[48,49] To redefine death in this way may be philosophically arguable, but it would not be publicly acceptable. If the argument that neocortical death was equivalent to actual death were adhered to, individuals in such a state might be buried while still breathing,[50] and the general public would not accept the thought of treating someone who could move his or her body and eyes as dead. However, it is reasonable to suppose that most people would not want to live in a permanent VS and that they would be willing to accept the concept of withdrawing life support in order to allow an individual in a permanent VS to die with dignity, despite the logical incongruities.

But the specter that haunts the medical and ethical analysis of the VS is uncertainty. Outcomes are based on probabilities. Trust is required for the public to believe that the diagnosis of permanence is most likely correct and that recovery from this nonsentient state will not occur. The permanent VS is not a common condition. Very few develop the expertise, or have the time, to make reliable diagnoses. This deficit is deepened by the lack of expertise of teachers in academic institutions who are unable to adequately train future physicians in this area of neurology. But despite its rarity in teaching hospitals, its social importance is clear. Training in the clinical evaluation of awareness is thus an ethical imperative, as is research on more objective methods of evaluating consciousness. The effect of this inexperience is compounded by the fact that most physicians see patients with neurological injury only in an acute hospital setting at the onset of their disorder. As Borthwick and Crossley write when discussing the outcome of a VS, "[O]ne patient at least had some difficulty convincing her medical practitioners of her recovery of sentience even when speaking to them over the telephone. It is not surprising that misdiagnosis occurs. Indeed it is predictable."[51]

Recently various investigative measures have appeared to demonstrate that, in some patients who seem to be in a VS, evidence of complex cortical processing function can be found.[52] Presently it is difficult to be certain whether this represents consciousness or any form of awareness. The medical importance of this lies in whether these findings are useful prognostic indicators. Its philosophical importance is whether the knowledge that the finding of, for example, an event-related potential that implied complex information processing in the association cortex in a patient clinically in a VS triggers our moral sense and intuition with respect to our actions concerning the individual. A recent report from the University of Cambridge claimed to demonstrate that functional magnetic resonance imaging revealed cognitive functions and conscious awareness in a young woman who was clinically vegetative (diagnosed after repeated, prolonged expert evaluation). Her traumatic brain injury had occurred five months earlier, and therefore she did not fulfill the criteria for a permanent VS. However, the report suggests, as stated by the lead author, "a means for detecting conscious awareness when existing clinical techniques have been unable to provide such information."[53,54] It also appears that false negative results may confound such investigations. That is, a patient may fall asleep or may not have heard or understood correctly.[55] There now appears to be a distinct possibility that robust and reproducible methods will be available in the future to demonstrate conscious awareness and the ability to follow complex instructions despite fulfilling the clinical criteria for a VS.[56] If these methods are found to be reliable and generalizable, the clinical ethical questions would have to be redefined. In the case of children in a VS or incompetent incapacitated adults, the question for parents or surrogates becomes whether we should withdraw life-sustaining treatment when the possibility of complex conscious awareness exists but the likelihood of any meaningful motor or behavioral recovery does not. However one may respond to this question, the new knowledge affects ethical analysis. At the moment, we rely on what we believe is the natural history of a VS. Despite the apparently firm definition of a VS, the statement by Plum and Posner[57] still holds: "The limits of consciousness are hard to define satisfactorily and we can only infer self-awareness of others by their appearance and acts." Just as the borders of the VS may be difficult to recognize and quantify, so may its prognosis early in its course. Its diagnosis requires serial observations by an experienced observer using a methodical and meticulous approach. Its prognosis needs to take into account its etiology and length of time following injury. Even with this approach, recovery from a diagnosed permanent VS is not impossible, but it is improbable.[58]

Could individuals in a permanent VS become beneficial sources of organs for transplantation after they die? If life support, in the form of hydration and nutrition, is withdrawn, cardiopulmonary death would be expected to follow in about one to two weeks. By that time, the organs would most likely not be in good enough condition for successful transplantation. Thus, to obtain useful viable organs for transplant, death would have to be accelerated, which is unlawful, but the alternative is that the organs would not be usable.[59] Anencephalic babies are born with a total absence of upper brain and the presence of a rudimentary brain stem and have a short life span. They are in a developmental VS, and they have been considered sources for organ transplantation. In 1987 Paul Holc had a successful heart transplant from an anencephalic baby. This is the only reported instance in which this has happened. The donor, Baby Gabriel, was declared dead before the donation and kept on a ventilator. The dead-donor rule was not broken, and the whole-brain death criteria were followed. Would it be ethical to harvest organs from anencephalic babies before brain stem death? It could be argued that great good could come from this and that it would provide some meaning to the short lives of anencephalic babies. But this commodification of a baby would defy the important Kantian principle of respect. Despite the good that might come from taking organs from anencephalic babies before they are declared dead, by present standards, the mindset that allows organ donation would require a change. That change is that morally and legally we would need to justify killing an innocent individual in these circumstances. The argument does not necessarily flounder on a right-to-life doctrine or on the interests of the anencephalic baby. It is reasonable to say that his or her interests would not be damaged. The argument involves boundaries, the definition of biological death, and the circumstances that allow us to perform certain acts, which we do not allow if the agreed-upon conditions are not met. This is the foundation of the dead-donor rule, which aims at maintaining the deontological imperative to maintain respect and dignity for the dying, but allow organ donation once that individual is accepted as dead, using the criteria for brain death. As Koppelman writes, "[T]his means that living persons cannot donate vital organs and cannot donate nonvital organs if doing so would lead to death."[60]

What about creating circumstances where the organs of an anencephalic baby could be harvested immediately after death? This method was successful for Paul Holc and avoids the need to change the definition of death, putting anencephalic babies in a special legal category or recognizing them as nonhumans.[61] The circumstances are that the anencephalic infant would be placed on ventilatory support to preserve the organs and the baby would be removed from the support at regular intervals to evaluate whether spontaneous respiration was occurring. But this would be a nontherapeutic procedure performed on a patient who was in no position to consent.[61] Even so, we keep adults "alive" after brain death to facilitate organ donation. In 1987 this strategy was attempted at the Loma Linda University Medical Center. Of 12 subjects, none proved suitable for organ donation, for various reasons, and it was concluded that providing intensive care while awaiting the patient's brain death was not worthwhile.[62] Another reason for terminating the Loma Linda protocol was the stress it placed on the health professionals involved. Adverse publicity and the knowledge of being part of an ethically ambiguous (although reasonable and arguable) situation surely undermined morale. Cold philosophical reasoning in clinical ethics is inevitably challenged and colored by emotion and qualms. There now seems to be a general consensus concerning whether anencephalic infants should be sources of transplantable organs. This is reflected by a recent position statement from the Canadian Paediatric Society:[63]

- Organ donation from anencephalic infants should not be undertaken due to serious difficulties surrounding the establishment of brain death in these infants and the lack of evidence to date supporting successful organ transplantation.
- There should be no alteration or modification of standard infant brain death criteria to include infants with anencephaly.
- Families who request the opportunity to donate organs from their infant with anencephaly should have information and educational material provided that explain why this practice is not supported. The option of tissue and stem cell

donation should be discussed using the ethical principles and medical practices applied to other donors.

- The practice of using medical therapy and mechanical ventilation to maintain organ function pending the declaration of death in infants with anencephaly is not supported.

THE MINIMALLY CONSCIOUS STATE

There are patients who demonstrate behavior consistent with a VS but inconsistently show limited, though clearly discernible signs of cognitive function.[64] This state has been termed a minimally conscious state (MCS) and is believed to be transitional and to represent an improvement or worsening of the degree of consciousness. Because of its inconsistency, it may be responsible for the misdiagnosis of chronic disorders of consciousness. Evidence for the presence of an MCS include[58] (1) simple command following; (2) gestural or verbal yes/no responses to questions (regardless of accuracy); (3) episodes of intelligible verbalization (regardless of accuracy); and (4) behaviors that occur in response to specific environmental stimuli and cannot be accounted for by reflexive activity. There are indications that early recognition following brain injury may be associated with a more favorable prognosis, although it may also represent a permanent outcome.[58] Thus, patients in an MCS demonstrate behavioral evidence of consciousness but are unable to reproduce this behavior consistently.[65] Individuals in an MCS may improve or the condition may remain permanent. Apart from its medical significance, use of the concept of the MCS could have ethical consequences, particularly if the courts recognize the state as a separate dire disorder of consciousness worthy of lesser moral consideration, akin to the permanent VS. Formal recognition of this state in a child with a static encephalopathy might trigger management choices that would be less acceptable if the diagnosis were one of severe disability. We would argue that the term is a useful operational one that may suggest a change in clinical condition and presumes consciousness. We are still unable to adequately define or recognize this state reliably or to discern what degree of awareness it implies. A full understanding of consciousness remains ineffable, but this is not an argument against attempts to recognize and categorize its disorders, provided that the dangers are also recognized. MCS is considered by some to be a neurological state whose recognition allows special legal and moral consideration. The interpretation of "minimal" becomes "hardly different from [that of] vegetative." But the term was coined to recognize that a VS may be misdiagnosed and that repeated observations may recognize a variable state that implies awareness.[66] Making quality-of-life judgments about these patients is also difficult. Certainly, obvious pain should be treated, but otherwise it is not always clear who is suffering intractable discomfort: the observer or the observed. The appearance of the severely disabled, poorly communicative individual, at least initially, may cause discomfort and moral distress (how could you let someone live like that?), even among health professionals. Perhaps this is why many might be surprised that patients in a locked-in state (i.e., who are conscious and aware but with very severe motor impairment) typically report that their quality of life is meaningful and that demand for death is infrequent.[67]

What ethical obligations are owed to the child in a VS or MCS? These obligations must be assessed from the perspective of health professionals, families, and the state. For health professionals, there is the requirement that they show respect and that they exercise and maintain all their skills with diligence. Ongoing care should be delivered with purpose and skill. This care also includes early and ongoing communication with and counseling of families and with others who are involved in the care of a most vulnerable population. Parents or principal caregivers are morally obliged to provide care for their child and seek necessary professional help. The state is morally obligated to support families, in its *parens patriae* role, by providing adequate physical, social, economic, and psychological services. These include services in the home or adequately staffed nursing and rehabilitation facilities. Adequate staffing includes not only experienced health professionals, but also social workers, psychologists, and therapists. There should be equity and justice from the state with respect to the allocation of resources. Whether private or public, the nature of these resources is a moral as well as an economic issue. It is unethical to expect caregivers and health professionals to make decisions at the bedside based on distributive justice and economics rather than on the perceived immediate needs of the child.

References

1. Kaufmann SR. Dying and death. In: Ember CR, Ember M, eds. *Encyclopedia of Medical Anthropology.* New York: Kluwer Academic; 2003:245.
2. Adams N. *Dead and Buried.* Aberdeen: Impulse Publications; 1972.
3. Singer P. Is the sanctity of life ethic terminally ill? *Bioethics.* 1995;9:307–343.
4. Mollard P, Goulon M. Le coma depassé [in French]. *Rev Neurol.* 1995;101:3–15.
5. A definition of irreversible coma: report of the Ad Hoc Committee of the Harvard Medical School to examine the definition of brain death. *JAMA.* 1968;205:337–340.
6. Bernat JL. The biophilosophical basis of whole-brain death. *Social Philosophy and Policy Foundation.* 2002;12:324–342.
7. Veatch RM. The whole-brain oriented concept of death: an outmoded philosophical formulation. *J Thanatol.* 1975;3:13–30.
8. Laureys S. Death, unconsciousness and the brain. *Nat Rev Neurosci.* 2005; 6:899–909.
9. Wijdicks EFM. Brain death worldwide: accepted fact but no global consensus in diagnostic criteria. *Neurology.* 2002;58:20–25.

10. American Academy of Neurology Quality Standards Subcommittee. Practice parameters for determining brain death in adults. *Neurology.* 1995; 45:1012–1014.
11. Canadian Neurocritical Care Group. Guidelines for the diagnosis of brain death. *Can J Neurol Sci.* 1999;26:64–66.
12. Haupt WF, Rudolf J. European brain death codes: a comparison of national guidelines. *J Neurol.* 1999;246:432–437.
13. Wijdicks EFM. The diagnosis of brain death. *N Engl J Med.* 2007;344: 1215–1221.
14. Paolin A, Manuali A, DiPaola F, et al. Reliability in diagnosis of brain death. *Intensive Care Med.* 1995;21:657–662.
15. Report of Special Task Force: guidelines for the determination of brain death in children. *Pediatrics.* 1987;80:298–300.
16. Ashwal S, Schneider S. Brain death in the newborn: clinical, EEG, and blood flow determinations. *Pediatrics.* 1989;84:429–437.
17. Ashwal S, Serna-Fonseca T. Brain death in infants and children. *Critical Care Nurse.* 2006;26:117–128.
18. Rix BA. Danish ethics council rejects brain death as the criterion of death. *J Med Ethics.* 1990;16:5–7.
19. Hoshino K. Legal status of brain death in Japan: why many Japanese do not accept "brain death" as a definition of death. *Bioethics.* 1993;7:234–238.
20. Morioka M. Is it morally acceptable to remove organs from brain-dead children? *Lancet Neurol.* 2007;6:90.
21. Miller G. Ten days in Texas. Hastings Cent. Rep. 2007;37:27.
22. Baron L, Shemie SO, Teitelbaum J, Doig CJ. Brief review: history, concept and controversies in the neurological determination of death. *Can J Anaesth.* 2006;53:602–608.
23. Wijdicks EFM. The clinical criteria of brain death throughout the world: why has it come to this? *Can J Anaesth.* 2006;53:540–543.
24. Greer DM, Varelas PN, Haque S, Wijdicks EFM. Variability of brain death determination guidelines in leading US neurologic institutions. *Neurology.* 2008;70:284–289.
25. Hornby, K, Shemie SD. Teitelbaum J, Doig C. Variability in hospital based brain death guidelines in Canada. *Can J Anaesth.* 2006;53;613–619.
26. Mejia RE, Pollack MM. Variability in brain death determination practices in children. *JAMA.* 1995;274:550–553.
27. Joffe AR, Anton N. Brain death: understanding of the conceptual basis by pediatric intensivists in Canada. *Arch Pediatr Adolesc Med.* 2006;160:747–751.
28. Mathur M, Petersen L, Stadfler M, et al. Variability in pediatric brain death determination and documentation in southern California. *Pediatrics.* 2008;121;988–993.
29. Shewmon AO. The brain and somatic integration: insights into the standard biological rationale for equating "brain death" with death. *J Med Philos.* 2001;26:457–478.
30. Seifert J. Is "brain death" actually death? *Monis.* 1993;76:175–202.
31. Shewman DA. Chronic "brain death": meta-analysis and conceptual consequences. *Neurology.* 1998;51:1538–1545.
32. Kantor JE, Hoskins I. Brain death in pregnant women. *J Clin Ethics.* 1993;4:308–314.

33. Loewy EH. The pregnant brain dead and the fetus: must we always try to wrest life from death? *Am J Obstet Gynecol.* 1987;157:1097–1101.

34. Feldman DM, Borgida AF, Rodis JF, Campbell WA. Irreversible maternal brain injury during pregnancy: a case report and review of the literature. *Obstet Gynecol Surv.* 2000;55:708–714.

35. Taylor RM. Re-examining the definition and criterion of death. *Sem Neurol.* 1997;17:265–270.

36. McMahan J. Brain death, cortical death, and persistent vegetative state. In: Kuhse H, Singer P, eds. *A Companion to Bioethics.* Malden, Mass: Blackwell; 2001:250–260.

37. Truog RD, Robinson WM. Role of brain death and the dead-donor rule in the ethics of organ transplantation. *Crit Care Med.* 2003;31:2391–2396.

38. Dagi TF, Kaufmann R. Clarifying the discussion on brain death. *J Med Philos.* 2001;26:503–525.

39. The Multi-Society Task Force on PVS. Medical aspects of the persistent vegetative state. *N Engl J Med.* 1994;330:1499–1508.

40. Zeman A. Persistent vegetative state. *Lancet.* 1997;350:795–798.

41. Burnell GM. *Final Choices: To Live or to Die in an Age of Medical Technology.* New York: Plenum Press; 1993:165–166.

42. Ashwal S, Bale JF, Coulter DL, et al. The persistent vegetative state in children: report of the Child Neurology Society Ethics Committee. *Ann Neurol.* 1992;32:570–576.

43. Ashwal S. Recovery of consciousness and life expectancy of children in a vegetative state. *Neuropsychol Rehabil.* 2005;15:190–197.

44. Aswal S, Eynian RK, Call TL. Life expectancy of children in a persistent vegetative state. *Pediatr Neurol.* 1994;10:27–33.

45. Strauss DJ, Shavelle RM, Ashwal S. Life expectancy and median survival time in the permanent vegetative state. *Pediatr Neurol.* 1999;21:626–631.

46. Strauss DJ, Ashwal S, Day SM, Shavelle RM. Life expectancy of children in vegetative and minimally conscious states. *Pediatr Neurol.* 2000;23:312–319.

47. Crandford RB, Smith DB. Consciousness: the most critical moral (constitutional) standard for human personhood. *Ann J Law Med.* 1987;13:233–247.

48. McMahan J. The metaphysics of brain death. *Bioethics.* 1995;9:91–126.

49. Wickler D. Not dead, not dying? Ethical categories and persistent vegetative state. *Hastings Cent Rep.* 1988;3:41–47.

50. Powner DJ, Ackerman BM, Grenville A. Medical diagnosis of death in adults: historical contributions to current controversies. *Lancet.* 1996;348:1219–1220.

51. Borthwick CJ, Crossley R. Permanent vegetative state: usefulness and limits of a prognostic definition. *Neurorehabilitation.* 2004;19:381–389.

52. Machado C. Can vegetative state patients retain cortical processing? *Neurophysiology.* 2005;116:2253–2254.

53. Owen AM, Coleman MR, Davis MH, Boly M, Laureys S, Pickard JD. Detecting awareness in the vegetative state. *Science.* 2006;313:1402.

54. Owen AM. When thoughts become actions: functional neuroimaging in the vegetative state. *Future Neurol.* 2006;1:693–695.

55. Owen AM, Coleman MR, Boly M, Davis MH, Laureys S, Pickard JD. Using functional magnetic imaging to detect covert awareness in the vegetative state. *Arch Neurol.* 2007;64:1098–1102.

56. Coleman MR, Rodd JM, Davis MH, et al. Do vegetative patients retain aspects of language comprehension? *Evidence from fMRI. Brain.* 2007;130:2494–2507.

57. Plum F, Posner J. *The Diagnosis of Stupor and Coma.* 3rd ed. Philadelphia: FA Davis; 1982:3.

58. Giacino JT. The vegetative and minimally conscious states: consensus-based criteria for establishing diagnosis and prognosis. *Neurorehabilitation.* 2004; 19:293–298.

59. Hoffenberg R, Lock M. Should organs from patients in a permanent vegetative state be used for transplantation? *Lancet.* 1997;350:1320–1323.

60. Koppelman ER. The dead donor rule and the concept of death: severing the ties that bind them. *Am J Bioethics.* 2003;3:1–9.

61. Ahmad F. Anencephalic infants as organ donors: beware the slippery slope. *Can Med Assoc J.* 1992;146:236–244.

62. Peabody JL, Emery JR, Ashwal S. Experience with anencephalic infants as prospective organ donors. *N Engl J Med.* 1989;321:344–350.

63. Bioethics Committee, Canadian Paediatric Society. Use of anencephalic newborns as organ donors. *Paediatr J Child Health.* 2005;10:335–337.

64. American Congress of Rehabilitation Medicine. Recommendations for use of uniform nomenclature pertinent to persons with severe alterations in consciousness. *Arch Phys Rehabil.* 1995;76:205–209.

65. Giacino JT, Ashwal S, Childs N, et al. The minimally conscious state: definition and diagnostic criteria. *Neurology.* 2002;58:349–53.

66. Ashwal S. Medical aspects of the minimally conscious state in children. *Brain Dev.* 2003;25:535–545.

67. Laureys S, Pellas F, Van Eeckhout PV, et al. The locked-in syndrome: what is it like to be conscious but paralysed and voiceless? *Progr Brain Res.* 2005;150:495–512.

19

The Forgoing of Life-Sustaining
Treatment for Children

Sadath A. Sayeed and Geoffrey Miller

In antiquity, sick or disabled children were often left to die in the open,[1] and even infanticide was not unusual up until the 20th century.[2,3] These morally questionable practices were at least partly informed by the heritage of our Greek ancestors, who obligated physicians to not provide treatment of no perceived benefit. Hippocrates wrote:

> Whenever therefore a man suffers from an ill which is too strong for the means at the disposal of medicine he surely must not even expect that it be overcome by medicine. [Treatment in such a situation was] ... allied to madness.[4]

And Plato in *The Republic* advised the physician:

> For those whose bodies were always in a state of inner sickness he did not attempt to prescribe a regime ... to make their life a prolonged misery ... medicine was not intended for them and they should not be treated even if they were richer than Midas.[5]

Following along with our rapid advancement in the biological understanding of human health and disease and our vastly improved ability to effectively treat "inner sickness," our normative ideas about benefit, harm, and misery have evolved. Nowadays, because of an abundance of resources available in the most economically developed countries, it is often medicine's first instinct to try to save the seriously ill or disabled before we start to worry about contributing to unacceptable suffering or prolonging misery.[6,7]

    As the Greeks accurately perceived, questions about which human lives are worth extending through medical efforts and which are better off being let go are inescapable; theirs was a first attempt at ethically answering an enduring dilemma for the medical profession. In this chapter, we will focus on issues raised when we consider forgoing life-sustaining treatment for a child, a matter complicated by the fact that children are often unable to intelligibly and reliably speak for themselves. We note from the outset a variety of sources that have come to inform this kind of a discussion, including some that are more conceptual, like religious doctrine and moral philosophy, and some that are more pragmatic, like law and professional and institutional guidelines. Not surprisingly, these sources are prone to occasional disagreement, and in canvassing them, we do not pretend to definitively reconcile all controversy. Still, we argue that some operational consensus is required to effectively manage the real decisions that must be taken at the clinical bedside. This requires basic agreement with respect to moral and legal boundaries. And while law and ethics are not coincident with each other, they often share similar goals: preventing harm and promoting good.

We also think it vital from the outset to stake an independent claim to the moral importance of virtue in medicine. We need not unconditionally adopt a "virtue-based" ethic or philosophy, but the argument in this chapter is informed by a professional commitment to the values of truth and trust. Aristotle described truth as "the proverbial door which no one can fail to hit."[8] By this, he meant to emphasize that almost every belief formed from human experience possesses an element of truth. We agree that there is an irreducible empirical quality to truth, even while acknowledging that some kinds of understanding are superior to others. Few question the importance and value of trust in medicine as an essential ingredient in any moral relationship between physicians and patients. In pediatrics, this trust, which extends to parents, must also exist between parent and child and, because of the unique vulnerability of the child, between state and child, and physician and state.

As we address the ethical issues related to the consideration of forgoing life-sustaining treatment in children, a number of questions immediately surface: What pathological conditions could potentially qualify for the cessation or noninstigation of life-sustaining treatment? When should this occur? How should it occur? Perhaps most importantly (if not pragmatically), who should decide these things? With respect to the last question, we have long granted parents the authority to make medical decisions for their children. Indeed, as a moral matter, we oblige them to do this because of their special relationship; we presume that, as naturally affectionate caregivers, they will attempt to do right by their children. This deference is also partly justified on practical grounds; as preadolescent children are assumed to be cognitively incapable of making acceptably informed decisions about their lives, a reliable and dependable surrogate is needed, and few are better positioned to fill this role than parents. However, experience shows that not all parents are deserving of a grant of decision-making authority. That thematic concern runs throughout this book.

Decisions to not provide medical care for children that result in their death are usually uncontroversial if all parties involved in the decision agree. Empirically, we typically see a lack of ethical controversy (or conversely, general agreement) when any of the following clinical conditions manifest: terminal illness (or alternatively, unpreventable death); unmanageable pain and suffering: and the so-called permanent vegetative state. We observe here, as an important aside, that very few pediatric disease states can immediately and confidently be classified as resulting in unmanageable pain and suffering. When such states of existence do manifest, it is typically only after much effort has been made over extended periods of time to treat the condition or conditions. We also note the difficulty of diagnosing a permanent vegetative state in an infant or young child who has any cortical brain that is capable of ongoing development.

Regarding the more resolute classification of terminal illness, we note that most ethical controversy here revolves around the characterization of the inevitability of death. While there is rarely anything like true certainty in medical prognosis, we consider a pathological condition to be properly regarded as terminal when that determination is based on the best available knowledge at hand, and expert medical opinion is such that no treatment can be offered that will prevent the condition from causing biological death in some predictable time period (days, months, years). Here, it is worth spending a little time distancing this term from a close cousin, "futility," whose use has fallen out of favor (though we believe it still does some inappropriate dirty work at the bedside). The essential problem with the word "futility" is its multiplicity of intended meanings. One can speak of physiological futility, which comes closest to resembling terminality, as an inability to produce a desired physiological response by a proposed intervention.[9] One can speak of quantitative futility as the probabilistic failure of any intervention derived from previous knowledge, experience, and/or available statistical data.[9] Finally, one can speak of qualitative futility as applying to an intervention whose outcome is deemed not worthwhile for a host of considerations, most frequently quality-of-life concerns.[9] Significantly, the use of the term "futility," even so narrowly defined and qualified, does not automatically prescribe the next therapeutic moves, nor does it lead to consensus decision making. Its qualified use does, however, provide a basis for removing misunderstanding. For example, when the forgoing of life-sustaining treatment is considered, providing further intervention may be classified as futile in terms of the chance of short-term survival or in terms of its leading to a worthwhile life. Such a key qualification sets the stage for a better discussion of the empirically derived physiological facts and the moral arguments that might justify a particular action, assuming the veracity of those facts.

We note discouragingly that futility is often unintentionally interpreted in a pejorative manner at the bedside. If parents resist the withdrawal of medical care but are told that treatment is futile, what they sometimes hear is that treatment is not worthwhile or that it is a waste of time, which may quickly be refashioned into a bothersome waste of time. Such misunderstanding might only serve to entrench differences of opinion regardless of their ultimate validity. As such, without clear qualifiers in place, we argue that the word is best avoided in negotiations with families about end-of-life care. Professionals can find alternative language to argue why they are not obliged to provide treatment they consider useless or harmful. Invoking an easily misconstrued word like "futility" threatens to change the debate from one focused on when it is right to forgo life-sustaining treatment to one concerning power and influence, that is, the right of parents to control what is happening to their child over a perceived professional or institutional authority.

On this note, we argue that the use of tactful language is as much a part of the practice of medicine as it is of political diplomacy. That physicians, in practice, have a determining role in recognizing when it may be appropriate to forgo life-sustaining treatment does not constitute the final step in the process. The next step is one of counseling, which is a complex, sociological exercise that critically depends on the skill of the provider. We all are familiar with model counselors and those who should have never been granted the privilege. We argue that professional skill in the counseling process is ethically obligatory. In addition to constituting a virtue, conscientious negotiating more often than not leads to a lessening of harm to all vested parties, a lessening of conflict and misunderstanding, and the promotion of good ends based on justifiable principles.

For this reason, we are wary of the recent enthusiasm of many providers to promote futility legislation across the country, much like the ongoing experiment in Texas. We are especially wary of its potential effect in pediatrics. The desire to expeditiously circumvent the hard moral work involved in ending seriously compromised early human life is quite understandable, but it risks undercutting trust by creating time-insensitive bypasses. We argue that there is independent moral value for the profession in avoiding actions that have the appearance of coercion, subtle or otherwise, in order to affect a desired nontreatment outcome.[10] The exercise of professional virtues such as patience, prudence, and empathic counseling more often than not resolves the situation, even if the time frame for doing so is exasperating and longer than most physicians would prefer.

Having touched on "easy" cases, like terminal conditions, we now turn to what we perceive to be the most enduring moral problem faced in end-of-life decision making for children: the issue of when it may be appropriate to forgo life-sustaining treatment when the prospects for a child's physical and mental flourishing are seriously jeopardized. Many thoughtful providers, parents, and child advocates have attempted to forge an acceptable ethical path that appropriately weighs the "inherent value" of a child's life with, as Walter writes,[11] "a life that, on balance, does not warrant aggressive treatment." Not surprisingly, considerable disagreement remains the norm, and actual decisions often depend on the attitudes and inclinations of the case-specific players. A hallmark conceptual difficulty lies in our inability to sensibly weigh the binary outcomes faced. At least in secular terms, death is ineffable and cannot be compared with a life of profound disability, as the two outcomes are incommensurable.

Recognizing this, we often turn to a seemingly more amenable calculus and attempt to weigh the perceived benefits of life extension accruing to a severely disabled child as compared with its burdens. But here we run into a deep problem of perspective, so provocatively identified by Robertson:

[T]he essence of a quality of life judgment is a proxy's judgment that no reasonable person can prefer pain, suffering, and the loneliness of, for example, life in a crib with an IQ level of 20, to an immediate painless death. ... [A] standard based on healthy normal development may be entirely inappropriate to this situation. One who has never known the pleasure of mental operation, ambulation, and social interaction surely does not suffer from their loss as much as one who has. ... [L]ife and life alone, whatever its limitations, might be of sufficient worth. ... [O]ne should always be hesitant to accept proxy assessments of quality of life because the margin of error in such predictions may be very great. ... [E]ven if the judgment occasionally may be defensible, the potential danger of quality of life assessments may be a compelling reason for rejecting this rationale for withholding treatment.[12]

Children incapable of expressing their own interests must rely on another's assessment. We follow Robertson in worrying about the ability of any surrogate to adopt the proper perspective. We acknowledge the ethical importance of honoring what appear to be reasonable parental wishes in cases of ambiguity and uncertainty, and also recognize the practical impossibility of policing parental motivations for their decisions. Nevertheless, we are reluctant to wholeheartedly endorse such deference.

We are also seriously concerned about the quality of information transactions between parents and providers. In medicine, health professionals determine facts, frame arguments, and present choices,[13] especially where life-sustaining treatment is concerned. As Meyers writes:

[A]utonomy undercutting power asymmetries prevail and decision making in routine care relies much more on assent than on consent. ... health care in general, and critical care in particular, represent profoundly difficult contexts for genuinely autonomous choices.[14]

Of course, to counteract the inevitable, and in some sense insurmountable, knowledge asymmetry between physicians and parents, the former have a duty to recognize those misunderstandings that significantly increase the risk of medical decisions that are, all things considered, uninformed. Some physicians take this responsibility more seriously than others. In addition, physicians have a duty to recognize when their own understanding and knowledge are incomplete. Nowhere is this more critical than in the forecasting of another's quality of life, a quintessential value judgment, which if we are honest, no physician has expertise in solely by virtue of his or her medical training.

We argue that it is easy to conflate value judgment with medical or physiological fact. In doing so, we do not deny physicians, parents, or others the right to opine about another's quality of life, but it is another step to equate this interpretation of another's posited human existence with something like authoritative truth. Most physicians, by virtue of their professional attainment in life, cannot claim personal, subjective understanding of the seriously cognitively impaired life of a disabled child; we are readily capable of genuine sympathy, but rarely true empathy. As such, prognostications informed by our view from "normalcy" are fraught with ethical risk and can lead to inappropriate recommendations.[15–19] Parents, who are not in a position to know differently and are often unexpectedly thrown into an emotional crisis by life-or-death circumstances, are vulnerable to persuasion, even if unintentionally.

As an example, consider a recent study by Laureys and colleagues.[19] The investigators asked 17 individuals who were in a chronic locked-in state (mean six years) and could communicate only by eye movement or blink, but otherwise could not move, their views on the quality of their lives. For many of us, such a state of existence might, without the vantage of authentic experience, appear to be a condition worse than death. However, the patients interviewed typically reported a meaningful quality of life, and they seldom demanded euthanasia. Measures of mental well-being and psychological distress were not significantly lower than those of age-matched controls. The researchers concluded that "to judge a book by its cover is unfair."

Such empirical data, which suggest a possible disconnect between our perception of profound disability and the actual experience of it, fundamentally challenge physicians involved in end-of-life decision making for children: Are we really capable of adequately distinguishing for parents the physiological facts that we rightly bear expertise on from the moral meaning of those facts? If not, how can we improve our counseling with respect to end-of-life care, when the decision involves choosing between a predicted "poor" quality of life and death? Such provocation is not meant to deny that most, if not all, of us agree that our rational preference is to avoid lives filled with disability, mental incapacity, chronic pain, and the like. Furthermore, we ought not prefer such a life for our children as well. This is not prejudice, nor is it discriminatory. However, even as we can and should maintain such preferences, we should not presume the easy and simple transposition of this preference to an incompetent who has never experienced life as we do.

Having set forth some of our ethical concerns about forgoing life-sustaining treatment for children, we now turn to describe how expert professional panels in pediatrics and bioethics have approached the issues in three English-speaking countries (the United States, Canada, and the United Kingdom). Not surprisingly, there are numerous thematic similarities among these national-level organizational pronouncements, but there are also areas of distinctiveness. At the outset, we note that almost all professional- or institutional-level guidelines are by necessity the product of compromise, as the end goal is to achieve a reasonably broad consensus across a diversity of opinion. While admirable in aim, the diplomatic aspiration to achieve consensus predictably forces a conceptual concession to provide less specificity, so that the language itself contained within recommendations can remain open to individual interpretations.

Starting in the United States, in 1994 the Bioethics Committee of the American Academy of Pediatrics (AAP) published guidelines on the forgoing of life-sustaining treatment.[20] They prominently rely on the best-interests standard (which animates much discussion throughout this book) to provide a principled means to direct ethically minded decision making by surrogates. In essence, the best-interests standard has pragmatically come to act as a balancing test measuring perceived benefits and burdens, weighing them against each other in some reasoned fashion, and on the basis of that metric, providing a decision about treatment. We hope that the reader will recognize that, morally, everything depends on our first accepting the commensurability of the proposed comparative variables.

In fact, many do agree with the list of considerations that ought to be included in the calculus. For example, the AAP Bioethics Committee's list of benefits includes prolongation of life with the proviso that "continuation of biological existence without consciousness may not be a benefit"; a reduction in pain and disability; and an increase in physical pleasure, emotional enjoyment, and intellectual satisfaction. Why there needs to be an increase in these pleasures is not explained, and we note it does not follow ipso facto that, because something is not a benefit, it must constitute a burden. Strictly speaking, if a human being happens to be nonsentient, it makes little sense to speak of burden to that individual, in the absence of demonstrable physiological pain. The burdens include (on cue) intractable pain, irremediable disability or helplessness, emotional suffering, and invasive and inhumane interventions or other activities that severely detract from the patient's quality of life. Again, we pause here to question the acceptability of irremediable disability or helplessness, without further elaboration by the AAP. Regardless, it should be apparent that each of these assessments is somewhat wooly, that is, to some extent they are invariably subjective determinations, and as such provide ample opportunity for personal preferences and value judgments to slip into the calculus. To be fair, the committee emphasizes that quality of life should be interpreted from the patient's point of view and rejects its use to reflect social worth.

In 1996, the committee updated its published position by acknowledging that different people may interpret, value, and weigh benefits and burdens differently:

[P]hysicians should recommend the provision or forgoing of critical care services based on the projected benefits and burdens of treatment, recognizing that parents may perceive and value these benefits and burdens differently from medical professionals.[21]

This is an important concession insofar as it parallels a general normative trend in medicine away from the long-prevalent paternalistic model of doctors knowing what is best for their patients. Nevertheless, as a pragmatic matter, heightened recognition that there is room for reasonable disagreement in the net benefit–burden calculus has largely complicated decision making, as it has provided surrogates with conceptual footing to stake more controversial claims; so-called vitalists can now argue that it may be in the best interests of an irreversibly nonsentient child to remain alive so long as there is no overwhelming pain or suffering, and the problem becomes, how are we to convincingly refute this position? As such, a few physicians have openly lamented and criticized the steady march away from a more physician-centered model for defining best interests, though this is hardly a predominant sentiment in the 21st century.

In 2000, the AAP published its recommendations for forgoing life-sustaining treatment in abused children.[22] Not surprisingly, these guidelines mirrored the aforementioned benefits–burdens–best interests calculus, but also included that decisions to forgo treatment in cases of severe brain injury need not be limited to children in a vegetative state. This publication offered no further elucidation. The AAP also recommended, following legal precedent, the appointment of a *guardian ad litem* in all cases of child abuse requiring life-sustaining treatment in which a parent or guardian may have a conflict of interest. Finally, in 2004, the AAP published guidelines for "do not resuscitate" (DNR) orders for children who require anesthesia and surgery.[23] These state that DNR orders are ethically appropriate "when the burdens of resuscitation exceed the expected benefit." Such orders do not have implications for other therapeutic interventions that might be appropriate for the patient. DNR orders may be written for children when "in the judgment of the treating physician an attempt to resuscitate the child would not benefit the child and the parent or surrogate decision maker ... expresses his or her preference that CPR be withheld in the event that the child suffers a cardiopulmonary arrest, as long as this is in accordance with the child's best interests."

The Canadian Paediatric Society is more specific in its recommendations.[24] At the outset, a strikingly different tone is noticeable:

[A]ll children, regardless of handicap either actual or potential, have a justified claim to life and therefore to such medical treatment as is necessary to either improve or prolong life.

Not surprisingly, this high-minded language is qualified by a statement that the decision to use life-sustaining treatment must be guided by the best interests of the child, which are defined as the balance of potential harm or distress resulting from the pursuit of a given treatment. Like the U.S. guidelines, these state that the interests of the infant should override those of the community, health profession, or family but, in notable addition, that the best interests of the child will usually favor the provision of life-sustaining treatment even when a chronic physical or mental handicap will continue to be present.

The Canadian emphasis on children's rights and surrogates' obligations is further seen in its setting forth specific exceptions to "the general duty of providing life sustaining or life prolonging treatment" as follows:

1. irreversible progression to imminent death,
2. treatment which is clearly ineffective or harmful,
3. instances where life will be severely shortened regardless of treatment, and where non-treatment will allow a greater degree of caring and comfort than treatment,
4. lives filled with intolerable pain and intractable pain and suffering.

The guidelines continue:

[If] the child's condition is incompatible with survival or where there is broad consensus that the condition is so severe that treatment would not provide a benefit in terms of being able to restore or maintain the patient's health, intervention may be unjustified. Similarly, where treatment would involve suffering and distress to the child, these and other burdens must be weighed against anticipated benefit, even if life cannot be prolonged without treatment.

Finally, our brief survey takes us to the United Kingdom, where, in 1997, the Royal College of Paediatrics and Child Health issued guidelines on forgoing life-sustaining treatment for children.[25] Five situations were given in which the forgoing of life-sustaining treatment might be considered:

1. Brain death
2. Permanent vegetative state
3. The "no chance" situation. The child has such severe disease that life sustaining treatment simply delays death without significant alleviation of suffering. Medical treatment in this situation may thus be deemed inappropriate.
4. The "no purpose" situation. Although the patient may be able to survive with treatment, the degree of physical or mental impairment will be so great that it is unreasonable to expect them to bear it. The child in this situation

will never be capable of taking part in decisions regarding treatment or its withdrawal.

5. The "unbearable" situation. The child and/or family feel that in the face of progressive and irreversible illness further treatment is more than can be borne. They wish to have a particular treatment withdrawn or to refuse further treatment irrespective of the medical opinion on its potential benefits.

In reviewing all of these professional guidelines, we observe, with admitted cynicism, that some question begging always follows the persistent reliance on fuzzy terms, like "best interests," "benefits," and "burdens," and that seems hardly diminished by attempts at further clarity with terms like "no purpose" or "unbearable." For example, just how much mental impairment need there be before we can conclude that it is unreasonable for a child to bear life? We hope it is not too difficult for the reader to see how such well-intended guidance can easily be manipulated by the craftier among us.

Recalling our earlier discussion regarding futility, we conclude by noting that any chosen language is only so helpful in solving these moral puzzles. These words describe situations that are unavoidably filled with value judgments about the moral meaning of human existence. With even modest introspection, we are bound to see their limitations and deficiencies. Indeed, nice-sounding words that "justify" our decisions cannot completely extinguish underlying intractable tension, regardless of their strategic value in making us feel psychologically better. Furthermore, there is a danger worth stressing: by seeking refuge in the safe-appearing meanings of such words and concepts, we always risk the possibility of collusive provider–parent agreement without adequate attention to the incompetent child. Anecdotally, we note that a recent official inquiry in Britain found that individuals with cognitive disability were abused, neglected, and discriminated against in the health care system.[26] As such, we should always feel obligated to closely scrutinize how specific biological details inform our rendering of the proposed benefit–burden analysis in each instance; in fully dispensing with our ethical professional duty, following Hume, we should be transparently prepared to defend how the "is" of life's biological details produce the "ought" in end-of-life decision making.

To complete this chapter's discussion of the issues related to ending life-sustaining treatment for infants and children, we now turn to a sampling of laws and legal decisions from several English-speaking jurisdictions. We do not attempt to provide an exhaustive legal history of the subject. All English-speaking democracies recognize a *parens patriae* function for the governmental authority, which is in its most generic form a sovereign power to protect the most vulnerable in society. However, modern states typically view their relationship to parents and children primarily in passive custodial terms, being prepared to intercede in family life only as a last resort when there is a compelling basis to question natural surrogates' child-rearing conduct. Pragmatically, governmental review of parental medical decision making nowadays almost never arises unless there is an intractable conflict between parents and providers about the ethically correct course of action or, in more operational terms, if there is fundamental disagreement about the best interests of the child.

Two classic sorts of cases present themselves to courts of law for ultimate disposition. The first pits parents who want to end potentially lifesaving treatment against providers who feel that such intervention is warranted, and the second pits parents who want to extend potentially lifesaving treatment against providers who feel that such intervention is inappropriate. Here we note an important mechanistic distinction between the two kinds of cases, particularly in the United States. The final move for U.S. health care providers in cases of the former type is to initiate formal involvement by the state's child protection services. This decision amounts to a conclusion by providers that the parents or guardians have taken a position that substantially threatens the child, and that at least temporary custody by the state is warranted. In cases of the latter type, the child neglect construct is far less often a suitable conceptual fit for analyzing the conflict. Parents who are committed to preserving a child's biological life and who insist on continuing medical care that others find objectionable are rarely appropriately characterized as neglectful or abusive (though we can imagine such a case when the pain and suffering of the child are incontrovertible). Thus, legal resolution in these kinds of cases does not necessarily imply a role for the state's child protective services.

Two factually similar cases recently adjudicated in the United Kingdom serve to illustrate the kinds of typical controversies just described. The British have largely eschewed legislative means, and instead follow a common law approach, to resolving disputes surrounding life-sustaining support for infants and children. Judges tend to rely heavily on the best-interests standard to evaluate the legal propriety of surrogate decisions. The two cases occurred about a decade apart and dealt with life-sustaining treatment for children with severe spinal muscular atrophy (SMA). In the more recent case, M.B. was an 18-month-old infant with SMA who was totally paralyzed apart from some eyebrow and eye movement.[27] Some providers assessed the child's condition as intolerable and therefore argued that life-extending treatment would be an unacceptable burden based on their perception of ongoing overwhelming discomfort, pain, and distress.[28] The hospital sought a declaration from the court to allow the withdrawal of life-sustaining treatment over the objections of the parents, who believed that their child was cognitively intact, able to enjoy the company and social interaction of others, and not excessively burdened by pain and suffering.

In deciding that it was in the child's best interests to continue medical treatment, Justice Holman stated he was unaware of a U.K. court ever being asked before

to approve, against the will of the parents, that life support may be withdrawn or discontinued, with the predictable, inevitable, and immediate death of a conscious child with sensory awareness and assumed normal cognition and no reliable evidence of any significant brain damage.

He also questioned the utility of "intolerability" as a meaningful measure when weighing the benefits and burdens for a disabled child:

I avoid reference to the concept "intolerability." It seems to me that it all depends on what one means by "intolerable" and the use of that word really expresses a conclusion rather than provides a test. If it is correct to say ... that life is literally "intolerable," then it is hard to see in what circumstances it should be artificially prolonged. If conversely it is "tolerable" then it is hard to see in what circumstances it should be permitted, avoidably, to end. ... the concept of "intolerable to the child" should not be seen as gloss on, much less a supplementary test to, best interests.

Consistent with his desire to avoid rendering terms ladened with subjective value judgment, the justice finally argued that his role was not to be concerned with ethical issues, only legal ones:

I myself am not concerned with any ethical issues which may surround this case. My task ... is to decide, and only to decide, where the objective balance of the best interests of M lies. If I decide that it is not in his overall best interests to continue with a given form of treatment ... then I must say so; and it will follow as a matter of law (and I will declare) that it is lawful to withdraw or withhold that form of treatment. The ethical decision whether actually to withdraw or withhold it must be made by the doctors concerned. Judges are neither qualified to make, nor required, nor entitled to make ethical judgments or decisions.

Whatever the merits of his substantive choice to decide for life extension for the child, we find Justice Holman's claim to neutrality under the guise of legal objectivity rather naive. To argue that his decision has no ethical bearing on how doctors should ultimately act is not only disingenuous (should they now risk liability for not following the command of the court?), it falsely dichotomizes an inherent task for the law when it is forced to resolve disputes involving the appropriateness of medically dependent life extension. His legal judgment, couched in the language of best interests rather than intolerability, still cannot escape expressing moral value; it represents a deliberate decision to put more weight on the "worth" of a gravely incapacitated human life over other presumably important considerations. We argue that it is a mistake to try to hide behind a purported legal neutrality in cases such as this; law and ethics cannot so easily be divorced when it comes to life-and-death matters.

The *MB* ruling stands in contrast to *Re C* (1998), which also involved a child with severe SMA.[29] The judge in this case ruled on whether objecting physicians would be legally required to initiate life-sustaining treatment if requested to do so by parents in the future. C was a 16-month-old child with severe SMA, who was placed on a ventilator following a respiratory arrest. Providers judged that life-sustaining treatment was simply a means of postponing death without significant alleviation of suffering and, therefore, sought declaratory relief so that they could avoid further intervention once the child was removed from the artificial respiratory support. The parents agreed that their child could be taken off the ventilator, but insisted on reintubation and mechanical ventilation should a further respiratory arrest occur. Independent medical expert opinion sided with the treating physicians, and the hospital sought leave from the court to manage the child as had been advised, that is, to extubate and not reintubate should there be further respiratory distress.

Justice Brown delivered the judicial opinion, referring to the disease as dreadful and the case as tragic. He found that the baby was in a "no chance" situation, using the term from the aforementioned Royal College of Paediatrics report[25] concerning life-sustaining treatment for children. He ruled that

[t]here be leave to treat the minor C, as advised by DrH, such treatment to include the withdrawal of artificial ventilation and non-resuscitation in the event of a respiratory arrest and palliative care to ease her suffering and permit her life to end peacefully and with dignity, such treatment being in C's best interests. ... [W]hilst the sanctity of life is vitally important, it is not the paramount consideration. The paramount consideration here is the best interests of little C.

Further substantive clarification of how the interests of C are definitively surmised by the court is lacking. Much as in the *MB* case, it is obvious that a core value judgment prioritizing certain factors over others underpins Justice Brown's opinion. Notably, the opinion draws some of its justification from overt policy considerations. Justice Brown argues that forcing providers to treat would be

[t]antamount to requiring the doctors to undertake a course of treatment which they are unwilling to do. The court could not consider making an order which would require them to do so.

Of course, judges and legal theorists across many jurisdictions have long found safe harbor in the act–omission distinction, even while ethicists and philosophers have criticized the distinction. We only identify the issue here for the reader and note the many nuanced problems in determining intention and causality in both moral and legal terms.

The contrasting judgments in *MB* and *C* decided only a few years apart in the United Kingdom serve our purpose of emphasizing to the reader the flexibility or fickleness of judicial interpretation of common law, depending on one's point of view. To be fair, the different decisions may also reflect changing social mores, attitudes, or awareness in Britian about aggressive life-sustaining treatment for a disabled child, which may be partly spurred by the increasing availability of improved technology and long-term care options. A decade ago, parents of a child with severe SMA type 1 would most likely never have been offered the option of long-term ventilation at a nursing facility, as that choice was not as economically or technically viable as it is now.

Turning now to U.S. law, as articulated by judges, legislators, and regulators, we see a tradition of the state favoring life-preserving outcomes rather than life-ending ones. This moral tilt is articulated by the majority United States Supreme Court opinion in the *Cruzan* case:

The choice between life and death is a deeply personal decision of obvious and overwhelming finality. We believe [a State] may legitimately seek to safeguard the personal element of this choice through the imposition of heightened evidentiary requirements. It cannot be disputed that the Due Process Clause [of the Constitution] protects an interest in life as well as an interest in refusing life-sustaining medical treatment. … We think a State may properly decline to make judgments about the "quality" of life that a particular individual may enjoy, and simply assert an unqualified interest in the preservation of human life to be weighed against the constitutionally protected interests of the individual.[30]

Cruzan is an important U.S. decision on the life-sustaining treatment issue, and its legal meaning is complex. We note it here but will not attempt further elaboration, particularly given its unclear effect on end-of-life decision making for children.

The United States has both statutory and common law sources to guide decision making that involves life-sustaining medical treatment for infants and children. The common law tradition flows from the *parens patriae* doctrine and, quite predictably, operationalizes in the form of a legal best-interests standard. Judges rely on a similar set of considerations that inform ethical analysis of when it may be permissible or obligatory to withhold or withdraw life-sustaining treatment from a child. Thus, in disposing of a contested case, judges usually rely on evidence about perceived benefits and burdens of treatment to the child. A comprehensive but inexhaustive list of factors to be considered includes the following: (1) the child's present level of physical, sensory, emotional, and cognitive functioning; (2) the quality of life, life expectancy, and prognosis for recovery with and without treatment; (3) the various treatment options and their risks, benefits, and side effects; (4) the nature and degree of physical pain, suffering, or serious complications resulting from the medical condition, from treatment, and resulting if treatment is withdrawn; (5) whether treatment would on balance be more beneficial than burdensome to the child; (6) whether pain and suffering resulting from removal of treatment could be minimized; (7) the degree of humiliation, dependence, and loss of dignity resulting from the condition and treatment; (8) the opinion of the family and their reasons and motivations for holding those opinions regarding treatment; and (9) the child's preference, if it can be ascertained.

As we have argued before, an inescapable set of value judgments must enter into this legal decision-making calculus. Numerous cases can be canvassed in order to demonstrate how state courts at various levels have mapped specific facts onto the benefit–burden analysis. Suffice it to say that despite relative consensus about animating principles for life-or-death medical treatment decision making, there is hardly uniform application across U.S. jurisdictions. This inconsistency simply reflects an ongoing thematic point: judges are human beings who bring their own predispositions, cultural commitments, and moral attachments to the task of legal interpretation. Cases often turn on the relative weight that individual legal decision makers choose to place on certain facts.

We do think it important here to emphasize a theme frequently evidenced in U.S. case and statutory law. As a child begins to mature and demonstrate the capacity to speak for him- or herself, courts will begin to seriously incorporate any such informed opinions into their final calculus. This is consistent with the robust moral and legal tradition in American society to prioritize individual autonomous choices in the absence of other compelling considerations. A paradigmatic illustration of judicial deference to an adolescent's expression of autonomy comes from Illinois, *In re E.G.*[31] The case involved a 17-year-old teenager diagnosed with leukemia who refused to consent to blood transfusions as a part of therapy due to her religious faith as a Jehovah's Witness. Her mother and she had consented to all other treatments and had signed a waiver of provider liability for failure to administer blood products. The treating physician testified that he was "impressed with her maturity" and felt the patient "competent to understand the consequences of accepting or rejecting treatment." Nevertheless, under advice from hospital counsel, child neglect proceedings were initiated and eventually resulted in the appointment of a temporary guardian who consented to transfusions, which the patient received.

The case continued and eventually the patient herself was allowed to testify; she "indicated that her decision was not based on any wish to die, but instead was grounded in her religious convictions." The trial court disposition of the case ended with the judge ruling that the patient was medically neglected, and a guardian was appointed to consent to further treatment. The patient and her mother appealed the decision, and before the state Supreme Court, the issue was "whether [an allegedly mature] minor like E.G. has a right to refuse medical treatment." In a divided decision, the court reversed the finding of neglect and held:

The State's parens patriae power pertaining to minors is strongest when the minor is immature and thus incompetent (lacking in capacity) to make decisions on her own. [It] fades, however, as the minor gets older and disappears upon her reaching adulthood. The State interest in protecting a mature minor in these situations will vary depending upon the nature of the medical treatment involved. Where the health care issues are potentially life-threatening, the State's ... interest is greater than if the health care matter is less controversial.

In deciding in favor of E.G. in terms of her medical decision, the court emphasized that, while the statutory age of majority in the state was 18, "that age is not an impenetrable barrier that magically precludes a minor from possessing and exercising certain rights normally associated with adulthood." The court detailed a list of circumstances in which both the legislature and common law had granted minors authority to make medical treatment decisions for themselves (e.g., sexually transmitted diseases, pregnancy) and stated that the chief role of the trial court in this case was to determine whether the minor was mature enough to make health care choices on her own. Notably, the court did not find the First Amendment issue of free religious exercise relevant to its disposition of the case.

However, the dissenting judge picked up on a not-so-subtle inconsistency in the majority's opinion:

The safeguarding of health and the preservation of life are obviously different conditions. ... I am sure that in a host of matters of far less importance it would not be held that a minor however mature could satisfy a requirement of being of legal age. It would not be held that a minor was eligible to vote, to obtain a driver's or a pilot's license.

Indeed, it is striking that the majority chose to respect the adolescent's "mature" choice when the stakes were highest and the consequences to her so final, despite the state legislature's having failed to grant the opportunity to find such maturity in less critical situations. This disconnect suggests that, at least under the circumstances of this case, the court has a distaste for an efficiency-driven argument that justifies a partly arbitrarily defined legal age of majority. We know that the age of 18 is merely an imperfect approximation; it necessarily includes some who shouldn't be included and excludes some who shouldn't be excluded. But from a policy standpoint, we cannot imagine society making individual maturity assessments on all teenagers from time to time to determine which decision-making capacities they possess and which they still need time to develop. Why the majority in the *E.G.* opinion felt obliged to grant individual evaluation under the circumstances presented remains a core legal controversy. We note that in a different state with a different set of judges' eyes, it is quite conceivable that this case might have been decided in the opposite manner (affirming the trial court's finding of neglect).

If deference to emerging autonomy is an important ethical and legal consideration in life-ending medical treatment choices for minors on the brink of attaining majority, it is important to contrast this construct with how life-ending decisions for infants have been viewed legally in the United

States for the past two to three decades. Heightened state and governmental scrutiny has been the norm and flows from the national politicization of common practices first publicized in the 1970s. Public reports from that time documented that some nonterminal infants died each year in U.S. hospitals as a result of the withdrawal or withholding of treatment,[32] and surveys demonstrated that a large percentage of physicians were willing to forgo life-sustaining treatment for disabled infants.[33] In one study it was revealed that 85% of pediatric surgeons and 65% of pediatricians surveyed were willing to honor parental wishes not to perform necessary surgery on an infant with Down syndrome, but less than 6% would deny similar treatment for a child without the disability.[33]

Some physicians made such life-ending decisions regardless of parental preference, even though such unilateral action generally was considered unlawful.[29] At the time these practices were gaining national attention, law professor John Robertson wrote:

In the case of a defective infant the withholding of essential care would appear to present a possible cause of homicide by omission on the part of parents, physicians, and nurses, with the degree of homicide depending on the extent of premeditation. Following a live birth the law generally presumes that personhood exists and that there is entitlement to the usual protections, whatever the specific physical or mental characteristics of the infant maybe. Every state imposes on parents a legal duty to provide necessary medical assistance to a helpless minor child. If they withhold such care, and the child dies, they may be prosecuted for manslaughter or murder. ... likewise physicians and nurses may face criminal liability ... even when all Parties, including the parents, are in agreement.[12]

Partly out of reaction to these events and rather infamous individual cases in Indiana, New York, and Maryland, the U.S. Congress amended the Child Abuse Prevention and Treatment Act (CAPTA) in 1984 (PL 98-457). These amendments and their administrative interpretation (often collectively termed the "Baby Doe rules") make conditional the receipt of certain federal funds for state child protective agencies dependent on the local adoption of federal reference criteria for defining medical neglect for children under a year of age (42 USC 5106 (b) (2) (B)).

Medical neglect was defined as the "withholding of medically indicated treatment" from disabled infants with "life threatening conditions." Medically indicated treatment was then defined as that

which, in the treating physician's reasonable medical judgment, will be most likely effective in ameliorating or correcting all [of the infant's life threatening] conditions, except that the term does not include the failure to provide treatment ... to an infant when, in the treating physician's reasonable medical judgment,

  (A) the infant is chronically and irreversibly comatose;
  (B) the provision of such treatment would (i) merely prolong dying, (ii) not be effective in ameliorating or correcting all of the infant's life

threatening condition, or (iii) otherwise be futile in terms of the survival of the infant; or

(C) the provision of such treatment would be virtually futile in terms of the survival of the infant and treatment itself under such circumstances would be inhumane.

These amendments were subsequently interpreted by the federal administration (through the Department of Health and Human Services). "Virtually futile" was interpreted as "highly unlikely to prevent death in the near future" on the basis of reasonable medical judgment (45 CFR pt 1340 app at 306). And a treatment was inhumane if

the treatment itself involves significant medical contraindications or significant pain and suffering for the infant that clearly outweigh the very slight potential benefit of the treatment for an infant highly unlikely to survive. ... the balance is clearly to be between the very slight chance that treatment will allow the infant to survive and the negative factors relating to the process of the treatment.

In the commentary to the amendments, the primary role of parents is made clear: "[E]xcept in highly unusual circumstances, [decisions to provide or withhold medically indicated treatment] should be made by the parents or legal guardian" (50 Fed. Reg. 14, 878 14, 880 (1985)). However, the legislative history also qualifies that "the parents' role as decision maker must be respected and supported unless they choose a course of action inconsistent with applicable standards established by law" (50 Fed. Reg. 14, 880).

We note that the CAPTA amendments and the Baby Doe rules are fundamentally passive legal instruments and do not compel state courts to any specific action. For states that desire federal funding as support for their local child protective agencies, there is an obvious attraction to adopting the federal language for defining medically indicated treatment for infants under a year of age. Thus, not surprisingly, almost all states immediately followed suit. But actual enforcement of these federal legal standards is strictly the business of state child protective agencies and interpreting state courts. CAPTA merely stipulates that local child protective services have the authority to pursue any legal remedies that may be necessary to prevent the forgoing of life-sustaining treatment[34] from an unqualified infant. The almost theatrical history of these notorious regulations, their minimal on-the-ground enforcement after an initial wave of conservative enthusiasm, and their mixed but enduring impact on clinical care from the 1980s until today is well documented. The reader is referred to a voluminous literature on the subject matter; almost needless to say, the Baby Doe rules remain highly controversial in the United States.

As the states were writing and modifying their statutes dealing with end-of-life issues, a number of landmark cases were heard that influenced these statutes and the action of health professionals. They have in common the drama of the law courts, intensive care units caring for the most fragile and moribund infants, and the actions and anguish of distraught parents. For example, in Illinois in 1991, the Health Care Surrogate Act was signed into law. It followed a well-publicized case that occurred at the Presbyterian-St. Luke's Center in Chicago.[35] In August 1988, Sammy Linares, an infant aged 6 months, had become asphyxiated by inhaling a rubber balloon and suffered a cardiac arrest. He was maintained on life support in a persistent vegetative state. In April 1989, following a refusal by the hospital and attending physicians to discontinue life support in the absence of a court order, the father, Rudy Linares, performed this act while keeping hospital workers at bay with a handgun. This followed an incident the previous December when the father had disconnected the baby from the ventilator but was physically restrained by security guards while the ventilator was reconnected.[35] Despite the manner in which the father acted, there clearly was much sympathy for him. A coroner found that asphyxiation from a balloon was the primary cause of death,[35] and a grand jury declined to issue an indictment for homicide. Mr. Linares did receive a suspended sentence for a misdemeanor arising from a weapons charge. The statutory law that followed made it clear that life-sustaining treatment could be withdrawn, without judicial involvement, from a patient without decisional capacity. The conditions that would allow this were that a surrogate could request withdrawal if two physicians certified one of the following:

a).   imminent death; that is, when death is inevitable within a short time, "even if life sustaining treatment would be initiated or continued";

b).   permanent unconsciousness, for which initiating or continuing life support, in light of the patient's medical condition, provides only minimal medical benefit;

c).   incurable or irreversible condition that imposes severe pain or an inhumane burden that will ultimately cause the patient's death and for which initiating or continuing life-sustaining treatment provides only minimal medical benefit.

The Act protects the parties involved provided they follow the legislation "with due care." Similar legislation exists in all the other states and they appear to eschew a best interests approach and quality of life judgments.

Finally, we turn to Australia, which also has a mixed approach. Somewhat like the U.S. CAPTA amendments, there is statutory law that supports physicians when an infant is terminal or in a persistent vegetative state; for example, the South Australia Consent to Medical Treatment and Palliative Care Act states that a physician who is responsible for the management of a terminally ill patient is

under no duty to use, or to continue to use, life sustaining measures in treating the patient if the effect of doing so would be merely to prolong life in a moribund state without any real prospect of recovery or in a persistent vegetative state.[36]

The *parens patriae* doctrine also animates common law and, as articulated by Justice Brennan in *Marion's Case,*

underlies and informs the law: each person has a unique dignity which the law respects and which it will protect. Human dignity is a value common to our municipal law and to international instruments related to human rights. The law will protect equally the dignity of the hail and hearty and the dignity of the weak and lame; of the frail baby and of the frail aged: of the intellectually able and the intellectually disabled. ... our law admits of no discrimination against the weak and disadvantaged in their human dignity.[37]

Much as in the United States and the United Kingdom, this state power is manifested through courts adopting a best-interests standard. Here again, we see an inherent tilt toward life preservation in case law and some evidence to suggest that quality-of-life decisions will generally be frowned upon judicially: "The law does not permit decisions to be made concerning the quality of life nor any assessment of the value of any human life"[38] (*F v. F* [unreported, 2 July Supreme Court of Victoria]).[39] This case involved a proposal to stop feeding an infant with spina bifida. Similar language is seen in a later judgment from the High Court of Australia involving a wrongful birth suit (which the court rejected):

[I]n the eyes of the law, the life of a troublesome child is as valuable as that of any other; and a sick child is of no less worth than one who is healthy and strong. The value of human life, which is universal and beyond measurement, is not to be confused with the joys of parenthood, which are distributed unevenly.[40]

CONCLUSION

In this chapter, we have attempted to survey a variety of arguments and sources to improve the reader's understanding not only of the issues involved in decisions to withdraw or withhold life-sustaining treatment taken on behalf of children, but also of the core moral tensions that resist resolution regardless of whether one looks to ethical reasoning, professional consensus, or law for answers. It is necessarily an incomplete treatment. Nevertheless, we believe a good accounting of the controversies should not shy away from a critical assessment of the inadequacies of any singular approach, however high-minded.

Moral value judgment is inescapable in this arena, and one must ultimately come to recognize one's own final commitments in any given case. The authors differ in this regard, as one (G.M.) is drawn much more to deontological, rights- and virtue-based arguments, while the other (S.S.) is an admitted mixed consequentialist who is comfortable living with some internal contradictions. Rather than try to settle our disputes, together we believe that it is more important for our readers to begin to appreciate the implications of adopting any moral rationale. We both agree that wisdom can be gained only when we start with a humble predisposition.

References

1. Boswell J. *The Kindness of Strangers: The Abandonment of Children in Western Europe from Late Antiquity to the Renaissance.* New York: Pantheon; 1989.
2. Lecky W. *History of European Morals from Augustus to Charlemagne.* Vol. 2. New York: Brazillier; 1955.
3. Langer WL. Europe's initial population explosion. *Am Hist Rev.* 1963;69: 1–17.
4. Selection from the Hippocratic Corpus: The Art (circa 5th century BC). In Reiser SJ, Dyck AJ, Curran WJ, eds. *Ethics in Medicine: Historical Perspectives and Contemporary Concerns.* Cambridge, Mass: MIT Press; 1977:6–7.
5. Plato. *The Republic.* Grube GMA, trans. Indianapolis: Hacket; 1974.
6. Wolraich ML, Siperstein GN, Reed D. Doctors' decisions and prognostications for infants with Down syndrome. *Pediatrics.* 1977;60:512–518.
7. Haslam RH, Milner R. The physician and Down syndrome: are attitudes changing? *J Child Neurol.* 1992;7:304–310.
8. Lear J. *Aristotle: The Desire to Understand.* Cambridge: Cambridge University Press; 1988:5.
9. Jonsen AR, Siegler M, Winslade WJ. *Clinical Ethics: A Practical Approach to Ethical Decisions in Clinical Medicine.* 5th ed. New York: McGraw-Hill, 2002:25.
10. Miller G. Ten days in Texas. *Hastings Cent Rep.* 2007;37(July/August):27.
11. Walter JW. Approaches to ethical decision making in the neonatal care unit. *Am J Dis Child.* 1988;9:293–308.
12. Robertson JA. Involuntary euthanasia of defective newborns: a legal analysis. *Stanford Law Rev.* 1975;27:246–261.
13. McHaffie HE, Laing IA, Parker M, McMillan J. Deciding for imperiled newborns: medical authority or parental autonomy? *J Med Ethics.* 2001;27: 104–109.
14. Meyers C. Cruel choices: autonomy and critical care decision making. *Bioethics.* 2004;18:104–119.
15. Morse SB, Haywood JL, Goldenberg RL, Bornstein J, Nelson KG, Carlo WA. Estimation of neonatal outcome and perinatal therapy use. *Pediatrics.* 2000;105:1046–1056.
16. Cook LA, Watchko JF. Decision making for the critically ill neonate near the end of life. *J Perinatol.* 1996;16:133–136.
17. Ginsberg HG, Goldsmith JP. Controversies in neonatal resuscitation. *Clin Perinatol.* 1998;25:1–15.
18. Campbell DE, Fleischmann AR. Limits of viability: dilemmas, decisions, and decision makers. *Am J Perinatol.* 2001;18:117–128.
19. Laureys S, Pellas F, Van Eeckhout PV, et al. The locked-in syndrome: what is it like to be conscious but paralysed and voiceless? *Progr Brain Res.* 2005;150:495–512.
20. American Academy of Pediatrics, Committee on Bioethics. Forgoing of life-sustaining treatment. *Pediatrics.* 1994;93:532–536.
21. American Academy of Pediatrics, Committee on Bioethics. Ethics and the care of critically ill infants and children. *Pediatrics.* 1996;95:149–152.
22. American Academy of Pediatrics, Committee on Child Abuse, and Neglect, and Committee on Bioethics. Forgoing life-sustaining medical treatment in abused children. *Pediatrics.* 2000;106:1151–1153.

23. American Academy of Pediatrics, Section on Surgery, Section on Anesthesia and Pain Medicine, and Committee on Bioethics. Do not resuscitate orders for pediatric patients who require anesthesia and surgery. *Pediatrics.* 2004; 114:1686–1691.

24. Canadian Paediatric Society, Bioethics Committee. Treatment decisions for infants, children, and adolescents. Reference No. B86-01. Available at: http://www.cps.ca/english/statements/B/b86-01.htm

25. Royal College of Paediatrics and Child Health. *Withholding or Withdrawing Lifesaving Treatment in Children: A Framework for Practice.* London: RCPCH; 1997.

26. *Health Care for All: Report of the Independent Inquiry into Access to Healthcare for People with Learning Disabilities.* 2008. Available at: http://www.iahpld.org.uk.

27. *An NHS Trust v. MB and Anor.* 2006 EWHC 507 (Fam).

28. Tibballs J. Withdrawal of futile treatment from children: implications of *NHS Trust versus MB. J Paediatr Child Health.* 2006;42:563–564.

29. *Re C (a minor) (wardship: medical treatment)* [1998] 1 FLR 384.

30. *Cruzan v. Director, Missouri Department of Health,* 497 US 261, 1990.

31. *In re E.G.* 549 N.E. 2d 322 Ill., 1989.

32. *Medical Ethics: The Right to Survival, 1974.* Hearings before the Subcommittee on Health of the Senate Committee on Labor and Welfare, 93d Cong 2d Sess 26 (1974).

33. Saw A, Randolph JG, Manaard B. Ethical issues in pediatric surgery: a national survey of pediatricians and pediatric surgeons. *Pediatrics.* 1977;60:588–599.

34. Smith SR. Disabled newborns and the federal child abuse amendments: tenuous protection. *Hastings Law J.* 1986;37:765–827.

35. Lantos JD, Miles SH, Cassel CK. The Linares affair. *Law Med Health Care.* 1989;17:308–315.

36. Consent to Medical Treatment and Palliative Care Act (1995) (SA) section 17 (2).

37. *Secretary Department of Health and Human Services v. JWG and SMB,* 175 CLR 218 *Marion's Case* (1991–1992).

38. *F v. F. The Age* (Melbourne), July 3, 1986.

39. Skene L. *Law and Medical Practice.* 2nd ed. Sydney: Lexis Nexis; 2004.

40. *Cattenach v. Melchior,* HCA 38 (2003).

Index